Western Herbs in Chinese Medicine
Methodology & Materia Medica

WESTERN HERBS IN CHINESE MEDICINE

METHODOLOGY
&
MATERIA MEDICA

Thomas Avery Garran

Passiflora Press
www.passiflora-press.com

Note to the reader: This book is intended as an informational guide. The remedies, approaches, and techniques described herein are meant to supplement, and not to be a substitute for, professional medical care or treatment. They should not be used to treat a serious ailment without prior consultation with a qualified health care professional.

Garran, Thomas Avery.
   Western herbs in Chinese medicine : methodology & materia medica Thomas Avery Garran.

Includes bibliographical references and index.
ISBN-13: 978-0-9915813-0-6
1. Herbs – Therapeutic use. 2. Medicine, Chinese. 3. Materia medica, Vegetable. I. Title. [DNLM: 1. Phytotherapy – methods. 2. Materia Medica. 3. Medicine, Chinese Traditional – methods. 4. Plants, Mediicnal

10 9 8 7 6 5 4 3 2 1

Text design and layout by Thomas Avery Garran
This book was typeset in Gentium Book Basic.

To contact the author of this book, please visit his website at www.sylvanbotanical.com

Other than the intial writing done in MSWord, I am proud to write here that all the layout, formatting, art work, and other aspects of this project were done on free open source software, including, Open Office, Scribus, GIMP, and Inkscape.

DEDICATION

To all those who have loved, inspired, and criticized me.
Thank you!

This book is dedicated to Autumn Reine Garran (吳嶸曉), who's brief but brilliant life has done more to shape this work than could possibly be measured.

Contents

Foreward

A westerner seeking higher education and academe within the terrain of China, Thomas Avery Garran earned his credentials practicing both eastern and western herbal medicines. His experience ranges from mentorship within graduate programs, to his role as herbal department chair in a school of Chinese medicine. I believe this background situates our author well for the work at hand.

His writing, as practical as it is cosmopolitan, provides a considerate exercise in bridging cultural divides. My thoughts, as I read this book, are that he has achieved a work that is mature, methodological, important and creative. I would like to approach his work from the viewpoint of integration, as it provides us with an exemplar of cross-cultural knowledge production. In addition, it seems important to address the methods employed herein, as well as the creative features of this book.

Integration

We speak of integration, what that means, how it occurs and who should care about the implications. In a social and cultural context, integration is presented through the eighteenth century terms *cosmopolitanism* and *world citizenship*. The cosmopolitan value serves no particular authority, unbiased by particular loyalties or cultural prejudice yet is fond of travel, cherishing a network of international contacts. Such social containers form the views that become integrated and blended. Garran proves himself to be such a syncretic thinker.

Predating the Silk Road, shared thought between East and West has infiltrated the practices of Hippokratic, Stoic, Unani, Ayurvedic, Tibetan and Chinese medicine in ways that are impossible to sort. The human tendency to incorporate other indigenous knowledge remains today. Contemporary evidence of integration is shown in Beijing via the slogans used in the development of Traditional Chinese medicine by Chairman Mao. They included:

The Cooperation of Chinese and Western Medicine from 1945-50
The Unification of Chinese and Western Medicine from 1950-58
Chinese Medicine Studies Western Medicine from 1950-53
Western Medicine Studies Chinese Medicine from 1954–58
Integration of Chinese and Western Medicine from 1958 – Present

The net result of these campaigns is a highly synthesized – read integrative - practice of Chinese and Western medicine that is currently taught in the major university medical systems throughout China. Such forms of integration are present at cognitive and practice based concerns of the practitioner. They also take place in the form of institutions of hospitals, governmental policy and the professional domain of education.

Creativity

Taken as a mode of transformation, preparing members of society for professional service, we consider four areas of scholarly inquiry. They include: personal transformation, improvement of professional practice, generation of knowledge, and the appreciation of the complexity, intricacy, structure and beauty of reality. Garran has participated in all four areas his story reveals the personal transformation of this journey. The generation of knowledge clearly emerges from a seasoned practitioner in deference to important historical personalities. As for improving professional practice, for me, insights have already accrued for my own practice in the brief time I have had to enjoy the pages of this book. Thus, by extension, in this work remains a transformative impulse at the heart of creative endeavor.

Arthur Koestler's theory of creativity involves uniting opposite pairs (1964). Having performed research on creativity, Koestler's coined the term *bisociation*, that is, to join unrelated, often conflicting information in a new way. While much of the knowledges built in this book are congruent, Garran manages to resolve disparate ideas through resourcing historic authority East and West.

The ability to tolerate chaos and seemingly opposite information is characteristic of creative individuals. Garran has tolerated chaos well and we benefit. Our way of knowing and acting in our world, continually reinforced by our cultural conditioning, has established a complex interlocking system. Underlying this great superstructure are our concepts, beliefs, assumptions, values, and attitudes, which are linked together like an underground network of pipelines connecting across a vast continent. Garran has effectively synthesized these ideas into a trans-cultural exercise.

Method

Herbal medicine transgresses both cultural and historical bounds. Presenting more than a catalog of findings, Thomas Avery Garren has furthered the discipline in terms of method and thought. The roots of this work can be considered from the worldview called 'constructivism', where reality is apprehended in the form of multiple, intangible mental constructions, the elements of which are often shared among individuals and across cultures. The methods of constructivism are hermeneutic in that the interpretation of texts has an important role, but also dialectical in terms of critical and comparative analyses which, in this case, have roots in dialogical forms of direct knowledge transmission along lineage.

This brings us to bear upon the problem that the historical record of herbal energetics is messier than the often-homogenized contemporary English language *materia medicas* would suggest. Garran demonstrates the problem deftly and succinctly. From the remains, he extracts a method to assign meaning. Crossing over the heuristic plateaus of genus, species, taste, effects and classifications, I believe that this work will stand as the most serious effort to date and over time for the purposes of a common nomenclature between eastern and western herbal practices.

Axiology

The reason we should consider this book – axiology – who should care and why? Aside from the academic contributions of method and practice; this book digs into some important terrain. This is the latest in recent transcultural efforts to construct western botanical medicine into the Chinese medical cognitive frame. In my opinion, it is the most rigorously performed work to date and deserves a seat as a clinical reference for both western and eastern practitioners of botanical medicine.

We live in a world where political changes can quickly alter access to plant medicines. Take, the removal of Ma Huang (Ephedra) from the market place in the US for example. While the plant is illegal for interstate trade, the over the counter agent Ephedrine is readily available in drug stores everywhere. Considered by many to be one of the more important agents in the pharmacopeia, this is not the first or last time such precipitous actions will take place under the purview of governmental agencies and legislative bodies.

We also consider the values of bioregional herbalism. There remains good cause for selecting a plant that grows nearby. Plants grow close by for health conditions taking place in the person at that moment. This thought stems from deep indigenous 'knowledges' and experiences. But there are other reasons to move in the direction of bioregional herbalism. The tyranny of commerce increasingly elevates cost and impact upon the environment. The notion of 'daodi,' the impact of the terrain upon the qualities of a medicinal, is a value that controverts the notion of bioregional herbalism.

Here, an ecology of soil, plant and other life along with weather create the possibilities of a plant having special functions. American ginseng has a cooler nature than Chinese or Korean and it is the taxes that were levied upon it that formed the basis of the Boston Tea Party.

Lastly, this book is useful to practitioners of herbal medicine east and west. For the eastern practitioner, patients will self-prescribe herbal agents and expect a degree of expertise from their practitioner on the topic. This book takes those agents and places them into the cognitive frame of the eastern practitioners. For the western clinical herbalist, the transformation of western pharmacopeia into the disciplined approach of energetics is a move towards a reasoned and reliable scaffolding for thought in practice. It could easily find its way into the curriculum of both eastern and western schools of herbal medicine. I would like to see such content taught in the entry level programs of Chinese medicine here in the US.

William Morris, PhD, DAOM, LAc
Author: *Path of the Pulse and Li Shi Zhen Pulse Studies: An Illustrated Guide*

Preface

At the time of the publication of what is essentially the first volume of this book, Western Herbs According to Traditional Chinese Medicine: A Practitioner's Guide, there were many monographs that were in various stages of development, – but we only published the material that I felt I could prepare within a reasonable timeframe. For many years, my students and colleagues had been urging me to publish the material and I just wanted to get it out there. Now, 5 years later, I am presenting you with the second volume, and there are plants that didn't make the cut this time either...

Encompassing both volumes, the total number of medicinals covered is 52, and yet there are so many more out there that need to be discussed. However, my interests have shifted a bit and I am no longer practicing full-time; my energy is increasingly devoted towards research, teaching, and writing about how plants are used in different cultures and in different ways, as well as other subjects of interest to me. I do continue to see patients and will likely develop more monographs, however it is likely that this 2nd volume will be the last in the series for some time.

As I look back across my more than 20 years of working with plants I see that I have learned much and yet know little. Understanding the plants and how to use them in the clinic is more challenging than most of us realize. Considering that people have been using plants for tens of thousands of years, and yet there is still much sickness and suffering in the world, is truly humbling. In considering this and other aspects of humans' interactions with plants, I decided to delve into the understanding of our interactions with plants in the past, present, and future, and try to interpret what I see are the commonalities that bring us together in how we work with and understand plants, and when there are differences to try to parse out what the roots of those differences are so that I might gain a better understanding of both humans and the plants they interact with.

I believe that I have the opportunity to gather data from a perspective that is somewhat unique based on my experience as a practitioner of Western herbal medicine, training in botany and ethnobotany, and my training and practice of Chinese medicine. It is my hope that this unique perspective will yield some answers and also pose interesting questions that may go unanswered in my lifetime, but perhaps will inform future generations.

There are a number of monographs that were created for the first volume but never completed in time for publication. An advantage of this is since that time my experience has evolved to enable me to better understand the plants and how to use them in the clinic. Concurrently, my language skills have improved significantly, which allows me to find and process far more Chinese language data than I could when I wrote the first volume. The result of this is significant improvement in these "left-overs" from the first volume.

There are some herbs that one might find in the Chinese literature such as European Angelica (*Angelica archangelica*). When one reads this material it is obvious that it is merely a translation of the English language material into Chinese, rather than material that is originally written in Chinese from the perspective of a practicing Chinese medicine doctor. This material is of little use to us, but it is worth noting here because I have been questioned about this type of literature and believe it is important that readers understand that when I use Chinese literature to help with this project, I am using literature that comes from Chinese sources which are clearly discussing the plant from a clinical usage point of view, not simply a translation of the English language literature. Other forms of Chinese literature that I have used, and sometimes included are source material that discuss diseases, patterns of disease, theoretical constructs, etc. Thus, in order for me to include literature citations from original Chinese I am using one of two types of literature. 1) Literature that discusses a medicinal covered or one that is closely related either botanically or by virtue of usage; 2) Source literature discussing any theoretical construct that I am using to explain how or why to use any medicinal within the book.

Another advantage of having five more years is that the internet has opened doors into pre-modern literature that has allowed me access to some of the storied greats of Western herbal medicine such as Parkinson and Salmon, just to name two. This has dramatically altered the way I have presented the Commentary section of each monograph. In the commentary you will find many quotes from authors of Western herbalism's past such as Dioscorides, Gerard, Parkinson, Culpeper, and

Salmon; as well as material from the masters of American herbal medicine from the late 19th and early 20th Century, primarily from the Eclectic and Physiomedical currents. Although I had access to some of this material while writing the first volume, I am very happy to be able to offer you a far wider breadth of information on many of these medicinals from the last 500–600 years, and occasionally (in the case of Dioscorides) 2000 years!

In the front matter of the first volume I discuss the main reasons for writing that text such as influences I had from teachers, my feelings around using more locally derived medicines (sustainability), potential hazardous plant material coming from abroad, and the fact that I believed that although there was some good literature out there in this area, I thought I could do it better by sticking with (in a pretty strict manner) Chinese medicine; none of those reasons have changed. There is little more to say in this regard other than to express that my goals are to explore this path, expound on what I learn as best I can, and hope that those who encounter this material will gain from it and be better able to help relieve the suffering of those they encounter.

I can be contacted through www.sylvanbotanical.com

Acknowledgements

There are so many people to thank for their teachings and support that I wil undoubtedly forget some of you, but you know who you are. This work is a culmination of my experience and that of some of my teachers and colleagues, but also my students, who have continuously pushed me to look at plants and medicine through different lenses and from different perspectives.

However, there are a few people I would like to acknowledge here in print. First, to my friend, colleague, and business partner, Benjamin Zappin for his unbridled support and constant questioning of my ideas along with offering some fine ideas of his own. This book could not possibly have been accomplished without you.

There are several people who read and commented on the text and inparticular I would like to thank William Morris for his encouragement and honest assessment. Also, Will McClatchey for his review of the *Reasoning and Methods* chapter. Will offered a great deal of insight and some good ideas for both more literature to help with the writing and more importantly for ideas and encouragement to turn that chapter into a bonafied research paper.

Of course there is a long list of teachers both here in China and back home in the USA. However, I would like to give a big thanks to Wú Bō-lín (吴波林) for being the teacher that every student should have. His experience, patience, and gentle giving nature have taught me more than he will ever know.

Finally, but certainly not least, I would like to thank my family for their constant support. In particular my friend, partner, and lovely wife Wú Jiāng-hóng (吴江洪) for being the best partner in this life a man could ever ask for, and more. We have travelled farther in this life together than many will travel their entire lives, over-come adversity no couple should ever have to bare, and through it all there has never been a doubt in my mind that asking you to marry me was the best decision I have ever made in my life.

Of course, it goes without saying, any and all mistakes found in this text are completely my doing and I take full responsibility for them.

Explanation of Text

I have done my best to make this text as similar to the first volume, Western Herbs According to Traditional Chinese Medicine: A Practitioner's Guide, as possible so that those familiar with that text will easily be able to segue into this text.

The first part of this text "*Reasoning and Methods*" and "*Using Botanical Classification as a Means of Understanding Relationships of Medicinal Plants*" is significantly different in this text than the first (Part One "*Methods and Measures*"). The current text has a far more developed theoretical construct to help the reader deepen their understanding of how this work has been accomplished. I am honored to say that the latter part was written with a co-author, my dear friend and colleague Benjamin Zappin. In this material we have outlined and discussed the tools we use to translate information from a myriad of sources to transform a plant from a Western botanical medicine and make it a Chinese medicinal. This process is in fact a significant question within the Ethnobotany field of science, how does one tradition, when given a new set of tools, fit those tools into their own cultural context. In this case, we are taking our tools and transplanting them in a different cultural tradition, Chinese medicine (zhōngyī 中醫). There is a dearth of literature on this subject, although there are many clear examples of it being done, even, as I explain in that portion of the text, within Chinese Medicine. The reason for this is that people, even in a literature society like Imperial China, for reasons unknown, have never discussed their process, and modern Ethnobotany has only scratched the source of this phenomenon through field study of non-literate societies.

Names of herbs are always capitalized, except for the Chinese *pīnyīn* (the modern phonetic spelling of Mandarin Chinese) names, which has been left without capitalization but has been italicized. For the most part, I have left Chinese characters out of the text with the exception of including them as alternate names of medicinals, and where the name only comes once and are of unusual medicinals, this latter point is almost exclusively in the Commentary or more commonly in the Translation of Available Texts section of the monographs. Names of Chinese formulas are capitalized with tone marks to represent the Chinese as best as possible. Names of books are Capitalized and generally presented in an English format (a translation of the Chinese), except for words such as place names found within the title, or in a few cases where the original Chinese book title is so well known that the majority of the readers should recognize it, e.g. *Shén Nóng Běn Căo* or *Nèi Jīng*. All other Chinese words have been, except author's names, italicized and given tonal marks, except place names, which have been left without tonal marks. Any time Chinese characters are used in the text, the full traditional characters are represented. Although many authors decide to use the simplified characters, mostly because it is the most common presentation these days since essentially all literature coming from the PRC is in simplified characters. However, although I have fallen into the simplified trap myself, I still believe the traditional characters are both easier to learn to read and are, quite honestly, more interesting; one might say beautiful. I have not included an index to render the characters as simplified since the characters are always accompanied by the pínyín pronunciation. Most Chinese word are italicized to conform with the standard of rendering foreign terms in this manner, and tonal marks have been added for those that either understand this reference, or are students/interested persons. However I have decided to leave a few terms that I deem both untranslatable and/or so well established in English as to essentially be borrowed into the language, the primary example is qi (qì 氣) have kept the remaining format of the book the same as the first volume, with heading of Common name, Botanical Latin name, Family name, Pharmaceutical name, Other names, Flavor and Qi, Channels entered, Actions, Functions & Indications, Dosage & Preparation, Major Combinations, and Commentary.

I have attempted to give better reasoning with Chinese medical theory within the main text (Functions & Indications) as well as in the commentary to help to deepen the understanding from the Chinese medical paradigm. This process has been the fruit of learning to read Chinese source literature, and also helped me to gain a greater understanding of Chinese herbal medicine and the traditional approach of presenting medicinals in a materia medica format. Thus there are quotes from source text in both the main monograph and within the commentary.

Another change in the presentation of this material is the shift in the way the Commentary section is approached. As I said in the Introduction, I have more information readily available to me now, source material from both pre-modern English and the entire word of Chinese.

A note on quoting from European sources of the 15ᵗʰ–17ᵗʰ Century. These authors wrote in a language that is what is commonly known as "Old English." Reading these texts is sometimes challenging for a modern person, so I have "generally" chosen to quote the original with a gentle editorial hand to render the text more easily readable for the readers of this text. Primary changes are spelling and use of more modern terms for diseases or conditions, but there are also occasional grammatical changes or sentence structure changes to help with readability. This should in no way hinder the reader's understanding of the quote, and has the sole purpose of allowing the reader to focus more on the meaning of the material and less of attempting to decipher the language.

The selected quotes help give context regarding historical use of the plant from its native tradition. I have attempted to assist the reader in understanding what the authors meant from the Chinese perspective by offering my own commentary to tie together what they wrote with the primary monograph. It is my wish that these commentaries will offer the reader a fuller, more complete understanding of each medicinal and how to apply it in a clinical setting.

There are a few clinical histories and clinical notes in this text. The primary reason there are not more is that, until recently, for the last 5 years I have had no access to most of these medicinals and also do not have access to my patient files from prior to that time. However, I will be including regular case histories on the blog at Sylvan Institute of Botanical Medicine (www.sylvanbotanical.com) attached to this material, as well as others. Nevertheless, I trust that the few that can be found here will greatly benefit the reader.

With regards to citations, in most cases I have left page numbers out of the text when the citation is from a book. The reasoning for this is two-fold, one is to attempt to save space, the other is that materia medicas are always categorized by herb, and occasionally larger headings such as "Herbs that Course the Exterior," thus I believe that the information would be very easy to find for anyone who chooses simply by looking up that particular medicinal in the given book. Furthermore, I have omitted books in the notes and left them to be found in the bibliography.

There are three Categories found in the text that were not found in the first text including: Open Orifices, External Application, and

Eliminate Parasites. And, there are three categories from the first text not found in this text, including; Warm the interior and Expel Cold, Stabilize and Bind, and Extinguish Wind. That there is three new chapters exchanged for three not present from the last book is completely by chance.

There are three appendices. Appendix I is some brief information about several plants found in *Western Herbs According to Traditional Chinese Medicine: A Practitioners Guide* from Chinese sources. Appendix II is some brief information about a few plant used in Chinese medicine and can be found growing outside of China, primarily in North America. This is not meant to be exhaustive, that material alone could be an entire book. Appendices III, IV, & V are indices of the plants found in the book by Common name (III), Botanical Latin Binomial (IV), and the phonetic Mandarin Chinese *pínyín* name (V).

Terminology of Chinese medicine and including all translation generally follows A Practical Dictionary of Chinese Medicine by Nigel Wiseman and Feng Ye (Paradigm 1998), with the noted exception of the word "constraint" instead of "depression" for the character 鬱 (pronounced *yù*).

NOTE: In the translation section of each monograph, when I say there are a given number of species used in Chinese medicine, this is based on the information I have available to me. It is quite possible there are other species used.

Introduction

Through the years a few things have sung to me with regards to this work, here are just a few of what I think relate to the material you are about to read.

> *"Far fetched and dear bought, is best for ladies. Yet it may be more truly said of fantastical physicians, who when they have found an approved medicine, & perfect remedy near home against any disease; yet not contented with that, they will seek for a new farther off, and by that means many times hurt more than they help. Thus, much I have spoken, to bring these new fangled fellows back again to esteem better of this admirable plant [Golden Rod] than they have done; which no doubt has the same virtue now that then it had, although it do grow so near our own homes in ever so great quantity."*

On the shift in both price and use of Golden Rod from the New World compared to that of the native species in English. — John Gerard (1597)

> *"Chinese herbal medicine is a treasure trove, great effort should [be used] to explore it and additionally [it should be] improved. Uniting new and old, Chinese and Western, every medicinal and healthcare worker, to form a strong united front, becoming a solid united front for great people to carry out the work and struggle of health."*

Selected Herbs From Shanxi, Gan Su, Ning Xia, and Qing Hai (1971)

While I have my doubts that using Western herbs in Chinese medicine was in the mind of the authors of this passage, and my translation may reflect my bias to some extent, I do believe that the authors would have been happy to integrate Western herbs if it would help to enhance and preserve Chinese medicine, and, of course, help in the struggle for health.

> *"No doctor has reliable knowledge of the curative power of a drug, except where he has proved it in his own practice, A remedy may appear to have cured in a given case, but no opportunity occurs for him to verify the cure, but if his experience is recorded, other observers may verify it and it thus becomes a standard remedy in similar cases..."*

Preface of *Medicinal Plants of North America* (1914)

When starting with an established system of medicine, how do we integrate new medicinals into that system? What characteristics have people considered when deciding what particular plants to use, and how? How have travelers learned about and adopted plants into their life when faced with new flora and only the knowledge of their own tradition to guide them? Likewise, when travelers brought plants to a new land, how did the native people develop those plants into the framework of their own cultural context and medical system?

The questions surrounding how humans have integrated plants from outside their bioregion are many. The goal of this work is not necessarily to answer these questions so much as to investigate some possible ideas about how this has been done in Chinese medicine and offer a methodology for us to build on in the future. We will specifically explore these questions through the lens of Chinese medicine and incorporate a number of tools that may or may not have been employed, or even been accessible, by past physicians in China. Additionally, we will explore how botany and ecology might assist us in this process, and we will touch on chemistry as a potential tool.

The ultimate purpose of creating this work is four-fold. First, I hope that this work will help practitioners to better serve their patients, more quickly and completely relieving their suffering. Second, from an ecological point of view, using plants that are geographically closer to where you live makes a great deal of sense and helps to relieve the pressure on fossil fuel resources used to distribute medicinal plants around the world. Also, there is a growing concern for the land, both agricultural and wild land in China; a land under enormous ecological pressure, as some 20% of the world's population go from poor farmers to modern sociolytes. Third, and somewhat related to the second reason, is that there is, rightly or wrongly, a deep concern for the cleanliness of the source material coming out of China. Some of these concerns are well founded, while others are not. As an example, there is a lot of talk about herbicides and pesticides on Chinese herbs, but the fact is that most Chinese herbs test either clean or well within FDA standards. Even heavy metals are rarely an issue, as long as you get your herbs from a reliable source.[1] This is not to say that there isn't a problem, there most definitely is; one that we all need to maintain consciousness around. That said, and I have visited herb farms from *rénshēn* farms in Heilongjiang province in the far Northeast of China to *shíhú* farms in Yunnan province in the far Southwest, and from what I can gather there is generally a lack of understanding of the ecosystems these farmers work in, and a general lack of care taken to preserve or manage them. However, there is often an interest and a trend seems to be starting. There are also some governmental policies that may help transform this issue and educate farmers to better understand their ecosystems. By doing this they should be able to develop farming practices that are relative to a particular medicinal, which should lead to better management,[2] not to mention better quality medicinal plants. And, fourth, perhaps most importantly, I hope to inspire other practitioners to further this work and the work of so many before me and get excited by the freshness, vitality, and beauty of the plants that grow within their own bioregion. Attached to this notion is the fact that I just really dig doing this work, which has more or less consumed me for the last 20 years; so naturally I want to share it with others (did I mention that I really dig it?)!

After publishing the first volume of this work, one of the most common questions I was asked is, "How did you come up with the flavor and qi, and the channels entered for the medicinals in your book?" Somehow, the functions and indications seem to be easier for people to swallow, but perhaps that is just my perception. Like so many other things in Chinese medicine there is much debate over detail; flavors and qi, and channels entered, as they pertain to a specific medicinal, is certainly no exception. Although I did lay out some methodology in the first book, this is an attempt to better clarify and elucidate this methodology with the hopes that others will be able to use it as guide to further this work.

1. Sturgeon, Skye, (2013). Chinese Herbs & Pesticides. The Mayway Mailer. October 2013.
2. Zhang, Ben-gang, et al., (2010). GAP Production of TCM Herbs in China. Planta Medica. 76: pp. 1948-1955.

Reasoning and Methods

Before introducing this complex of ideas, let's take a look at some of what has been done in China, as documented over the past 2000 or so years, to get a sense of how past physicians approached and tackled this issue. To the authors' knowledge there has never been any methods set forth by any Chinese physician about how to incorporate new medicinals into their practice, although they have obviously done it for well over 2000 years as evidenced by the fact that even the *Divine Farmers Classsic on Materia Medica* (*Shén Nóng Běn Cǎo Jīng*, 神農本草經), or simply *Běn Cǎo Jīng*, circa 200 BCE, has medicinals in it from outside of China. In order to do this, we need to understand the essential tools that every doctor of Chinese medicine has had over the last 2000 years or so.

The fundamental information that all Chinese physicians have had over the last 2000 years came from the *Yellow Emperor's Classic of Medicine* (*Huáng Dì Nèi Jīng*, 黃帝內經), or simply *Nèi Jīng*. Although there have been discussions, modifications, additions, etc. to the theoretical construct of Chinese medicine, the fundamental concepts of Flavors, Qi [temperature], and Channels (organ systems) and how they relate to each other, and the therapeutics associated with each of these were laid out in this classic work, which has remained the ultimate source of foundational information since it was first published more than 2000 years ago. I will explore this theoretical framework and how it relates to the use of medicinal agents (specifically plants), and later I will explore ways to use this framework, along with a wider scope, to incorporate plants from outside Chinese medicine into your everyday practice.

Brief History

When medicinals are added to the materia medica in Chinese medicine there appears to be no discussion of a methodology used in the incorporation process; it just happens. There have been many medicinals added, and yet there is no discussion of a methodology and rarely any mention that it comes from a foreign land; a clear exception to this is the *Hǎi Yào Běn Cǎo* "*Medicinals from the Sea,*" written by Lǐ Xún, a Persian born in China. Although this book does not discuss any sort of method for determining uses, it does mention the origin of the plant (often in a very non-specific manner such as "from the East Sea"). The author is known to have been born in Guangdong and lived in Chengdu, nothing is known of his medical background. However, it is suggested that he is likely from a royal family, and he is known to have strong connections to the royal court of the time (Tang Dyansty).[1] While it is plausible that Li had some training or understanding of Persian medicine, we have no records to show that he did have such training and thus we can't be sure if he might have used that understanding to influence his writing that became a work of significant influence on later authors. (Note: Li's work is not the only text to notate that plants came from outside China, it is merely offered as an example.)

Throughout the historical literature, authors say this or that about a particular medicinal, and then someone else says something different with perhaps some overlap. And that's the way it goes! Over time, the differences about most of the critical data become fewer and fewer and it is easier and easier for people to add any particular medicinal into their repertoire based on available literature. *Páozhì* and *duìyào* are established, formulas are modified with the medicinal, and finally, perhaps, the medicinal is used in a major formula or even becomes a leading medicinal in a formula or two. (NOTE: *Páozhì* is technically any preparation of a medicinal, whether it be drying, slicing, or soaking in wine. The term here is used in a more specific manner that is generally understood by Chinese medicine practitioners to mean special preparation techniques used to change the therapeutic action of the medicinal, i.e. stir-frying in wine or baking until calcined. Although not unique to Chinese medicine, there is little doubt that Chinese medicine has one of the most advanced systems of this type of preparation. *Duìyào* is a term that essentially mean "combination of medicinals" with an implicit meaning of "two medicinals." However, *duìyào* is not *always* two medicinals and can be three or four. Chinese herbal medicine, and its formulas and modifications, is based on these combinations with volumes of books written specifically on this subject alone.)

So, what method did those who first came in contact with a new medicinal, say Myrrh (*mòyào*, 沒藥) or American Ginseng (*xīyángshēn*, 西洋 蔘), use to ascribe what we now, more or less, consider the characteristics about these medicinals? Since we cannot answer that question, we can, instead, ask, "What method can WE use when assessing medicinals that are not already part of the Chinese materia medica?" In the following chapters, I offer some tools I believe can be used to develop a reasonable and repeatable method.

Although references to botanical medicine are nearly absent from the *Nèi Jīng* it is this paradigm that was adopted by those that came after, and is the theoretical construct that is the backbone of the materia medica literature. This foundational information has been distilled to its essence and over the centuries has become the structure of how medicinals are categorized and how they are used therapeutically. These basic categories of information, although not laid out in the *Nèi Jīng* as such, or even the *Běn Cǎo Jīng* for that matter, assist us in our decision making process when determining how to use a medicinal in the construction or modification of a formula in an attempt to relieve human suffering. The most basic of these are the *Flavor* and *Qi*, *Channels Entered*, *Functions*, and finally *Indications*. Furthermore, *Dosage*, and *Cautions* or *Contraindications* are quite important for us as practitioners to guide us to "first do no harm." The importance of these latter two heading, and this adage is paramount. This phrase is often attributed to Hippocrates and likely comes from the book *Of the Epidemics* and reads, "The physician must be able to tell the antecedents, know the present, and foretell the future–must mediate these things, and have two special objects in view with regard to disease, namely, to do good or to do no harm."[2] Within Chinese medicine there are similar sayings. This one from from Sūn Sī-miǎo, typical to Chinese medicine, uses dichotomies to exemplify his point, "To add to what is already full or to decrease what is already deficient, to penetrate further into what is already flowing freely or to congest what is already blocked, to cool what is already cold or to warm what is already hot, this is only doubling the disorder. Where there was still hope for the patient's life, I now see their death!" This statement is similar to Hippocrates' statement, but interestingly, unlike Hippocrates, Sūn Sī-miǎo did not practice herbal medicine, or even acupuncture, at least there is no evidence that he did, but he was no less a wise scholar than Hippocrates.[3] Finally, *Major Combinations* (duìyào, 對藥), and suggestions of formulas that can be modified by the medicinals, are also helpful in guiding our use of the medicinal. With this information, coupled with our understanding of the fundamental theories of Chinese medicine and good diagnostic skills, we have the tools necessary to practice herbal medicine.

This book assumes a working knowledge of Chinese medicine. For those who do not have this knowledge, please refer to the first volume of this book, *Western Herbs According to Chinese Medicine: A Practitioners Guide*, or any fundamental Chinese medicine book, for an overview of the theories.

The next several pages will be an introduction to the major categories of *Flavor*, *Qi*, and *Channels Entered*. This is an exploration of the history of these categories in the materia medica literature and the methods used in this work to arrive at the information presented in the materia medica section of this book. It is my hope that this will serve as a jumping off point (and perhaps inspiration) for others to continue this work, hopefully advancing it beyond my humble offerings.

Flavor

According to the *Nèi Jīng* there are five primary flavors (sweet, bitter, acrid, sour, and salty; plus bland) found in both medicinals and foods. These flavors are said to have an effect on the human body that translates as one or another type of physiological transformation. Each of these flavors is also said to "enter" a particular organ system, and thus has a primary effect on that organ system. The five flavors are also said to have an action that is inherent in them that governs, to one extent or another, how they act within the human body. Most were said to have only one flavor, although this has evolved to allow for more than one flavor.

The idea of flavors as a classification system, or at least the idea that they relate to certain physiological actions contained in a medicinal is not unique to Chinese medicine. There is evidence that in both literate and non-literate societies the use of flavors to describe actions of medicinal substances was/is common and some have suggested that this may in fact be a deeply embedded "sense" in humans used as a method to understand our environment. Messer (1991) wrote, "Taste and smell, visual and tactile characteristics, and physiological effect are all "sensory" information by which people recognize, evaluate and classify plants. People in every culture learn to use these sensory cues to identify, group and use the plants in their environments according to certain culture-specific taxonomic nomenclatural principles and functional classifications."[4] Other traditions such as Ayurveda from India, Unani from Eastern Europe and West Asia, and even the Galanic tradition from Greece all have codified flavors in similar ways that Chinese medicine has within their own medical paradigm. As an example, "In Āyurveda, this complex relationship between flavor and physiological function is well established, and as such, each rasa [flavor] has a specific activity upon the doṣāḥ [humors], dhātavaḥ [tissue] and agni [digestion]."[5] Here the author is suggesting that the physiological functions, as understood by Āyurveda are understood within the context of that system of medicine.

Acrid: enters the lung, can dissipate and move
Bitter: enters the heart, can drain and dry
Sour: enters the liver, can contract and astringe
Sweet: enters the spleen, can supplement and relax
Salty: enters the kidney, can soften and cause moist precipitation
Bland: can disinhibit water

The five flavors, plus bland, as explained by Chinese medicinal theory.

Chinese medicine diverges to some extent on this idea. The idea of flavor affecting a particular organ system or having a particular action has roots in the *Nèi Jīng*, and perhaps before, but early materia medicas generally only assigned one flavor to a medicinal. When we look at these flavors they are generally "easy" to see as the taste of any particular medicinal. For example, *gāncǎo* (*Glycyrrhiza uralensis* Frisch. ex DC.) is sweet, *mùxiāng* (*Aucklandia costus* Falc.) is acrid, and *huánglián* (*Coptis chinensis* Franch.) is bitter. These are fairly obvious tastes that anyone who chews on one of these plants would likely find. While *mùxiāng* is the only one of these three that has changed (most modern books say that it is acrid and bitter), the other two are extreme examples of their respective flavors and most other medicinals have been assigned a second or third flavor over the history of their use. Why is this? Has the ability of the Chinese people to perceive flavors changed over time? Although there is evidence of people's (culture's) taste perception changing over time, the five flavors (not including bland) have been laid out in the theories of Chinese medicine since at least the time of the *Nèi Jīng* and so therefore the awareness of these flavors being present has been well established since at least this time. However, what has changed is the way people have interacted with the core theoretical construct that we call Chinese medicine. This change has led to an ever-more complex system that prides itself on using its historical texts (often called "Classics") to legitimize any new idea or treatment method. While there is nothing inherently wrong with this methodology, it does tend to lead to a web that continues to draw lines from these central texts, often using horizontal or diagonal lines to join new and old points; by its very nature creates a labyrinth that can be confounding and laborious to navigate.

Therefore, keeping in mind that *flavor* and *taste* are not necessarily the same; your ability to taste a flavor when you put the plant in your mouth does not mean that the plant would or would not be ascribed that flavor within the framework of Chinese medicine. More accurately, while it is likely that if you taste bitter that medicinal will be considered bitter in Chinese medicine, while it is also likely to have other flavors assigned to it that you cannot perceive. This is easily witnessed by putting any number of Chinese herbs into your mouth and trying to taste the flavors ascribed to them in the materia medica.

Knowing that a flavor has an affinity to a particular organ system, or has a particular action on the qi or blood or other aspect of the body, i.e. heart, liver, etc., helps us to understand both why a particular medicinal acts in the way it does, and how to ascribe a flavor to a medicinal if we understand how that medicinal works within the body. As an example, we are told in the Chinese materia medica that *huánglián* is bitter. Therefore, it is likely to act on the heart and have a draining action. Of course, not all bitter medicinals act on the heart and not all medicinals that act on the heart are bitter. Likewise, not all medicinals that are bitter have a draining action and not all medicinals that have a draining action are bitter. Or, at least, these actions are not prominent in the actions of all medicinals. However, understanding these principles creates for us a helpful guide and we can assess medicinals that we know to either act on the heart, or have a draining action and decide whether or not this is, at least in part, because they are bitter. One key might be to consider whether or not the medicinal is actually bitter to the taste. As I mentioned in the *Materials and Methods* chapter of my first book (Garran 2008), when looking at Chinese references on medicinal plants the idea of taste and flavor can be a bit confusing for those not trained in Chinese medicine. The idea that any medicinal has a particular flavor which cannot obviously be tasted might be a little confusing. (Factoid: >95% of the medicinals in the *Shén Nóng Běn Cǎo Jīng* are classified as having only one flavor; 1.6% are ascrided two flavors; 1.4% are not classified; and 0.5% are classified as *píng* (平) "level".) In a random modern textbook (462 medicinals) 56.7% are assigned one flavor, 40.9% two flavors, 2.4% three flavors. (Note: The latter does not include "level" but does include "bland," thus this numbers are slightly skewed. I also did not include astringent in the latter because it was not used in the *Běn Cǎo Jīng* and would have skewed the numbers significantly.)

An early example of flavor and function being seemingly incongruent can be taken from the *Shén Nóng Běn Cǎo Jīng*. In that text the medicinal *chēqiánzǐ* is classified as sweet (this classification has been maintained to the present day), but the functions/indications give for the medicinal are to "treat strangury, stop pain, disinhibit water and free urination, and expel water impediment." I chose this example because based on the information above, which comes from the *Nèi Jīng*, sweet "enters the spleen, and can supplement and relax." The *Shén Nóng Běn Cǎo Jīng* information for how to use this medicinal is not congruent with the tenents of flavor laid out in the *Nèi Jīng*, or at least it appears to be that way.

Chén Xiū-Yuán offers an explanation in his Shén Nóng Běn Cǎo Jīng Dú (early 19th Century):

> "*Chēqián grows well on the side of the road, although oxen and horses trample it, it does not die, there is no doubt it is able to be used [to treat] the qi of earth [spleen/stomach]. [When there is] qi dribbling [of urine], the qi of the urinary bladder is blocked. [When there is] block then there is pain, [when there is] pain then the waterways are inhibited. Chēqián is able to be used for earth qi, [when] earth qi moves, then the waterways also move. Furthermore, [when there is] no dribbling, then [there is] no pain, and urination is long! [When the] earth qi moves, then dampness evil disperses, [when] dampness-evil disperses, then dampness impediment certainly is eliminated! Taking [chēqián] for a long time upbears earth qi and distributes water qi, therefore it makes the body light and the patient can endure old age.*"

What we can see from the quote above is the author using the theoretical construct of Chinese medicine to explain how the medicinal works. Although he does not mention the flavor in this passage, he does classify it as sweet, and because sweet enters the spleen/stomach he is offering an explanation of how this medicinal performs the functions ascribed to it through this understanding. The following anecdote may help to elucidate the difference between flavors and taste, how they are perceived and what this might mean for the process I am discussing.

While studying ethnobotany at the University of Hawai'i at Manoa, I did a survey of 20 people (admittedly small) about what flavors they perceived in *wŭwèizĭ*, which literally translates as "5 flavor seed." Chinese medicine generally considers this fruit to possess all five flavors (see below for further explanation). Indeed, all five flavors were perceived in the study, but only one person chose sweet and 85% of participants chose either two (35%) or three (50%) flavors. Furthermore, the data showed that only 35% percent of the participants perceived either acrid and/or salty, while bitter and/or sour were perceived by 90% of the participants.

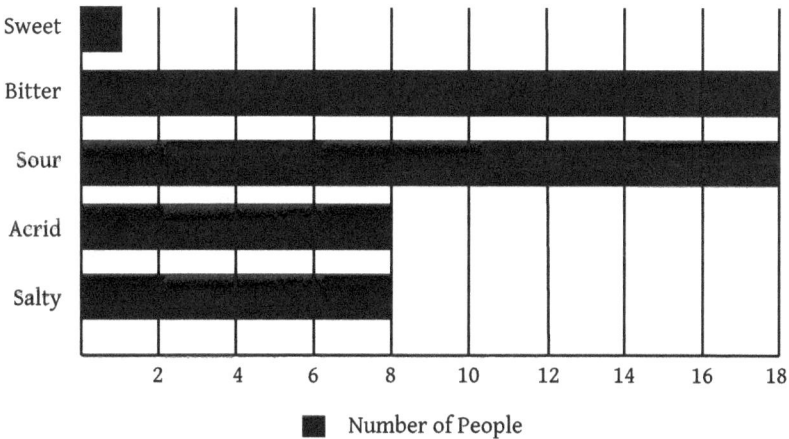

Number of People

What does this study show? It shows that of the five flavors ascribed to this medicinal, three of them (sweet, acrid, and salty) weren't well perceived. This tells us that although a medicinal is ascribed a particular flavor or grouping of flavors, any one of them may or may not be easily perceived simply by tasting that medicinal. This further exemplifies that flavor and taste are only somewhat related and should help to demonstrate that flavor is specifically associated with how the medicinal acts in the body, while taste is merely a perception. This point is important! Chinese medicine has, over the last 2000 or so years built a very complex theoretical construct which it uses to explain, or attempt to explain, health, illness, birth, death, etc., basically the entirety of the human experience. As a classification system, flavors (and other senses such as olfaction) are used to help explain medicinal substances and how they intercept at various points in that human experience. Like many other cultures around the world, this is built on the complexity of the Chinese cultural milieu.[6,7]

Could we do this study with trained Chinese herbalists? No, because they would recognize the herb, and their answers would be biased by the fact that they know that all five flavors are ascribed to this particular medicinal. However, not all books agree! Several books only ascribe sour including the *Shén Nóng Běn Cǎo Jīng* (cira 200 BCE) and *Grand Dictionary of Chinese Medicinals* (2009), as well as a major textbook used by students in China, *Zhōng Yào Xué* (2002), while other books say it is sour and sweet; sour, slightly bitter, salty; etc. There is no consensus! Two books, *Newly Revised Materia Medica* (659) and *Yào Yì Míng Biàn* (1793), clarify this issue somewhat and tell us that the flavors ascribed are only found in different parts of the fruit, and to different degrees. The *New Revised Materia Medica* says the skin and flesh are sour and sweet, the seed is acrid and bitter, and all parts are salty. However, in the opening part for the monograph for this medicinal it only ascribes the flavor of sour. It is not until the Cautions and Solutions (謹案) section that an explanation is given for this apparent problem. The *Yào Yì Míng Biàn* gives even more detail. "The skin and flesh is sour and sweet, sweet to a lesser extent while sour to a greater extent; the kernel is acrid and bitter, acrid to a lesser extent and bitter to a greater extent, while the entirety of the fruit is salty."

If we look at the functions and indications for *wǔwèizǐ*, it is not terribly difficult to understand why/how it has been ascribed all five flavors. Taking the *Newly Revised Materia Medica* as our marker, since it appears to the first to discuss this issue, it gives the following information about the functions/indications of *wǔwèizǐ*: "Governs[:] boosts qi, cough upward-counterflow qi, taxation damage with marked emaciation, supplements insufficiency, strengthens yin, and boosts male essence. Nourishes the five organs, expels heat, and engenders yin inside the flesh." So, the five flavors are represented in this medicinal as follows:

sour: restrains lung qi and yin in general
sweet: nourishes
acrid: moves the lung qi, courses qi generally
bitter: draining
salty: enters the kidney

Interestingly, the book says this medicinal is warm, yet says that it expels heat; perhaps this is part of the functional combination of acrid and bitter, or simply acrid, which can course the exterior and thus release heat, or the bitter flavor can drain. (For more on qi/nature/temperature see the next section.)

So, whether we start with known flavors, or known functions and indications we can derive assumptions about the other. It is very likely, although we don't know, that prior to the writing of the *Běn Cǎo Jīng* plants were more commonly only assigned functions, i.e. treats cough with phlegm, and later, as medicine developed into a more complex study, flavors were added. Thus, in the case of adding Western herbs into the Chinese materia medica we have herbs with known and often well-developed classifications regarding their indications with functions from the modern physiological and classical humoral perspective well understood. Furthermore, we often have well established traditional Western functions that predate modern physiology. These might include functions[†] such as diaphoretic, carminative, diuretic, etc. These functions may be quite different than Chinese functions to one extent or another and we must understand their meaning if we are going to be able to assess them in terms of Chinese medicine. We also have indications, i.e. stops dry cough, stops diarrhea, etc. These types of data do not vary much from one tradition to the next in terms of how they are expressed, it is generally only the mechanism explained using different tradition's understanding of health and disease that tends to differ.

A process we can use to help understand and explain the native Western functions and indications is to ascribe medicinals flavors, which builds on the theoretical constructs of Chinese medicine and helps to elucidate their functions and indications. We can see that adding flavors, with descriptions of how those flavors help us understand the medicinals within the constructs of Chinese medicine, is done in traditional Chinese literature. This is not a new concept and has been documented in other societies. In the Mapuche community of Northwerstern Patagonia it has been "observed how there is a process of trial and experimentation which is seen mainly in the countryside, where plants with similar smells and tastes to those of known medicinal value are considered potentially useful as a replacement for the first [known medicinal species]."[8] Sometimes, this is relatively easy, for example a medicinal that has a very limited therapeutic scope where certain flavors couldn't really be ascribed to the medicinal, e.g. an herb like Goldenseal has no supplementing action, tastes extremely bitter (it is similar to *huánglián*) couldn't possibly be ascribed the sweet flavor. But to what extent this information is important to us as practitioners when deciding whether or not to use a particular medicinal

---

[†] In the body of the materia medica bio-medical functions are called "actions" to differentiate them from Chinese functions.

is debatable. As a learning tool for students, the relatively small amount of information regarding flavor can be a key to remembering how a particular medicinal works, e.g. "bitterness clears heat and drains fire."

This final note on flavors may, in fact, be its most important attribute. While it is true that the fundamental theories of Chinese medicine regarding flavors originated in the *Nèi Jīng* more than 2000 years ago, the use of flavors to describe the functions of medicinals did not come until several centuries later, and, as mentioned earlier, there is no consensus in the literature. Thus, although there is undoubtedly physiological responses[9] in the body when tasting certain flavors, these do not necessarily correspond to the tradition of the *Nèi Jīng*, and are therefore most useful as tools (mnemonics) for students to use while studying and likely help practitioners remember how to use them.

Qi

Qi, or "nature" or "temperature," (from here simply termed "qi") is perhaps the most fundamental of all the qualities ascribed to a medicinal. This idea is found in many traditions of herbal medicine around the world, although Chinese medicine very clearly includes qi (temperature) as part of every monograph, which was also true of Classical European, Greek, Arabic, Unani, and Ayurveda, and is common in pre-literatate societies.[4,7,8] American herbal medicine traditions used this to some extent and there was some further development of it in the 19th and early 20th Centuries, but this concept has lost considerable attention over the last 100-200 years, in favor of a more modern physiological view. Qi, is essentially a simple dichotomy (hot vs. cold) where there is a spectrum of temperatures from cold to cool to neutral to warm and finally to hot, ascrided to each medicinal. This was even further dissected in the traditional Western scheme, which originated with Greek medicine (the origins of Greek medicine were also influenced by Arabic medicine) where the format was hot and cold in four degrees, as well as moist and dry often being used in tandem to describe a medicinal. But what does it mean when we say *huánglián* is cold? Or that *ròuguì* is hot?

The qi of an herb is only relevant when we consider how a particular medicinal might affect a patient's condition, i.e. if they have a condition of heat we generally will use cooling medicinals and vice versa. So, the idea of the qi of a medicinal is very important, but these ideas are not always so firm that there isn't a little wriggle room. There are five main categories used in most Chinese materia medicas and this one is no different. These five categories are easy to understand and the ideas about how to use them are fairly simple.

Qín Bó-wèi (2003 p. 257), who was a modern master (1901-1970) and was known for his ability to distill classical Chinese medicine and present it in ways that made him a famous teacher and practitioners explains the qi, or nature, of herbs this way:

> *"There are four different natures (性) of medicinals, cold, hot, warm, cool. These can be seen as two [main] aspects. Hot and cold nature are two extremes, warm is not as 'hot' as hot, cool is not as 'cold' as cold, therefore [one should] meticulously say [if one has] cold natured medicinals, cool natured medicinals, and hot natured medicinals, warm natured medicinals, [one could] also simply say [one has] cold/cool medicinals and warm/hot medicinals. Taking medicinals and dividing them by the four qi is the medicinals uses in the human body, so it leads to each type [of qi/nature in both the body and the medicinals] reacting and that inducing emergence of a result, this is a gernalization of the nature of medicinals. For example, shígāo, zhīmǔ, etc. can treat hot diseases, keeping that in mind; therefore [these medicinals] are cold/cool in nature. Fùzǐ, ròuguì, etc. can treat cold diseases, keeping that in mind; therefore [these medicinals] are warm/hot in nature. What this means is that cold and cool natured medicinals posses the therapeutics of clear heat and drain fire; hot and warm medicinals posses the therapeutics of dispelling cold and returning yang."*

Qín Bó-wèi actually starts the discussion with a note about the "fifth" qi of medicinals, neutral. He continues this discussion by correlating this with yin/yang theory, then, after discussing the 5 flavors, he ties qi and flavors together using yin/yang theory to do so. Later, he also discusses the concepts of upbearing, downbearing, floating, and sinking.

Qi of Medicinals According to Chinese Medicine:

Cold: mostly minerals (e.g. talc); medicinals from the sea are cold, along with very bitter herbs *huánglián* and Goldenseal
Cool: many herbs *shíhú* and Lemon Balm
Neutral: mostly seeds *huǒmárén* and Stinging Nettle seed
Warm: many herbs *chuānxiōng* and Osha
Hot: few herbs, most are also considered acrid *ròuguì* and Cayenne

Salmon (1710), who is largly considered to have written the last of the great English language materia medicas (herbal) of the Early Modern Era in Europe, explains temperatures this way:

> *"The temperature of medicaments are five-fold, considered, 1. As they are perfectly temperate, neither hot nor cold, dry nor moist; 2. As they are hot; 3. As they are cold; 4. As they are dry; 5. As they are moist. In the four last of which, there are said to be 4 degrees, receding from their principal. An herb which is hot, may be hot in the first, second, third, or fouth degree of heat. Again, from the four prime qualities, these also proceed such that a medicament, 1. As it is hot, may be hot and dry, or hot and moist; 2. As it is cold, also cold and dry, or cold and moist; and these likewise in all the four degrees of temperature. Hot medicaments (and so also cold) are considered in respect of our bodies, and not of themselves; for those simple are called hot, which heat our bodies.*
>
> *Their uses are, 1. To make the offending humour thin, to be expleed by sweat, or through the pores; 2. To help concoction [digestion]; 3. To warm and comfort the viscera; 4. And by outward application, to discuss tumors; 5. Or raise blisters, make cauteries, etc. according to the degrees of heat.*
>
> *Cold medicaments are such as cool our bodies being over-heat, by any adventitious or accidental causes. Their uses are, 1. To cool the parts or bowels; 2. To condense vapours; 3. To thicken humous; 4. To abate the heat of fevers; 5. To refresh the spirits almost suffocated; 6. Allay inflammations; 7. Repress sweating; 8. Ease violent pains."*

Salmon actually goes on at length about moist and dry, the various degrees of each (hot, cold, dry, moist) and how those different qualities of medicinals act in the body and can be used therapeutically.

When looking at new plants, the process of deciding what qi to assign to any particular plant is relatively simple. However, they are not always as obvious as one might assume, and over the more than 100 medicinals I have published monographs for, there are a few with with I have struggled. One can assume that a plant which is always used for heat conditions is cool or cold, but what about an herb that treats both heat and cold conditions? Taking an example from the first book, *Ligusticum grayii* and *L. porterii*, was a pair I struggled with for some time to rectify the contradiction in qi verses therapeutics of these plants. On one hand, they are most famous for treating conditions of heat mostly infection of the upper respiratory tract, but on the other hand they also are known to treat conditions related to cold, specifically wind-damp-cold patterns. Furthermore, although they are most famous for treating conditions of heat, they belong to a botanical genus well-known in Chinese medicine being represented by at least five species, including the herbs *chuānxiōng* and *gǎoběn*; ALL these Chinese species are considered warm. Furthermore, the experience of ingesting these medicinals give a distinctive warming feeling, both in the mouth and throughout the body while under their influence. In the end, I settled on a designation of warm, and this was influenced by the botanical relationships with the species within the Ligusticum genus in Chinese medicine. I struggled to rectify the fact that these two medicinals, which are more or less used in the same way, have a primary function of clearing heat, yet are considered warm. However, my use of botanical relationships helped me reach the characterization found in the first volume, warm!

Channels Entered

Finally, to complete the trifecta we have *Channels Entered*. The "*Channels Entered*" categorization is to my way of thinking of less importance. (Note: This is a topic that is argued in China amongst scholars, with some saying it is important, while other say it is not.) However, I have given this heading significant consideration. In doing so I have explored the Chinese literature in an attempt to better understand the history and context of this heading. My work here is not meant to be exhaustive as there has been much research into this subject in China and it is beyond the scope of this essay to delve into all of it. Channels ascribed to Chinese medicinals have long been, and is likely to continually be, a point of great debate. Even the most famous medicinals often have a range of ascribed channel entries across the source literature. Proponents primarily argue that if a medicinal's primary action is to treat an illness in a particular organ, then that medicinal goes to that organ and the assignment should be made. They also say that herbs with different qi and flavors, that enter the same channel, will have different actions on that channel, essentially saying that qi and flavor are the key characteristics to understanding the action of the medicinal.

Going back to assignment of *Channels Entered* by any particular medicinal, it is my opinion that one first needs to understand the channel flow, i.e. the parts of the body any particular channel has a direct association with or effect on, as the basis for understanding how to assign a medicinal to any particular channel. The *Líng Shū* Chapter 4 clearly lays out the areas each channel is associated with and anatomically where the channel flows, including both internal and external areas of the body and the organ systems. Likewise, we know that certain types of diseases affect certain channels systems, i.e. external wind attacks the *tàiyáng* channels. Thus, understanding the channel system allows us to gauge what channels a particular medicinal may enter. And, better understanding of both the channel systems and the medicinal will likely lead us to a more honed understanding of the channels any particular medicinal will enter. This type of understanding has been part of every Chinese medicine doctor's training over the millennium and yet there is still little agreement, why?

Historically, herbs were not assigned channel entries until the Tang Dynasty materia medica the *Běn Cáo Shí Yí* (741), before that time they were only assigned nature and flavor along with indications; and even those classifications were certainly not standardized. Functions, which are frequently represented with a four character set in modern materia medicas, i.e. quickens the blood and stops pain (活血止痛) or clears heat and resolves toxin (清熱解毒), were also not generally part of materia medicas at this time; or at least they were not standardly written in this format. Instead the medicinals were said to have specific indications such as stops cough. However, looking at older texts helps one to realize that even some of these assignments were not always written in any particular materia medica regarding any particular medicinal. For example, the *Běn Cáo Yǎn Yì* (1116) makes no mention of channels entered through the entire book. However, just over 100 years later in the *Tāng Yè Běn Cáo* (mid-13th Century), qi and flavor are always assigned, but sometimes channel entry information is left out. Later in the Ming Dynasty the *Běn Cáo Měng Quán* assigns channels entered for some, but not for all. Using this book as an example, *huángqí* and *dāngguī* are assigned channel entries, while *rénshēn* and *gāncǎo* are not. These are four of the most famous medicinals used in Chinese medicine, why is *rénshēn*, arguably the most famous Chinese medicinal, and *gāncǎo*, likely the most used Chinese medicinal, not assigned channels entered? Still later, in 1840, the *Běn Cáo Fēn Jīng* was published and says that *gāncǎo*, *niúbàngzǐ*, *mòyào*, and *fùzǐ* all enter the 12 channels and yet makes no mention of whether or not *rénshēn* enters any channels. What I find so striking about this is that a medicinal such as *mòyào*, which was introduced in the *Yào Xìng Lún* (original book lost, but the first mention of it is in the *Táng Běn Cǎo* (659) from a foreign land, is said to enter all 12 channels, while *rénshēn*, a native and exceedingly famous medicinal, has no channel entry assignments! However, what we know about the *Yào Xìng Lún* (the first book to mention *mòyào*) suggests that it assigned *rénshēn* to the lung channel and *mòyào* is not given a channel assignment, but rather a function and 3 indications, "breaks blood and stops pain and removes eye screen and dizziness." So why does a book from the Tang Dynasty assign a channel entry to *rénshēn* but not *mòyào*, while a Qing Dynasty book assigns all 12 channels to *mòyào* but gives no channel assignment to *rénshēn*? A mystery indeed! However, I posit that, in fact, these channel assignments are not only a bit arbitrary, but also weighted quite differently by different writers, and perhaps just the idea was considered nefarious by some authors who seemed to not bother with it at all. It is not until sometime in the 20th Century, along with the "standardization" of Chinese medicine, that *Channels Entered* becomes standard in every materia medica. Why some authors assigned channel to some herbs and not to others remains a mystery.

There is no doubt that most, if not all, authors of materia medicas throughout China's history were well versed in the classics and fully understood channel anatomy and physiology. All these doctors/authors were part of the literate elite and as such would have been well versed in texts such as the *Nèi Jīng*. However, considering that there are only 13 formulas mentioned in that text, it seems reasonable to assume that these designations were originally designed to address qi flow in the body specifically directed at those treating illness with manual therapies rather than herbal medicine. But, qi flow *is* qi flowing and if it is affected by manual therapies, it can be affected by herbs, right?

As mentioned above, the evolution of the material describing the use of plants as medicine suggests that humans have chosen to create an ever more complex milleau to describe the medicinal use of plants. This context imparts a rich texture on the literature and it stands to reason that writers would look to draw on the original corpus to further elucidate each medicinal; bringing greater and greater sophistication to the literature. Therefore, if one is to buy into the theoretical underpinnings of Chinese medicine, then there should be no doubt that medicinals affect the flow of qi in the channels. Thus, there seems good reason to assign channel entry to medicinals, if only to help us understand, from a theoretical standpoint, how they work.

Therefore, when considering the *Channels Entered* heading it is important to look thoroughly at how, and specifically *where*, a particular medicinal acts in the body. We must understand where the qi flows throughout the channels and whether or not the medicinal has a specific action within that area, which includes the organs themselves. Although, as noted above, there is no standard for this classification system and even the heading itself has been called into question, there is little doubt in my mind that this information helps one to better understand and/or remember how the medicinal functions.

An Historical View at a Glance

As an example of the conundrum surrounding these three headings, I randomly chose 7 medicinals to set into the table below. The medicinals were choosen because of their inclusion in the *Běn Cǎo Jīng* so I could start with that text as a reference. The first three (*rénshēn*, *gāncǎo*, and *wǔwèizǐ*) are from the "superior" class of medicinals; the next two (*báisháo* and *dāngguī*) are from the "middle" class; and the final two (*fùzǐ* and *liánqiào*) are from the "lower" class. I then choose nine (9) other famous materia medicas, trying to space them out historically as much as possible, to illustrate the changes that have occurred over the last ~2000 years or so.

The listing of information in the table is in order given in the book looking at the flavor, qi, and channels entered. With only one exception (*Tāng Yè Běn Cǎo*) the flavor is always listed first; that book lists the qi first. Some books do not give some of the information, particularly channels entered, as noted above. Some text, particularly later text such as *Běn Cǎo Gāng Mù* and *Shén Nóng Běn Cǎo Jīng Dú* frequently quote other texts and include that information. However, I have omitted that information unless the author specifically mentions it in his own discussion of the medicinal. The term "level" is a bit ambiguous and could be referring to the flavor or qi of a medicinal, I have used semi-colons (;) to separate each category to the best of my ability, but there is a chance that the original author meant for that term to be used for a category other than where I placed it.

Even a cursory look at the information in the table clearly shows that there is very little agreement, even when it comes to presenting this information. First, it should be noted that the older books didn't generally

Historical View of Basic Categorizations of Seven Medicinals

	Shén Nóng Běn Cǎo Jīng (~200BCE)	Xīn Xiū Běn Cǎo (659)	Chóng Xiū Zhèng Hé Běn Cǎo (1116)	Tāng Yè Běn Cǎo (1298)	Běn Cǎo Yuè Yán (1520)	Běn Cǎo Méng Quán (1565)	Běn Cǎo Gāng Mù (1590)	Dé Pèi Běn Cǎo (1761)	Shén Nóng Běn Cǎo Jīng Dú (1803)	Zhōng Yào Dà Cí Diǎn (2009)
rénshēn 人參	sweet; slightly cold	sweet; slightly cold, slightly warm	sweet; slightly cold, slightly warm	warm; sweet; (sweet/sl.) bitter, sl. cold)‡	sweet, slightly bitter; warm, sl. cold; lung	sweet; warm, slightly cold	sweet; slightly cold	sweet, sl. bitter; sl. cool (raw), slightly warm (processed); lung	sweet; slightly cold	sweet, sl. bitter; sl. warm; lung, spleen, heart, kidney
gāncǎo 甘草	sweet; level	sweet; level	sweet; level	level; sweet; liver, spleen, lung, heart, kidney	sweet; level, cold/warm; liver, spleen, lung, heart, kidney	sweet; level; raw cold, honey mix-fried warm; lung, spleen, heart, kidney, liver	sweet; level; all 12 channels	sweet; heart, stomach, lung, spleen, liver, PC	sweet, level	sweet; level; spleen, stomach, heart, lung
wǔwèizǐ 五味子	sour; warm	sour; warm; (skin & flesh: sweet, sour, seed: acrid, bitter, whole fruit: salty)†	sour; warm	warm; sour, slightly bitter; lung, kidney	sour; warm; (sour, bitter, sweet, sl. acrid)‡	sour; warm	sour; warm;	skin & flesh: sweet, sour; seed: bitter, acrid; warm; lung, kidney	sour; warm	sour; warm; lung, heart, kidney
báisháo 白芍	bitter, level	bitter, sour; level; slightly cold	bitter, sour, level; slightly cold	slightly cold, sour, bitter; kidney, lung	bitter, sour; sl. cold; lung, spleen, liver	bitter, sour; level, slightly cold; lung	bitter; level	sour, bitter, sl. sweet; sl. cold; lung, spleen, liver	bitter; level	bitter, sour; slightly cold; liver, spleen
dāngguī 當歸	sweet; warm	sweet, acrid; warm, great warm	sweet, acrid; warm, great warm	warm; acrid, sweet; spleen	sweet, acrid; warm; heart, spleen, liver	sweet, acrid; warm	bitter; warm	sweet, acrid; warm; heart, liver, lung, spleen	bitter; warm	sweet, acrid; bitter; warm; liver; spleen
fùzǐ 附子	acrid; warm	sweet, acrid; warm, great hot	acrid, sweet; warm, great hot	great hot; great acrid; sm. intestine, TB, stomach, large intestine	great acrid; extremely hot	acrid, sweet; warm, extremely hot	acrid; warm	great acrid; great hot; heart	acrid; warm	acrid, sweet; warm; heart, kidney, spleen
liánqiào 連翹	bitter; level	bitter; level	bitter; level	level; bitter; GB, small intestine	bitter; level, slightly cold	bitter; level, sl. cold; heart, GB, stomach	bitter; level	bitter; cool; spleen, large intestine, heart, liver, PC	bitter; level	bitter; sl. cold; lung, heart; GB

† in the cautions and answers   ‡ later in the monograph

create headings for this body of information, instead the author merely incorporated what he thought was necessary or important. Thus, there was no standard in either presentation or specifics offered. Furthermore, many authors who wrote commentaries on the *Běn Cǎo Jīng* did not deviate from what was written in that book in regard to these aspects of the medicinals; notably Chén Xiū-yuán, whose 1803 publication of the *Shén Nóng Běn Cǎo Jīng Dú* is widely considered one the best commentaries of that work. As far as I can tell, this style of presentation (using headings) didn't come until the 20th Century, and wasn't standardized until sometime in the 1960's or 1970's when there was a large push in China to create a standardized medicine that could be taught in a Western university style and with an eye on "legitimizing" Chinese medicine with the use of "modern scientific method."

It is easy to see from the information above that there really isn't consensus in Chinese medicine with regard to assigning these categories to any particular medicinal, even medicinals with a very long history of use.

That being the case, I don't necessarily think that everyone will agree with what I propose regarding these categories for the medicinals I present in this text. Furthermore, there is no system for evaluating new plants when they are introduced, and yet there have been many introductions over the centuries of Chinese medicine, and each of those substances has been assigned designations within these categories; and mostly people don't agree. So, how important are any of these categorizations? That is for you to decide, I will only say that I believe there are varying degrees of usefulness for any of these, in any given situation in a clinic. Ultimately, whether a medicinal is bitter or sweet, hot or cold, or enters the liver or kidney channels only matters insofar as you are able to make use of that information.

I am often asked by laypersons, students, and practitioners alike, "What does this herb treat?" or "What is that herb good for?" Rarely does anyone ask about any of the information I have been discussing here. Of these categories of information, qi is by far the most common subject of such questioning and it is often posed as a suggestive question such as, "So, it is cooling?" It may be interesting to note here that temperature is the primary link that is shared across most cultures' categorization of medicinal substances.

What practitioners and students are most interested in is how they can use the medicinal; specifically! Students are more likely to ask about these categorizations simply because they are constantly being reminded of them through their studies at school and they are, or can be, useful mnemonics for memorizing the vast amount of data required to gain even beginning proficiency in herbal medicine. In fact, it may actually be that the most important aspect of these classifications is their value as mnemonics, as has been suggested in other cultures by ethnobotanists and anthropologists.[7,9,10] Meanwhile many practitioners would likely fail a test concerning this material because they have long ago realized (either consciously or unconsciously) that most of this information has little use in the clinical setting, and any practitioner that has gained access to source literature in Chinese has learned that there is no standardization of this material.

A point on the convergence (one might say "standardization") of these ideas in modern times. It seems reasonable that much of why this has happened has to do with recent history within China that has allowed less descent and been more supportive of consensus, "towing the party line" so to speak. So, it seems interesting to me that although for nearly 2000 years there was little in the way of consensus, and yet since the early 1960's, or so, there has been wide consensus about these categorizations. It certainly gives one pause.

In conclusion, each of these main categories are important to the understanding of how and why a particular medicinal functions, to a lesser or greater degree. The simplicity of qi is not unique to Chinese medicine when it comes to either categorization or understanding the therapeutic nature of a medicinal substance. Using Gerard (1597) and his entry for Angelica as an example (All his monographs had a heading "*The Temperature*"): "Angelica, especially that of the garden, is hot and dry in the third degree, therefore it opens and attenuates, or makes thin, [assists in] digestion and procures sweat." Notice that he not only gives this medicinal a temperature (qi) but also states that it is "dry in the third degree," a quality that Chinese medicine never had and another dichotomy (dry vs. moist) that is used throughout Gerard's and many other books. He also gives more specific information, or functions, relevant to the "energetics" stated, showing a clear and coherent methodology of thought when it comes to the interaction between the medicinal and the human body; strikingly similar to that of Chinese medicine.

This "energeitic" model of understanding plants and how they affect health and disease is not foreign to Westerners. In the author's opinion this ligitimizes his assertion that trained Chinese herbalists from outside China may have, or can develop the ability to assign the qi of a plant within the therapeutic context of Chinese medicine. Therefore, although there are occasional questions, the process of assigning a "temperature" to Western plants using the Chinese classifications system of "qi" should not really be in question. While deciding whether any particular plant is cool or cold, or warm or hot, may be a bit of a debate, I hope that for the most part whether an herb is cool or warm is of less debate. That being said, I fully accept that even these will be debated. Looking at what a medicinal does clinically in the body, what types of diseases and patterns it treats, in most cases, pretty clearly lays out for us which side of neutral any particular plant should be classified.

Taste is a basic human capacity, and it can be said that most people understand the difference between bitter and sweet. As discussed above, "taste" and "flavor" are different in the context of Chinese medicine. When assessing *Flavor* one must both taste a medicinal and also understand how it functions in the context of health and disease in the human body if one is to designate flavors to it. We must fully understand what the therapeutic action of each flavor is, and base our decision on our knowledge of each of these factors. Assigning flavors to a medicinal is somewhat subjective and there is rarely agreement within the source literature (as noted above). It is also likely that this designation is most importantly a mnemonic rather than anything of particular therapeutic importance, therefore if an author can correlate the tastes assigned to a therapeutic action to help the reader better understand the medicinal, this may be the most important feature of this classification.

Channels Entered is a great debate and I will not suggest that what I have written here is "true" or "right," only that it is a starting place to understand how to use the herb. I have considered how the plant is used, i.e. Is it used for acute external invasions? Perhaps it enters the *tàiyáng* channels. Does it act on a particular area of the body? Perhaps is enters the channels that goes to that part of the body. Assigning *Channels Entered* follows the same logic as *Flavor*, in that this category most importantly helps the reader understand the therapeutic action of the medicinal substance, and proper understanding of both the medicinal and the theory of Chinese medicine offer us a reasonable ability to complete this task. And, like flavors, there is a high likelihood that *Channels Entered* is most importantly a mnemonic. Finally, this heading is the most debated assignment to medicinal substances in Chinese medicine, and agreement is rare in the traditional literature, thus its importance is questionable.

I have, and encourage others to ingest all the herbs you use in the clinic yourself (obviously there are some that you may need to be more careful with based on your particular constitution or the nature of the medicinal) and understand in *your body* what is happening when you ingest each one. The physical memory you gain in your body may be far more valuable than the memory you gained by reading this (or any) book.

I invite you to challenge any of these hypotheses via email or otherwise contacting me. I would very much like to hear what you have to say and I sincerely hope that you can contribute to the sum total of our understanding of how to use these plants within the system of Chinese medicine.

Addendum

When the herb known by Westerns as Senna and Chinese herbalists know as *fānxièyè* (*Cassia angustifolia*) came to China sometime near the end of the Qing Dynasty or the early Republican Period it was greeted like any other good medicinal and incorporated into the materia medica. The book that is recognized to have first included it is the Yǐn Piān Xīn Cān (1935), but Zhāng Xī-chún who died in 1934 first wrote about it in an article, which is now included in his collected works. I have been unable to find the original source, so I don't know exactly when he first published this short monograph, but it is illustrative of how a seasoned doctor and prolific writer of the late Qing and early Republican periods might try to characterize a non-Chinese herb so that Chinese medicine doctors could use it. The significance of this is that this is the only example of a non-Chinese medicinal that I can be fairly sure this is the first published work on it in the modern era. I have also included the information published in 1935 to show a slight evolution in how it is presented, particularly showing how it goes from an introduction to a more formalized presentation. I would suggest that this is potentially how non-Chinese medicinals have been evaluated over the millennia yet we only have records showing the more formalized presentation.

Zhāng Xī-chún on 旃那葉 [zhānnāyè] (Folia Sennae):

> *The shape of zhānnāyè* is like a small dànzhúyè, [it is] light
> green combined with a slight yellow color, [it has] no smell and
> no taste, [it is] produced in India and Iraq. It's nature it can
> increase the peristalsis of the large intestine, it can also increase
> the bile. So, it is good at freeing large intestine dry-binding, it is a
> mild downward draining medicinal, it's nature is neither fierce
> nor harsh, [and it is] unlikely to go so far as to injure the
> construction (qi) aspect. It is also used to treat menstrual block. It
> can be either decocted or steeped. Dosage used alone is 2-3 [qian],
> ground to a powder 1-2 [qian].*

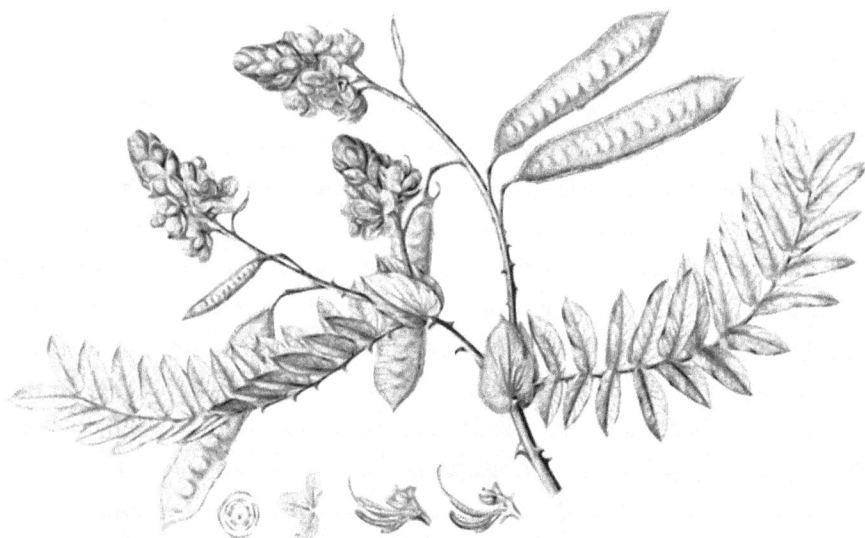

1. Chen Ming (2007). The Transmission of Foreign Medicine via the Silk Roads in Medieval China: A Case Study of Haiyao Bencao 海药本草. *Asian Medicine* 3: pp 241–264.

2. Adams, Francis, trans. *The Works of Hippocrates and Galen.* London: Encyclopaedia Britannica 1952.

3. Sūn Sī-miǎo, circa 650. *A Thousand Pieces of Gold Emergency Formulary* Vol. 1. Translated by Sabine Wilms, personal communication.

4. Messer, Ellen, (1991). Systemactic and medicinal reasoning in Mitla folk botany. *Journal of Ethnopharmacology.* 33: pp. 107-128.

5. Caldecott T. (2013). *Inside Ayurveda: Clinical Education for the Western Practitioner* (Course Notes). PhytoAlchemy Press: Vancouver

6. Etkin, Nina L. (1988). Cultural Constructions of Efficacy. **In** *The Context of Medicines in Developing Countries.* S. van der Geest and S. R. Whyte, eds. Dordrecht: Kluwer Academic Publishers. pp 299-326.

7. Shepard jr., Glenn H. (2004). A sensory Ecology of Medicinal Plant Therapy in Two Amazonian Societies. *American Anthropologist.* 106(2): pp 252-266.

8. Molares, Soledad & Ladio, Ana (2009). Chemosensory perception and medicinal plants for digestive ailments in a Mapuche community in NW Patagonia, Argentina. *Journal of Ethnopharmacology.* 123(3): pp 397-406.

9. Teff, Karen L. (2010). Cephalic Phase Pancreatic Polypeptide Responses to Liquid and Solid Stimuli in Humans. *Physiol Behav.* 99(3): pp 317–323.

10. Leonti, Marco, et al. (2002). Medicinal plants of the Popoluca, México: organoleptic properties as indigenous selection criteria. *Journal of Ethnopharmacology.* 81(4): pp 307-315.

11. Ankli, Anita et al. (1999). Yucatec Maya Medicinal Plants Versus Nonmedicinal Plants: Indigenous Characterization and Selection. *Human Ecology.* 27(4): pp 557-580.

解表藥

Resolve Exterior Medicinals

The exterior resolving category is a group of medicinals used to expel pathogenic factors from the exterior of the body. The category is often divided into warm and cool external resolving medicinals. However, I have not made that division here leaving it to the reader to understand when to use each based on the nature of the medicinal.

External pathogenic factors manifest in many ways and each medicinal has a range of specific uses; most are also used for other types of illnesses. Typical symptoms of externally contracted pathogenic factors are headache, avoidance of cold or wind, body aches, heat effusion, sweating may be present but is not necessary, and a floating pulse. Some of these medicinals can also be used for non-acute pathogens on the exterior such as sores, skin diseases, swelling, etc.

The acrid flavor moves and tends to move outward. Medicinals in this category generally have an acrid flavor and are often aromatic. One medicinal, Blue Curls, is both very acrid and very aromatic.

Most of these medicinals are considered diaphoretics in the biomedical sense and therefore cause sweating. These medicinals can also be used for stagnation of fluids with disinhibited urination with or without swelling. However, medicinals in this category DO NOT necessarily cause sweating because the term "resolving the exterior" in Chinese medicine does not specifically mean "diaphoretic." Ox-eye Daisy is an example of a medicinal in this materia medica that does not, at least very strongly, cause sweating.

Ambrosia

Ambrosia dumosa (A. Gray) Payne and others
Asteraceae
Ambrosi Dumosae herba seu flos
Other names: Ragweed
Favor and Qi: acrid, bitter, warm
Channels Entered: lung, large intestine, urinary bladder
Actions: diaphoretic, aromatic, decongestant

Functions & Indications:

Courses wind, diffuses the lung, and unblocks the nasal passages.
Ambrosia is used for sinus congestion due to external wind invasion
inhibiting the lung's ability to diffuse and downbear, causing an
accumulation of snivel in the nasal passages. It courses wind with
acridity, and downbears with bitterness. Although it is warm, it can be
used for warm conditions with the appropriate herbs.

Diffuses the lung, transforms phlegm and calms panting. Ambrosia is
used for wheezing and panting with hasty breathing, difficulty taking
full breaths, anxiety and even panic. This is mainly in the form of what
we know today as "allergic asthma." For a discussion on allergic asthma
and how it fits into Chinese medicine please see the Commentary
below. The commentary in the following monograph on Blue Curls also
relates to this discussion.

*Aromatically transforms dampness for damp accumulation due to kidney
and spleen vacuity.* This is a suggestion based on the scant literature
available about this herb. I have no direct experience using this
medicinal in this manner, but, based on my experience and the
literature cited below, it seems probable that there is room for
expanding its usage to this area. See the *Commentary* for further
discussion on this matter.

Cautions:

None noted, but it may be prudent to exercise caution with those known to
have "ragweed" allergies.

Dosage and Preparation:

Fresh plant tincture 0.5–3ml, light decoction 2–6g. The herb is best when prepared fresh as a tincture, however the dried plant is also very useful.

Major Combinations:

Combine with Yerba Mansa, *xīnyíhuā*, and Yerba Santa for sinus congestion with clear or white phlegm. This can be administered for phlegm that is either copious and runny or difficult to discharge. For yellow or green phlegm, add Echinacea, *huángqín*, and Goldenseal.

Use by itself for acute relief from seasonal allergies or hay fever.

Combine with tincture of *Cāng Er Zǐ Sān* for relief from seasonal allergies with clear or white discharge.

Combine with *Xiǎo Qīng Lóng Tāng* for non–diffusion of lung qi with chronic cold phlegm or rheum congesting the lung channel, with symptoms of panting, cough, sinus congestion, and copious clear or white phlegm and snivel. This fits neatly into what we often refer to in the clinic as allergic asthma.

Commentary:

The genus *Ambrosia* is native to North America but a couple of species are native in other places in the world, and several species have become successful weeds worldwide (see below). The common name, Ragweed, is well known to those who suffer from allergies because the pollen from many of the species in this genus is the culprit for seasonal (mostly spring and early summer) allergies. Ironically, this plant appears to be, in the author's experience, the most potent plant available for the effective amelioration of symptoms associated with hay fever, including itching eyes and sinus congestion, sneezing, scratchy throat, etc. Some Western herbalists swear by the prophylactic application of Ambrosia sp., providing a moderate dose (15–45 drops) of the tincture a couple of months prior to the patient's allergy season.

The primary plant in the monograph, *Ambrosia dumosa*, is the species with which I have the most experience, and I consider it to be more potent than other species. Nevertheless, many of my colleagues who have more experience with other species have suggested that those species are more than adequate for the above use. One of these, *A.*

artemesiifolia, is probably the most commonly used species, and I have also found it to be useful in the same way as the primary species described above. However, my experience with *A. artemesiifolia* is far too limited to compare them in specific ways. This species (*A. artemesiifolia*) has the added benefit of having a far greater range, including naturalization in China. While *A. dumosa* is only found in the southeastern portions of California, southern Nevada, most of western Arizona, and only the furthest southwestern portion of Utah, as well as northwestern Mexico, *A. artemesiifolia* is found throughout the United States, and *A. psilostachya* can be found throughout much of North and Central America, part of South America, as well as Western Europe, Australia, and South Africa.

The use of organoleptic observation will provide insights into the potency of the various species. From my observations, the more acrid and aromatic species tend to be more drying and fast acting, both in the treatment of phlegm and in coursing wind. The species listed in descending order from most to least bitter and acrid are *A. dumosa*, *A. psilostachya*, and *A. artemesiifolia*. However, differences in growing conditions, ecologies, etc. may pruduce higher or lower levels of any of the bitter and acrid compounds.

"Allergic asthma" is a disease name that more or less fits a mixed repletion and vacuity panting pattern in Chinese medicine. According to The Asthma and Allergy Foundation of America, "Allergic asthma is the most common form of asthma, affecting over 50% of the 20 million asthma sufferers. Over 2.5 million children under age 18 suffer from allergic asthma. Many of the symptoms of allergic and non–allergic asthma are the same (coughing, wheezing, shortness of breath or rapid breathing, and chest tightness)."

The term *chuǎn* (喘) in Chinese medicine is translated as "panting" and is defined as, "Hasty, rapid, labored breathing with discontinuity between inhalation and exhalation, in severe cases with gaping mouth, raised shoulders, flaring nostrils, and inability to lie down." (Wiseman & Ye 1998) There is both vacuity and repletion panting, and in Zhāng Jǐng-yuè's (張景岳) late Ming Dynasty book *Jing Yue's Complete Compendium* (1624) he differentiates them as follows:

> "I suggest that repletion panting has an evil, an evil qi repletion; vacuity panting is without evil, a yuan qi vacuity. In

repletion panting the breath is long and there is enough, in vacuity panting the breath is short and is not continuous. In repletion panting the chest is distended and the breathing is rough, there is a loud voice and turbulent breathing, and expanding as if the lungs are unable to contain the breath with a rapid exhalation; in vacuity panting there is flusteredness and timidity, the voice is low and the breathing short, there is a state of panic as if the breath will be cut off..."

He goes on to say,

"In repletion panting patterns, the repletion evil lays within the lungs, [this is] repletion evil of the lungs, without wind–cold then it must be fire evil. I suggest the evil of wind–cold must be received from the body hair [exterior], so it enters the lung and becomes panting, in intense fire, metal must receive damage, therefore also is disease of the lung becoming panting. The treatment of repletion panting of wind–cold, it is suitable to use warming and dissipation; the treatment of repletion panting of fire–heat, treat using cold and cooling. On the other hand, it is said if there is phlegm panting, those who came before us all said 'treat phlegm,' if you don't know phlegm, how could you have panting?"

Zhū Dān–xī, in his *Zhū Dān–xī's Heart Methods* (mid–14th Century) states of panting, "Although, phlegm–fire internally constrained can never not be the cause, yet [it is] wind–cold externally binding that is the trigger."

Allergic asthma tends to have similar symptoms as outlined in the vacuity panting above, but this is certainly not always the case. However, it clearly has an acute nature about it, which suggests an external attack, and we know there is an external trigger. So, I suggest that whether the internal pattern is vacuity or repletion, it is the invasion of wind–cold that is the trigger, which can be treated with Ambrosia. See *Commentary* in Blue Curls monograph for further discussion.

The following passage is from William Cook's 1869 classic Physio–Medical Dispensatory:

"The leaves are stimulating and astringing, bitter, and permanent in action. An infusion is useful in diarrhea and dysentery of a passive character; in uterine, gastric, and pulmonic hemorrhages; and in degenerate leucorrhea as an

injection and drink. A use of a strong decoction influences the kidneys considerably, sustains the tone of the stomach, and slowly elevates the circulation; and these actions render it useful in the treatment of chronic dropsies, especially when combined with hepatics and stimulating diaphoretics. A very strong decoction, used freely, is reputed among the people in some sections to be a reliable antiperiodic; and many of the actions of the agent certainly suggest properties analogous to Cinchona. It is said to be useful in poultices to phagedaenic ulcers—checking putrescence; and I do not doubt but such is the case. The article is too much overlooked by the profession."

The above quote is specific to *A. artemisiafolia*, but Cook also states that *A. trifida* is likely analogous. This offers an extension of the use of this medicine beyond my experience with it, but may also support the monograph above, particularly the last function and indication to "aromatically transform dampness." Although we can't be exactly sure what Cook was seeing when he says, "diarrhea and dysentery of a passive character" and "degenerate leucorrhea", these symptoms do suggest a vacuous nature to the pathology, such as "spleen vacuity with damp encumbrance", or perhaps even "spleen–kidney yang vacuity." I mention the latter specifically because Cook lists a combination of Ambrosia 30g and Ginger (*gānjiāng*) ~3.5g to be infused in a quart (nearly 1 liter) of water to be used for these conditions. Further evidence from this quote suggesting Ambrosia's action on the spleen is that it is used, "in uterine, gastric, and pulmonic hemorrhages." This could, in fact, be due to the spleen unable to manage the blood. Finally, this medicinal may prove useful in conditions that include both spleen vacuity and liver constraint. This combination pattern could originate from either spleen vacuity or liver constraint. Cook notes that "dropsies" (an old name for a condition that include swelling and excessive fluid in the tissues and abdomen) are treated with this medicinal, "especially when combined with hepatics and stimulating diaphoretics." Many herbs that Cook used as "hepatics" are herbs that resolve constraint, such as Barberry bark, Chelone, Boneset, and others. Use of a stimulating diaphoretic, such as the use of *guìzhī* in *Fú Líng Tāng*, is not an unusual methodology employed by Chinese medicine to improve a formula's ability to rid the body of dampness.

Cook finishes his monograph by noting that this medicinal is "too much overlooked by the profession," which, to a certain extent, is still true nearly 150 years later. However, there have been recent mentions of it by a number of herbalists, and it may be that Ambrosia has found its time in the history of herbal medicine to shine.

While there are a number of research papers on other species in this genus, I could only find one species, *A. maritime*, that is known to treat asthma.1

1. Ghazanfar, S., (1994). *CRC Handbook of Arabian Medicinal Plants*. CRC Press, Boca Raton, pp 265.

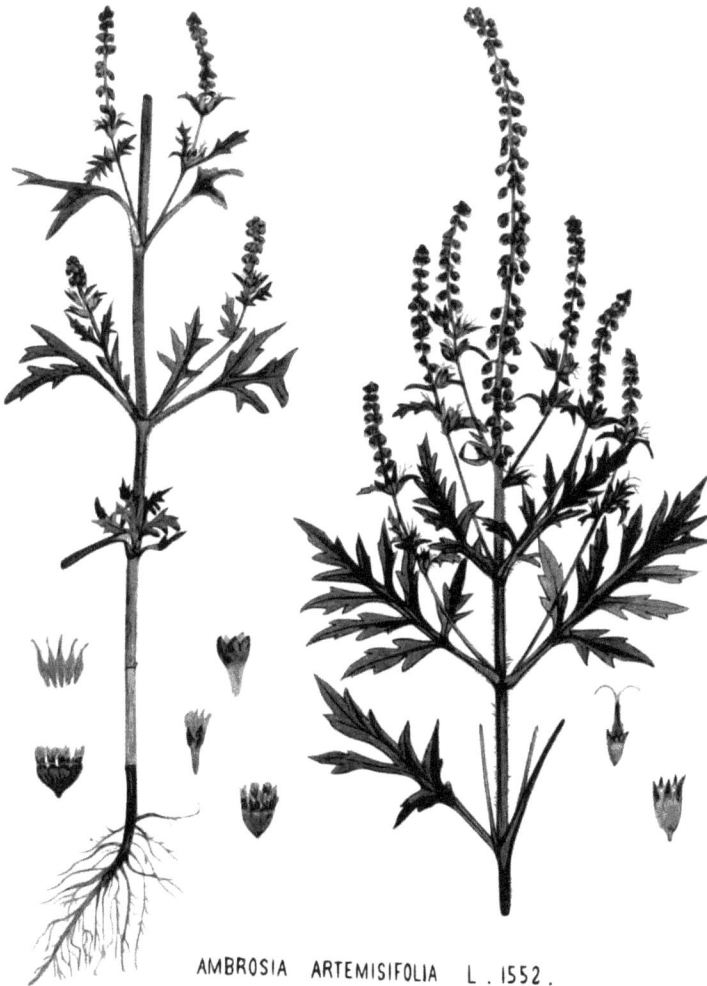

AMBROSIA ARTEMISIFOLIA L . 1552.

Blue Curls

Trichostema lanceolatum Benth., *T. laxum* A. Gray
Lamiaceae
Trichostemae herba
Other Names: Vinegar Weed, Turpentine Weed
Favor and Qi: aromatic, acrid, bitter, cool
Channels entered: lung
Actions: aromatic, diaphoretic, antiinflammatory, antitussive

Functions & Indications:

Diffuses and downbears lung qi and stops panting. Blue Curls can be used in all forms of acute asthma. Blue Curls uses aromatic, bitter acridity to diffuse the lung qi and restore the depurative downbearing function of the lung, and restore easy and steady breathing. Although this herb is cool, it is not overly so, and can be used either alone as a simple, or combined with other herbs in both heat and cold patterns. However, as noted below in the commentary, Zhāng Jǐng-yuè seems to favor a phlegm-fire pattern (repletion) as the primary acute pattern.

Opens the orifice of the nose and transforms phlegm. Blue Curls aromatically penetrates and opens the orifices of the nose. Blue Curls is strongly aromatic and acrid, flavors that easily penetrate the sinuses and open the orifice of the nose to transform phlegm. Blue Curls is also bitter and cooling, which, along with its aromatic and acrid flavors, allows for a draining of turbid phlegm from the upper orifices and clearing of associated heat. Although this medicinal is cooling, it can be used with warm medicinals for cold patterns.

Cautions:
None noted

Dosage and Preparation:
Fresh plant tincture 1–4ml. Although the dried plant retains some action and the infusion can be used, the fresh plant tincture is far and away a superior medicinal for use in acute asthma and obstruction of the orifices of the nose. For acute asthma attacks, administer the fresh plant tincture in 15–20ml hot water. May be repeated as necessary, but rarely requires more than 1–2 administrations.

Major Combinations:

Use as a simple, administering 30–60 drop dosages of the fresh plant tincture in 20–30ml of warm water for acute asthma attack. Administration in this format rarely requires more than two doses, but there is no toxicity to this plant so, if needed, repeating the dosage should not be problematic.

Combine with Yerba Mansa, *xīnyíhuā*, and *báizhǐ* for sinus congestion due to cold phlegm congesting the orifices of the nose.

Commentary:

The two species in the monograph are closely related and to my knowledge, nearly interchangeable. However, they have not been well studied, and I know of only a few herbalists who have experience with these medicinals. There is very little information found in literature searches relating to either the ethnobotanical uses or chemical constituents, from which we could extrapolate information to better instruct us on how to integrate this plant into modern herbal medicine.

Trichostema is a genus within the Lamiaceae (Mint) family. Like many other mints which are aromatic, the two species mentioned in this monograph are exceptionally so. There are only about 17 species of *Trichostema*, all in North America, and 11 are found in California. I have also seen *T. dichotomum* (a species found throughout most of Eastern North America) in my home state of Massachusetts, but it is not aromatic like the species listed here.

Ethnobotanical literature is scant, which is true of many of the medicinal plants from California, and usages of medicinal plants by encroaching Europeans has often been relegated to species related to plants they were already familiar with from their place of origin, such as *Solidago* sp., with noted exceptions such as Yerba Santa and Yerba Mansa.

The two species listed are both native to California. *T. lanceolata* has the widest range, from Washington State to Baja Mexico, and is common throughout most of these areas (except the northern part of its range). It is found in dry, often disturbed, locations up to about 2200m in elevation, and can be quite abundant in some areas. The other species, *T. laxum* is found in the interior of the Coastal Range of Northern California. It is sparse, but locally abundant along streams or in sandy locations below 1700m elevation. I have the least amount of experience with this plant, but included it here because I believe it to be at least somewhat interchangeable with the other species. A third species (not listed above because it is not nearly as aromatic, and beause the author has much less experience with it), *T. lanatum*, is a coastal species and is found from Big Sur to Baja Mexico, staying within the coastal ranges. It is scattered, but fairly common within its range. Unlike the other two species mentioned in this monograph, *T. lanatum* is a perennial shrub and may have utility as a landscape plant, especially within its range. The Native people of the La Jolla tribe use this plant "as a flu remedy and to strengthen one's memory."[1] This plant deserves further investigation.

In describing acute panting, Zhāng Jǐng-yuè states:

> "*Panting and hasty breathing are not the same, panting is rough breathing and congestion, [the] congestion is acute, panting makes lung evils superabundant; breathing [is] hasty breathing and short, upper and lower [regions of the body; i.e. burners] are not interlinked nor replenished, hasty [breathing] makes the lung and kidney insufficient. These two; one is replete [the other is] vacuous, as opposite as ice and charcoal, if treated inappropriately, [the patient] will die, [one] must have comprehensive [pattern] discrimination [to treat properly].*

However, in the rest of his discussion under the Acute Panting heading, he only mentions it one more time specifically when he states, "*[If] phlegm is caused by fire stirring and from acute panting, the ruling [treatment] must be by clearing phlegm and downbearing fire.*" These statements outline the author's thoughts on acute panting. Although there are both replete and vacuous patterns of acute panting mentioned in the opening of his discussion, it is phlegm and fire that get the real attention in his later discussion.

Chén Xiū-yuán (陳修園) says, "*Repletion patterns without qi block [but with] failure to open promptly [leads to] lung distention [and qi] not constrained.*"

The idea of aroma in Chinese medicine is one that is usually associated with warm herbs that revive the spleen, such as *cāngzhú* and *huòxiāng*, or with transforming turbidity in the middle burner, like with *shíchāngpú* and *hòupò*. The unusually light nature of the aroma of Blue

Curls guides it to the lung, where other aromatic herbs do not so easily go. In the lung, it also affects the nose and throat, opening the orifice of the nose and transforming phlegm congestion to assist breathing.

1. Stout, Nathan F. Master's Thesis. 2011.

Hedge Nettle

Stachys spp. L.

Laminaceae

Woundwort

Stachyes herba

Favor and Qi: acrid, slightly bitter, cool, aromatic

Channels entered: lung, stomach, liver

Actions: expectorant, diaphoretic

Functions & Indications:

Disperses wind and clears heat. Hedge Nettle is used for wind–heat invasion with sore throat, sinus congestion, headache and fever. Hedge Nettle is acrid, slightly bitter, and cool. Acridity can outthrust and course the exterior while bitter can drain. The combination of flavors and coolness resolve the exterior of heat while gently draining to disperse wind and clear heat, to treat the symptoms of wind–heat invasions.

Clears the eyes and head. Hedge Nettle is used for external invasion by wind–heat with symptoms of headache, eyestrain, sore and inflamed eyes. Also for headaches in the liver channel due to excessive intake of alcohol or over–indulgences of greasy/fatty foods that may adversely affect the liver. Acridity disperses the wind and resolves the exterior and, combined with coolness, can treat wind–heat invasion affecting the head and eyes. This is especially true when combined with bitterness that drains downward. This combination of flavors and nature also work to move qi and clear the liver.

Expels wind and clears heat for wind–heat impediment with swollen, red, and painful joints. The root is also applied topically for this purpose. This is a traditional use for which I have no experience with, but it is noted frequently in the literature and I offer it here so that you are informed.

Cautions:

Use with caution with yin vacuity.

Dosage and Preparation:

Light decoction or infusion 3–10g; tincture 2–4ml. Mash the roots into a paste with Wintergreen essential oil and apply to inflamed joints.

Major Combinations:

Combine with *mànjīngzǐ* for wind–heat headache. Add *xīnyíhuā* and *bòhé* for headache with sinus congestion due to wind–heat.

Commentary:

Hedge Nettle is an erect perennial 6–10dm tall. It produces seed, but spreads mainly by rhizomes. It has opposite leaves that range from glabrous to soft or stiff–hairy, which may be glandular. True to the mint family, Hedge Nettle has a square, hollow stem. The flowers (tube 6–10mm) appear in whorled spike fashion and are pink (occasionally magenta to purple), with two distinct lips. The entire above–ground portion of the plant is gathered in the late spring and early summer, as it begins to flower. Good quality is light green, has few or no seeds, and has a pungent lemony aroma.

The genus is one of the largest in the mint family with estimates of 250–450 species around the world and 32 species found in the US and Canada.[1] There are a number of famous plants that most people recognize from within this genus, including Lamb's Ears (*S. byzantine*), which is a very common garden plant. Another species, Wood Betony (*S. officinalis*), is a well–known medicinal plant from Europe with a long history of use, which has been known to treat nearly all ailments, but is most commonly known in modern herbalism for treating stress and anxiety, especially associated with headaches. There are also a large number of *Stachys* used as garden plants for their attractive blooming spike (the name *Stachys* comes from the Greek meaning "a grain spike").

There is a significant number of species within the genus that are very common throughout Western U.S. and naturalized elsewhere in the U.S. They frequently have a lemony/minty odor combined with something that could only be described as a "*Stachys scent*." Many people familiar with this region especially enjoy the spring and summer scent of these species, which are commonly found along trails, on the edges of parks, and other locations frequented by humans. When the leaves are crushed, the smell is very strong, and I initially found it repulsive. To each their own! That being said, this plant is a sweet, gentle medicine that deserves a proper place in the materia medica. It is not particularly strong, but is an excellent addition to a formula that requires a gentle touch. I believe there is potential for this plant, when used in higher dosages, for more serious conditions and infections. Like other herbs in the Mint family (Lamiaceae), it has a pleasant taste and can be used in the summer as a refreshing and cooling sun tea. Furthermore, there are a number of species wild-harvested or cultivated for their edible tubers, including Japanese Artichoke (*S. sieboldii*).

While there are many research papers discussing both traditional uses and chemistry of a number of species around the world, I was unable to find any such research on the species known to me from California and surrounding Western United States. While there may or may not be relevance to these other species, I have included a brief look at some of the literature available on several species, including some Chinese species in the *Translation of Available Literature* section.

In Iran, following up on traditional usages for infections, rheumatism, and other inflammatory illnesses, researchers found that hydro-alcoholic extracts of *S. inflata* have significant antiinflammatory activity.[2] In Greece, *S. chrysantha* and *S. candida* have been found to exhibit both antiinflammatory and antibacterial properties in the laboratory.[3,4] And in Serbia, four native species have been shown to have significant antioxidant properties.[5]

Although this is a large genus and there may be significant differences between the species mentioned in this monograph and those in the literature cited above, said literature does suggest that the species described here are quite likely to be valuable and worthy of further investigation.

Translation of Available Literature:

There are eight species of *Stachys* listed in the *Grand Dictionary of Chinese Medicine* (2009). Of the eight, three are listed under the same Chinese name, but although they have some overlap in growing regions, they mostly grow in different areas of the country, which leads one to believe that they are, in fact, very similar in action. Their morphology is similar to that of *Stachys rigida* and other species, and it appears they have similar uses. The three species are *S. japonica* Miq., *S. chinensis* Benge ex Benth., and *S. baicalensis* Fisch. ex Benth., collectively known as *shuǐsū* (水苏) although *S. chinensis* is also called *huáshuǐsū* (华水苏) and *S. baicalensis* is also known as *máoshuǐsū* (毛水苏). These herbs were first listed in the *Shén Nóng Běn Cǎo Jīng* and have entries in many famous materia medicas, although, like so many of the medicinals in that text, they don't have the national attention enjoyed by so many other herbs. The *Grand Dictionary of Chinese Medicinals* says that they are acrid and cool, and enter the lung and kidney channels. They clear heat and resolve toxin, stop cough and free the throat, stop bleeding and disperse swelling, and are used to treat common cold, sand patterns, lung wilting and lung welling abscess, head wind with dizzy vision, throat pain with inability to speak, spitting and expectorating [phlegm], spontaneous bleeding, flood and leaking, malaria, strangury patterns, and pain and swelling due to external blunt trauma.

1. Mulligan, G. A., Munro, D. B. (1989). Taxonomy of species of North American *Stachys* (Labiatae) found north of Mexico. *Naturaliste Canadien.* 116(1): pp 35–51.
2. N. Malekia, A. Garjania, et al. (2001). Potent anti–inflammatory activities of hydroalcoholic extract from aerial parts of *Stachys inflata* on rats. *Journal of Ethnopharmacology.* 75(2–3): pp 213–218.
3. Skaltsa H, et al. (2000). Inhibition of prostaglandin E2 and leukotriene C4 in mouse peritoneal macrophages and thromboxane B2 production in human platelets by flavonoids from *Stachys chrysantha* and *Stachys candida*. *Biological & Pharmaceutical Bulletin.* 23(1): pp 47–53
4. Skaltsa, Helen D., et al. (1999). Composition and Antibacterial Activity of the Essential Oils of *Stachys candida* and *S. chrysantha* from Southern Greece. *Planta Medica.* 65(3): pp 255–256.
5. Jelena Kukic, Silvana Petrovic, Marjan Niketic. (2006). Antioxidant Activity of Four Endemic *Stachys* Taxa. *Biol. Pharm. Bull.* 29(4): 725—729.

Ox-eye Daisy

Chrysanthemum leucanthemum L. or *Leucanthemum vulgare* Lam. (alt. name)
Asteraceae
Chrysanthemi Leucanthemi flos or Leucanthemi Vulgare flos
Favor and Qi: bitter, acrid, cool
Channels entered: lung, liver
Actions: antipyretic, antiinflammatory, diaphoretic

Functions & Indications:

Courses and dissipates wind-heat. Ox-eye Daisy is used for external wind-heat patterns and warm disease defensive aspect (lung) patterns with symptoms of heat effusion, sore throat, sweating, and a rapid pulse. Ox-eye Daisy is bitter, acrid, and cool; its nature is light. Therefore, it can course the exterior and disperse wind from the defensive aspect (lung). Yè Tiān-shì (1777) states, "[The] lung along with the body hair belong to qi, therefore it is said [that they are] on the exterior. [When treating these diseases] first use acrid, cool, and light formulas." The examples he gives are actually medicinals (*bòhé* and *niúbàngzǐ*), not formulas. Ox-eye Daisy fits into the same category as these two medicinals and can be used in these patterns.

Clears liver heat and downbears liver fire. Ox-eye Daisy is used for liver heat/fire with symptoms of red eyes, breast pain, headache, sore throat, and mouth and tongue sores. Can also be used for heat in the liver channel affecting the genitals. Ox-eye Daisy is bitter, acrid, and cool. Cool bitterness can drain heat/fire that has risen from the liver into the upper burner. Although this is a not a strong medicinal for these patterns, it is effective as an assistant in formulas, and should be used in larger dosages.

Cautions:

Some people have allergies to Asteraceae family plants, therefore, those with such allergies should use this plant with some caution. However, in the author's experience, even those with allergies to Asteraceae family plants only rarely react to this species, and in those cases, the reaction is usually very minor and dissipates when the herb is discontinued.

Dosage and Preparation:

Infusion 6-20g; fresh plant tincture 3-6ml

Major Combinations:

This species may be used in place of *júhuā* in any formula.

Combine with *niúbàngzǐ* for wind-heat external invasions when the pathogen is still in the defensive aspect, with symptoms such as rapid, floating pulse, heat effusion, and sore throat.

Combine with *juémíngzǐ* and Feverfew for liver fire harassing the upper burner with red, painful eyes and headache.

Commentary:

Ox-eye Daisy is a member of the Sunflower family (Asteraceae). The plant is native to Europe, but has naturalized throughout much of North America, as well as India and Pakistan (having arrived there with the British colonization as an ornamental). Unfortunately, the naturalization of this plant in many places has led to a reduction in diversity of native species.1 This naturalization far from its native habitat is an advantage to herbalists wishing to use this medicinal. First, because it is so common in so many places, it is easy to find; second, because it is invasive, we do not need to be concerned with ecological damage when harvesting it within these areas of naturalization. In fact, we are likely doing the native habitat a favor by reducing the population of this plant. Also, there is no need for cultivation of this species because it is so easily harvested from the wild, thus reducing the need to use land for cultivation.

Gerard (1597) says, "Dioscorides says, that the flower of Ox-eye made up in a cloth, assage and waste away cold hard swellings; and it is reported that if they be drunk by and by after bathing, it makes them in short time well colored that have been troubled with the yellow jaundice." Here we have an external application that is somewhat contrary to what the author might expect, given the qi of this medicinal. However, Gerard clearly connects the use of this flower, albeit not from his personal experience, to the liver via his mention of jaundice.

Culpeper (1653) says that it, "doth much temper the heat and choler, and refresh the liver, and the other inward parts. A decoction made of them and drank, helpeth to cure the wounds make in the hollowness of the breast. The same cureth also all ulcers and pustules in the mouth or tongue, or in the secret parts." Culpeper's attention to what Chinese medicine would characterize as the liver channel, i.e. breasts and genitals, indicates that this medicinal enters the liver channel. In fact, Culpepper directly mentions the liver, which is a reasonable indication of a connection, although this is not always the case when "translating" from European medicine to Chinese medicine.

Salmon (1710) says little of the flower (and we can not be absolutely sure he was talking about the same species because he mentions four kinds) except the following, "The powder of the flowers. It may be given in white wine, from a dram to two drams morning and evening, and so it is helpful against the jaundice; or, it may be so given immediately after bathing, as Dioscorides says, and so it gives a good color to the skin." This further supports the use for this medicinal for liver complaints.

This medicinal has been given very little attention by modern herbalists, although the American herbal great Michael Moore wrote a monograph on it in his *Medicinal Plants of the West*. Moore (1993) discusses it as a mild antiinflammatory and overall gentle herb, and although I generally agree, I would suggest that significantly larger doses of this medicinal will yield a more "therapeutic" clinical result and would be more specific to the applications discussed within this monograph.

Translation of Available Source Material:

I was unable to find anything written about this medicinal in the Chinese literature. As mentioned elsewhere, this plant is closely related to *júhuā* and has similar medicinal properties. There is a plethora of other species that are closely related, most of which are used in similar ways.

1. Khuroo, Anzar A., et al. From ornamental to detrimental: plant invasion of *Leucanthemum vulgare* Lam. (Ox-eye Daisy) in Kashmir valley, India. *Current Science*, 98(5): 10 March 2010.

Medicinal	Nature	Flavor	Channels	Functions	Indications
Hedge Nettle	Cool	acrid, slightly bitter, aromatic	lung, stomach, liver	Disperses wind & clears heat; Clears the eyes and head; Expels wind and clears heat	sore throat, sinus congestion, headache & fever; headache, eyestrain, sore and inflamed eyes. Also for headaches; swollen, red, painful joints
Ambrosia	cool	acrid, bitter	lung, large intestine, urinary bladder	Courses wind, diffuses the lung & unblocks the nasal passages; Diffuses the lung, transforms phlegm and calms panting; Aromatically transforms dampness	sinus congestion; wheezing and panting; damp accumulation due to kidney and spleen vacuity
Blue Curls	warm	acrid, bitter, aromatic	lung	Diffuses and downbears lung qi and stops panting	acute panting (asthma); penetrate the sinuses and open the orifice of the nose
Ox-eye Daisy	cool	acrid, bitter	lung, liver	Courses and dissipates wind-heat; Clears liver heat and downbears liver fire; Clears heat, expels wind and courses the exterior	external wind-heat patterns & warm disease defensive aspect patterns; red eyes, breast pain, headache, sore throat, mouth & tongue sores; externally contracted wind-heat with heat effusion, sore throat, sweating, & a rapid pulse

清熱藥

Clear Heat Medicinals

The clear heat category is a large group of medicinals that are cool or cold in nature and are used to treat internal heat. Clear heat medicinals clear and drain internal heat from the bowels and viscera, however these are generally different in method and action. Medicinals that clear heat via the bowels do so, in part, by creating movement within those systems such as increasing the flow of urine from the urinary bladder or increasing the flow of stool from the intestines.

There are five sub-categories in this large category: clear heat and drain fire, clear heat and dry dampness, clear heat and resolve toxin, clear heat and cool the blood, and clear vacuity heat. While each one of these sub-categories is important, I have not made those divisions here. Instead, I have left it to the reader to read and understand each monograph clearly.

Common symptoms of internal heat include a sensation of heat, thirst, constipation, dark and/or scant urination, blood in the urine, boils, red tongue with a yellow coat, and a rapid pulse. There are, of course, many other symptoms that can be associated with heat.

From a biomedical point of view heat is often some sort of infection from a bacteria, virus, or other pathogen, but this is not always the case and treating heat as one of these infectious agents could lead to improper treatment and worsening of symptoms. Likewise, using clear heat medicinals for some types of infections, such as exterior pathogens that have not entered the interior of the body can lead to incomplete resolution of pathogenic factors and more serious problems in the future.

Black Walnut

Juglans nigra L., *J. californica* S. Watson, others
Juglandaceae
Juglans fructus paricarpium immatura
Favor and Qi: bitter, cold
Channels entered: stomach, large intestine
Actions: antibacterial, antifungal, vermifuge

Functions & Indications:

Clears heat, dries damp, and resolves toxicity. Black Walnut is used for damp and heat toxin with purulent abscesses or wounds. Used both internally and externally, this medicinal is a cold herb with strong heat-clearing, toxicity-resolving actions. With cold bitterness, immature Walnut husk clears heat, dries damp, and resolves toxicity. See note on external application of this medicinal in the *Cautions* section below.

Clears heat and kills worms. Black Walnut is a premier medicine for killing a variety of parasites, both internally and externally. Well known as an anti-parasitic medicinal, Black Walnut uses its cold bitterness to clear heat and kill worms.

Cautions:

Use with care with middle burner weakness. Although there may be some toxicity at very high doses, the use of this medicinal within normal therapeutic ranges is not known to cause any harm. This medical will stain skin, clothing, and anything else it comes in contact with, so caution should be used when applying it externally. Be sure to inform patients of this precaution. Stains on the skin will dissipate over the course of several days, but clothing, sheets, etc. may be stained permanently.

Dosage and Preparation:

Fresh plant tincture 10–60 drops; dried husk in decoction 2–6g; leaves in decoction 3–10g

Although the dried husks can be used for medicine, the fresh husk tincture is far superior. As such, I have no experience using the dried husks, preferring to always use the fresh plant tincture. When using the tincture externally, be sure to use it carefully on skin that is sensitive, and remember that it will stain the skin. In cases of sensitive skin, such as applying to the vagina or anus, the tincture should be watered down with sterile water or by adding to a decoction of other appropriate medicinals. The primary monograph above is referring to the fruit husk, however the leaves have also traditionally been used.

Major Combinations:

Combine with *kŭshēn* and *huángbái* as a wash for vaginal infections with inflammation, itchiness, and odorous discharge.

Combine with *kŭshēn*, Goldenseal, and Capsicum in tincture format as an external application to nail fungus. This is most effective when it is applied to a cotton ball or gauze and fixed in place with a bandage or medical tape. Application must be for at least two weeks, and often up to six weeks. Although this is not likely to completely eliminate the fungus, it will slow it significantly, and new nail growth often occurs.

Commentary:

Black Walnut and other species, such as the Persian (or English) Walnut, are well known trees, famous for both their fruit, which has been used since antiquity as food, as well as their wood, which is highly prized for its hardness. However, not all the *Juglans* species have the same hard wood for which the Eastern American species (the primary herb in the monograph) is so famous. Some species, such as the Asian *J. mandshurica*, have softer wood and, although they are used in building, are not valuable like the American and other species. The center for the genus diversity is the Americas, with only four species being native outside of the Americas (two in East Asia and two in Europe/Central Asia). The South American species, *J. australis*, measures as the 6th hardest wood known! This genus is significant economically as medicine, food, and building material.

Gerard (1597) discusses the kernels and several ways to prepare them as food and medicine. Interestingly, he warns that the newly gathered kernels are "a little cold" and are hard on the digestion. Conversely he states, "The dry nuts are hot and dry, and those more which become oily and rank, these be very hurtful to the stomach; and besides that they be hardly digested, they increase choler; they cause headache, and be hurtfull for the chest." Here he clearly confirms what Chinese medicine says about the qi of Walnuts. Also, he recognizes that those that have gone rancid are not to be consumed without considerable harm to the body. Later, he invokes Galen by saying: "The outward green husk of the nuts has a notable binding faculty," and that Galen specifically stated that the juice made from the green husks is good against all inflammations of the mouth. Again, by quoting Galen, Gerard draws upon the great physician from 17 centuries earlier, showing us now that this medicine has a long history of consistent, safe, and apparently positive therapeutic use.

Culpeper (1653) discusses the use of the common, or Persian, Walnut (also commonly called "English Walnut", *J. regia*) extensively, describing the virtues of the leaves (both young and old), the bark, the fruit, and the green hulls, but it is the green hulls that are most commonly used today. Furthermore, while I have not used this species, I believe that there is little difference between the two species when it comes to the uses I have discussed in the monograph above. Of the green hulls he says, "The juice of the other green husks, boiled with honey is an excellent gargle for a sore mouth, or the heat and inflammations in the throat and stomach." And, "The distilled water of the green husks, before they be half ripe, is of excellent use to cool the heat of agues, being drank an ounce or two at a time; as also to resist the infection of the plague, if some of the same be also applied to the sores thereof. The same also cooleth the heat of the green wounds and old ulcers, and healeth them, being bathed therewith." This clearly shows Culpeper understanding of this herb as a cooling medicinal that clears heat, dries dampness, and resolves toxin. Although he does not specifically state that the green husks are drying, he does say that the bark and leaves, "doth bind and dry very much". The medicinal virtues of the leaves and husks are similar, and the use of the husks for "green wounds and old ulcers" suggests that this part of the plant also addresses dampness (as he states about the leaves and bark), though perhaps to a lesser degree.

Research on the various *Juglans* species is scant when it comes to medicinal action. There has been some research on the antioxidant properties of the green husks, mostly of *J. regia*, but this research is aimed at creating food preservatives. However, a paper on the aqueous extracts of *J. regia* showed strong actions against several Gram-positive bacteria including *Staphylococus aureus*, which is a major cause of food borne illness.[1] The hydro-alcoholic extract was shown to have "important activity" against eight common fungal pathogens, including *Candida krusei* and two *Microsporum* species.[2] The former of these two fungi is a common pathogenic fungi of the vulva and vagina, as well as both the skin and nails. The latter genus is well know to cause ringworm, tinea, and a number of other fungal infections of the skin.

The major constituent thought to be responsible for this antifungal activity is called juglone and is in the class of consituents known as naphthoquinones. This compound is apparently present in all parts of most species within the family,[3] thus it is likely that many different species within this family would be useful in treating many of the illnesses described in this monograph.

Translation of Available Source Material:

There are several Juglans species used in the Chinese materia medica. The most famous is probably *J. regia* L. (*hútáo* 胡桃), but this and others are not used in the same way as the herb in the above monograph, with the exception of J. mandshurica Maxim. (hétáoqiū 核桃楸), of which the entire fruit is used. The *J. mandshurica* tree is native to Central and Northeastern China, into Russia, as well as the Korean peninsula. Yet another species growing in Southwestern China and into neighboring countries is J. sigillata (*pāohétáo* 泡核桃). The peel of the fruit (or sometimes the whole fruit) is used, and first appeared in *Journal of Medicinal Plants of the Northeast* [China] (1959); whether the information came from the West or had simply been an undocumented folk use is unclear. That book says to use the peel to make a tincture, and use this to treat stomach disease and abdominal pain. The *National Chinese Herbal Medicine Compilation* (2012) says the fruit is considered acrid, neutral, and toxic, and is used for stomach and duodenal ulcers and stomach pain; externally it is applied for neurodermatomyositis. The *Grand Dictionary of Chinese Medicinals* (2009) says it is used to move qi and stop pain, and kill parasites and stop itching. It is used for stomach duct and abdominal pain, and "ox-hide lichen," which is an episodic skin disease characterized by thickening and hardening of the skin that gives it the appearance of the skin of an ox's neck. It is used as a tincture in 10–15ml doses, or as a decoction in 6–9g doses.

1. Oliveira, Ivo, et al (2008). Total phenols, antioxidant potential and antimicrobial activity of walnut (*Juglans regia* L.) green husks. *Food and Chemical Toxicology*. 46: pp 2326–2331.

2. Rodrigues, L, et al (2010). Antifungal activity in *Juglans nigra* green husks. *Planta Medica.* 76: pp 444.

3. Clark, Alice M., Jurgans Tannis M., Hufford, Charles D., (1990). Antimicrobial activity of Juglone. *Phytotherapy Research.* 4(1): pp 11–14.

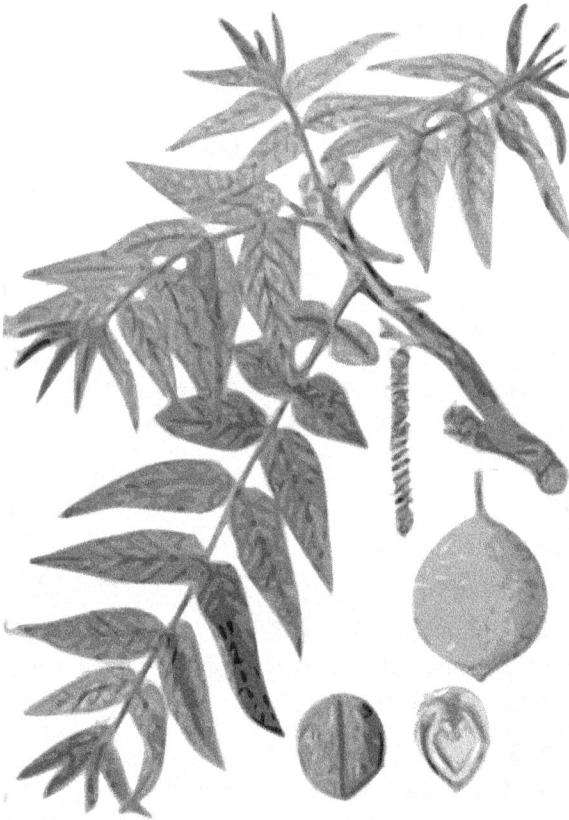

Juglans nigra

Blessed Thistle

Centaurea benedicta (L.) L. 1763 (Formally *Cnicus benedictus*)
Asteraceae
Cnici Benedicti herba
Favor and Qi: bitter, acrid, cool
Channels entered: liver, gallbladder, spleen
Actions: bitter, antibacterial, diuretic, diaphoretic

Functions & Indications:

Clears heat, dries dampness, and downbears fire. Blessed Thistle is used for liver heat/fire rising and liver/gallbladder damp–heat patterns. This medicinal treats dampness, but its virtue lies in clearing heat and downbearing fire. When liver heat/fire arises, from any cause, it will rise upward and affect the upper burner, manifesting as headache, red face, red eyes, vexation, dizziness, etc. Blessed Thistle is well known for treating these symptoms. Because liver fire can damage the fluids, it can cause reduced and bloody urination; for this, Blessed Thistle is also well–known and will be beneficial. Blessed Thistle is bitter and cool, which can clear heat and downbear fire; it opens the liver with bitter acridity which, combined with coolness, is very effective for reducing liver fire.

Courses the liver, resolves qi stagnation, and harmonizes liver and spleen. Blessed Thistle is used for patterns of liver stagnation leading to dizzy head, oppression in the chest, irascibility, pain and fullness in the stomach duct, aversion to food, glomus and fullness after eating, sloppy diarrhea, and string–like pulse. This pattern presents much like spleen vacuity but has the string–like pulse. This is a common pattern in the clinic, but the pulse is often either over–looked or misread, leading to an inappropriate use of formulae to supplement the spleen without coursing the liver and harmonizing Wood and Earth.

Courses the exterior, dissipates heat and abates fever. Blessed Thistle is used for *shǎoyáng* patterns with symptoms of alternating heat effusion and chills, fullness in the chest and rib–side, bitter taste in the mouth, dry throat, slight dizziness. With bitter acridity, it courses the exterior and dissipates heat. Entering the *shǎoyáng*, this herb's action is similar to *cháihú* but is more bitter and draining; it may be used as a substitute of *cháihú* in cases where that herb is inappropriate, such as during interferon treatment in hepatitis C therapy or when there is concern that its upbearing action is contraindicated, such as yin vacuity with exuberant fire, qi counterflow, etc. Although Blessed Thistle compares in many ways to *cháihú*, it does not have an upbearing energy.

Courses the liver and resolves constraint. Blessed Thistle is used for liver constraint qi stagnation causing painful, irregular, or stopped menstruation, breast distention, rib-side pain, and chest fullness. With bitter acridity, Blessed Thistle courses the liver and resolves constraint, moves qi, and stops pain, while also cooling the heat caused by constraint.

Moves qi, resolves constraint, and frees the breast milk. Blessed Thistle is used for inhibited flow of breast milk due to liver constraint and qi stagnation. Blessed Thistle is well-known by midwives for its ability to improve milk flow in postpartum moms, particularly first-time moms who might be anxious, nervous, or feeling pressure to perform. Blessed Thistle is acrid and bitter, and opens the liver to move qi and free constraint.

Cautions:
Use caution with spleen yang vacuity, or repletion cold in the stomach.

Dosage and Preparation:
Infusion or decoction 3–6g, tincture 1–3ml.

Major Combinations:
Combine with *Xiāo Yáo Sǎn* and *chēqiánzǐ* for fullness in the lower abdomen, frequent but scant urination due to liver constraint where the liver is unable to perform its free-coursing action.

Combine with *Lóng Dǎn Xiè Gān Tāng* for patterns of damp-heat in the liver channel with symptoms of red eyes, scanty yellow urination (possibly with blood), headache, vexation, and red face.

Combine with Skullcap and Lemon Balm for liver fire flaming upward with red eyes, red face, and headache due to excessive consumption of alcohol.

Combine with Fenugreek for inhibited or ceased lactation.

Commentary:

Blessed Thistle is a member of the Asteraceae family in the *Centaurea* genus. The *Centaurea* genus is large, with about 500 species worldwide, including many noxious or invasive weeds.[1] This annual plant is native to Europe, but has naturalized in North America. Typical of many thistles, Blessed Thistle is well-armed, but the spines are fairly soft and it can be harvested without significant problem, especially when compared to a plant like Milk Thistle, which requires gloves or mechanical harvesting to avoid self-imposed acupuncture.

This medicinal has been written about for over 2000 years. Dioscorides mentions it and he also offers the name used by the Egyptians, which suggests a much longer period of use. However, there is some question as to proper identity, owing to the fact that thistles are easily misidentified. However, based on Dioscorides' description, it seems likely that authors have mostly been discussing the same plant. It should be noted that this is not an uncommon problem, and also exists in Chinese medicine, where there are often questions regarding the specific plant about which the authors were describing, even in the famous *Shén Nóng Běn Cǎo Jīng*,.

Although not a popular medicinal in American practice, it remains a frequently used herb in European practice, where we have records from at least 500 years ago. Its use as a medicinal to improve milk flow for nursing mothers, however, remains a common use in both Europe and North America. Traditionally, this herb was prepared as a tea for this purpose, but many modern midwives have switched to tinctures as a more simple (read "easy") way to ensure that mom is getting what she needs without needing to work hard to get it (let's face it, she has enough on her plate as it is). In her classic *A Modern Herbal* (1937), Mrs. M. Grieve states, "It is chiefly used now for nursing mothers the warm infusion scarcely ever failing to procure a proper supply of milk. It is considered one of the best medicines which can be used for the purpose."

Gerard (1597) tells us that this medicinal, "is bitter, so it is also hot and dry in the second degree" as well as being "cleansing and opening." The connection here between bitter and hot and dry is interesting and curious; we mostly consider bitter to be draining (Gerard seems to agree with that by stating it is "cleansing and opening"), but most bitter medicinals, particularly those that are primarily bitter, are considered (in Chinese Medicine) to be cooling. However, the entirety of the monograph must be taken into account when considering the qi of the medicinal. Gerard writes that Blessed Thistle treats the following: deafness, giddiness of the head, expels worms, it is very good against fever, liver inflammation, pestilence, plague sores, poisonous bites, etc. Most of these symptoms are likely to be associated with heat, not cold, and a medicinal that treated these ailments in Chinese medicine would almost definitely be considered cooling.

Culpeper (1653) says of this medicinal, "It is an excellent remedy against the yellow jaundice, and other infirmities of the gall . . . [it] clarifies the blood . . . The continued drinking the decoction of it, helps the red faces . . . Also it provokes urine . . ." Culpeper was an astrologer, and the monograph he wrote for this medicinal clearly shows his deep understanding of both subjects. While he almost always discussed some facet of astrology when discussing a medicinal plant, within this monograph he equates every action to some astrological sign. This leads me to believe he had extensive experience with the herb and gave it considerable thought when writing the monograph.

Salmon (1710) says Blessed Thistle is hot and dry in the second degree, and "It is good against recurring fevers, malign and pestilential fevers, pleurisy, [kidney and/or] gall stones, urinary gravel, vertigo . . ." As with Gerard, Salmon calls this medicinal "hot and dry", but then goes on to describe myriad ailments that would call for cooling medicinals within the Chinese medicinal paradigm.

Modern research is scant, however there are several ethnobotanical papers that are available. None of them cover Blessed Thistle specifically, and few of them go into any depth on its traditional usage. In Algeria, the plant is used for urinary tract infections[2] and as a hypotensive.[3] And, in the Dominican Republic (far from its native range), a decoction is used externally for tumors.[4] Although it does not specify, this last citation is most likely for the treatment of tumors of the breast or vaginal area because the paper specifically covers medicinal plants used in the treatment of gynecological disorders.

1. *Jepson eFlora* http://ucjeps.berkeley.edu/cgi-bin/get_IJM.pl?tid=2297 accessed 2013–08–13.
2. Sekkoum, K. et al. (2010). Inhibition Effects of Some Algerian Sahara Medicinal Plants on Calcium Oxalate Crystalliztion. *Asian Journal of Chemstry*. 22(4): pp 2891–2897.
3. Amel, Bouzabata (2013). Traditional treatment of high blood pressure

and diabetes in Souk Ahras District. *Journal of Pharmacognosy and Phytotherapy.* 5(1): pp 12–20.

4. Ososki, Andreana L., et al (2002). Ethnobotanical literature survey of medicinal plants in the Dominican Republic used for women's health conditions. *Journal of Ethnopharm.* 79(3): pp 285–298.

Chaparral

Larrea tridentata (DC.) Coville
Zygophyllaceae
Larreae ramulus cum folium
Favor and Qi: bitter, acrid, cool
Channels entered: lung, urinary bladder, large intestine
Actions: antibacterial, antifungal, anti–inflammatory

Functions & Indications:

Clears heat, disinhibits urine, and resolves toxin. Chaparral is used for damp–heat in the urinary bladder (strangury) with symptoms such as scant, painful (burning), reddish (possibly) or yellow, malodorous urine. Chaparral is cool bitter, clears heat and resolves toxin, while its acrid flavor can disinhibit the qi dynamic of the kidney/urinary bladder, allowing urine to flow more freely.

Expels wind, clears heat, and resolves toxin. Chaparral is used for wind–warmth entering the upper burner and manifesting in fever, cough with thick yellow sputum, sore throat, sinus congestion with purulent discharge, etc. Chaparral is bitter, cool, and acrid, clearing heat and resolving toxin while coursing the exterior and expelling wind. Chaparral also has a secondary action to treat phlegm–heat accumulation and/or obstruction.

Clears heat, resolves toxin, generates flesh. Chaparral is used for use externally for a variety of toxic–heat skin conditions (either from external injury or of internal etiology). Chaparral can be applied using a variety of methods to treat external skin conditions. It is also used externally for painful, swollen joints.

Cautions:

Although there have been some reports of toxicity, these reports more likely involve users with previous significant health issues and/or inappropriate (mostly above normal) dosage range that would otherwise not be seen. "However, as far as we can conclude from these data, the reported toxic doses in humans and experimental animals always exceeded the traditional use of the plant and are often confounded with use of other herbs and potentially with lifestyle choices. Overall, prescribed appropriately traditional uses of other herbal medians appear safe."[1]

Dosage and Preparation:

Tincture 0.5–2ml; decoction 1–4g; oil used externally

Major Combinations:

Combine with *báimáogēn* and Plantain leaf for hot, scanty, painful urination with the prescence of blood.

Combine with Echinacea, *shìgān*, and *Yín Qiáo Sàn* for wind–warmth penetrating the upper burner with symptoms of sore swollen throat, fever, yellow tongue coating, and a floating rapid pulse.

Commentary:

This is one of the great, though little known and underutilized, North American medicinal plants. Although it has gained some fame, it was knocked down harshly in the early 1990s, with reports of toxicity surfacing after some people experienced serious liver damage while taking the herb. This has since been seriously questioned because of inappropriate usages and dosages (see caution section above). Despite these reports, the medicinal has a long history of safe and effective use, and should again find its way into common practice.

Chaparral is a desert–dweller with its own method of self–imposed birth control in the way it excretes a chemical in the seed coat and leaves which prevent it from growing too "thick." However, it is likely to sprawl across the desert floor for as far as one's eyes can see.

Some research indicates that this plant has shown significant activity against human papillomavirus, herpes simplex, and human immunodeficiency virus.[2,3,4] This modern research, combined with much of the traditional information (however fragmented), might lead a practitioner to consider using this medicinal when treating latent evil (*fúxié* 伏邪).

Moerman (1998) lists all of the Native groups living in the vicinity of this plant as having used it in medicine to cure nearly 50 diseases (according to their claim). Although this is, perhaps, a bit of an exaggeration, there is no doubt that continued use and understanding of this plant is warranted.

1. Arteaga S. et. al. (2005) *Journal of Ethnopharmacology* 98(205): pp 231–239.
2. Craigo, J. et al., (2000). *Antiviral Research* 47(1): pp 19–28.
3. Chen, HS et. al., *J. Med. Chem.*, 1998, 41(16): pp 3001–3007.
4. Gnabre, JN, *PNAS.* 92(24): pp 11239–11243.
5. Moerman, D. *North American Ethnobotany.* 1998.

Yellow Pond Lily

Nuphar luteum (L.) Sm., *N. polysepala* Engelm.

Nymphaeaceae

Nupar rhizome cum radix

Favor and Qi: bitter, slightly sweet, astringent, cold

Channels entered: kidney, lung

Actions: astringent, anti–inflammatory, antibacterial

Functions & Indications:

Clears heat and dries dampness. Yellow Pond Lily is used for damp–heat in the lower burner with symptoms of hot sloppy diarrhea, vaginal discharge with a strong odor, or hot, burning urination (with or without bleeding). Yellow Pond Lily is bitter, astringent, and cold. Bitter drains, while astringent restrains. This medicinal uses bitter flavor and cold nature to effectively clear and drain heat from the lower burner, while using astringency to restrain and stop excessive loss of fluids. This is an exceedingly effective medicinal for the treatment of these patterns.

Drains lung–heat and restrains the yin. Yellow Pond Lily is used for replete heat in the lung with symptoms of cough, shortness of breath, difficulty breathing, and sweating. Yellow Pond Lily is bitter, astringent, and cold. Utilizing bitterness and coldness, it effectively clears and drains heat from the lung, while its astringency helps to contain lung qi and yin fluids that are easily damaged by replete heat in the lung.

Cautions:

The only caution I could find comes from two disparate sources stating that excessive use of this medicine could lead to male sterility.[1,2] Since I feel confident that neither of these sources had access to the other, this could be a very real phenomenon. Yellow Pond Lily is cold in nature and should probably be used with caution in yang vacuity, cold in the middle, or spleen qi vacuity.

Dosage and Preparation:

The rhizome should be peeled. Use 3–10g in decoction or strong infusion; 2–4ml fresh plant tincture

Major Combinations:

Combine with *huángbái* and *fúlíng* for damp–heat pouring downward, with symptoms such as yellow vaginal discharge, yellow malodorous urination, or malodorous sloppy diarrhea. Add *huánglián* or Goldenseal for dysenteric conditions. Add *tànshānzhīzǐ* for blood in the urine or stool.

Combine with *tiānhuāfěn* and *màiméndōng* for dry cough due to either vacuity or replete heat in the lung.

Combine with Echinacea, Osha, and *huángqín* for cough with yellow or green phlegm. Add *yúxīngcǎo* for purulent green sputum. Add *bànxià* and Elecampane for excessive amounts of phlegm. Add Wild Cherry bark or *xìngrén* and *jiégěng* for unrelenting spasmodic cough; Wild Yam or Lobelia can also be a good choice in this situation.

Commentary:

Yellow Pond Lily, also known as Spatterdock, is a common water lily found in ponds, lakes, and sluggish streams throughout North America. It has a large rhizome with long roots which anchor it, usually deep in the mud. Although the roots are mentioned in a number of ethnobotanical sources, to the best of the author's knowledge, most herbalists only use the rhizome. This is a medicinal that is not commonly found in commerce, but is one that has excellent medicinal qualities and deserves further investigation. There are a number of related species throughout the world, including several in North America (see *Translation of Available Source Material* below for information about Chinese species). The White Water Lilies (*Nymphea* sp.) are only botanically related by family, but it is likely that, in a broad sense, many of these plants (both within the *Nuphar* and *Nymphea* genus) could be used interchangeably, based on literature sources that discuss other species in essentially the same way as this species. In fact, many sources, including Salmon (1710) and Felter & Lloyd (1905), clearly state that the Yellow Pond Lily and White Water Lily are interchangeable.

Yellow Pond Lily has been shown to have rather strong antibiotic activity.[3,4] This may account for some applications of this medicinal, particularly its use in the treatment of damp–heat conditions.

The functions and indications listed above are limited to my clinical experience but, based on a literature search of the genus there is likely a wider use of this medicine. For example, a Japanese species (precise species was not identified in the paper) is part of a traditional formula that was shown to be significantly better for pain relief, duration of healing, and cost, as compared to non-steroidal anti-inflammatory drugs (NSAIDs) for rib fracture.[5] *Nupar pulilum* (a Japanese species) has been shown to have strong anti-tumor activity against some types of cancer.[6]

Gerard (1597) does not say whether the medicinal is warm or cold, but states: "Both the root and seed...have a drying force without biting." He starts out *The Virtues* portion of the monograph with "Water Lily with the yellow flowers stop laskes, the outflowing of see [semen] which come away by dreams or otherwise..." This clearly shows a binding or astringent nature and, according to Wiseman & Ye (1998), there are five patterns that cause involuntary loss of semen. Of these five patterns, only two (heart vacuity and liver depression & noninteraction of the heart and kidney) do not call for securing the essence or downbearing fire (which is a form of clearing heat). Thus, it seems likely that this medicinal would be very helpful in most cases of this disorder. However, he also warns that the continued use of the medicinal will cause sterility in men. And, in support of this author's primary use of this medicinal, he says: "...the root of the yellow cures hot diseases of the kidneys and bladder, and is singular good against the running of the raines [excessive urination]."

Culpeper (1653) grouped the European Yellow Pond Lily (*Nupar luteum*) together with White Pond Lily (*Nymphaea odorata*), but the above monograph only focuses on the Yellow Pond Lily (*Nuphar luteum*), although their uses are essentially the same. Of the rhizomes, he said "[they are] cold and dry". He also said that the roots (presumably meaning rhizomes) are "most used [compared to the leaves], and more effectual to cool, bind, and restrain all fluxes in men and women; also running of the reins, and passing of the seed when one is asleep." This statement is in accord with the information presented in the Functions and Indications section, which uses terminology consistent with Chinese medicine. The phrase "running of the reins" refers to frequent urination, and the phrase "passing of the seed when one is asleep" is nocturnal emissions. He further states that, "The root is likewise very good for those whose urine is hot and sharp, to be boiled in wine and water, and the decoction drank."

Felter & Llody (1905) states, "The root is astringent, demulcent, anodyne, and antiscrofulous. Used in dysentery, diarrhea, gonorrhea, leucorrhea, and scrofula, and combined with Wild Cherry in bronchial affections." This description refers to the *Nuphar alba*, which is now known as *Nymphaea odorata*, but the text states that the two (White and Yellow Pond Lily) are interchangeable.

Translation of Available Source Material:

The root of a related species, *Nuphar pumilum* (Huffm.) DC. (*píngpéngcǎogēn* 萍蓬草根), first appeared in the Tang Dynasty materia medica, *Supplement to the Materia Medica* (741). This text attributes a number of supplementing actions to the plant: "it is sweet and without toxicity, it supplements vacuity, boosts the physical energy, and treats long–term eating with absence of hunger." The *Grand Dictionary of Chinese Medicinals* (2009) says "sweet, cold, and entering the spleen, lung, and liver channels. It clears heat and quickens the blood, and fortifies the stomach and disperses food. It is used for lung heat cough, static blood with irregular menstruation, menstrual pain, knocks and falls, and food accumulation."

As we can see, the latter text agreed with the former to some extent, but the emphasis of how to use this medicinal has certainly changed over time, which leads us to wonder about the identification of the original plant. However, Yellow Pond Lily is pretty easily identifiable, thus we can assume an evolution in understanding has occurred, rather than mis–identification.

1. Gottelsfeld & Anderson; (1988). Gitksan Traditional Medicine: Herbs and Healing. *Journal of Ethnobiology.* 8(1). pp 13–33.
2. Salmon, William. *The English Herbal or History of Plants.* (1710)
3. McCutcheon, A.R., et al. (1992). Antibiotic Screening of Medicinal Plants of the British Columbian Native Peoples. *Journal of Ethnopharmacology.* 37: pp 213–223.
4. McCutcheon, A.R. et al. (1997). Anti–Mycobacterial Screening of British Columbian Medicinal Plants. *International Journal of Pharmacognosy.* 35(2): pp 77–83.
5. Hajime Nakae, et al. (2012). Comparison of the Effects on Rib Fracture between the Traditional Japanese Medicine Jidabokuippo and Nonsteroidal Anti–Inflammatory Drugs: A Randomized Controlled Trial. *Evidence-Based Complementary and Alternative Medicine.* Volume 2012, 7 pages.
6. Hisashi Matsuda, et al. (2003). Potent anti–metastatic activity of dimeric sesquiterpene thioalkaloids from the rhizome of Nuphar pumilum. *Bioorganic & Medicinal Chemistry Letters.* 13(24), pp 4445–4449.

Willow Bark

Salix sp. L.

Chinese Name: *báiliŭ* (白柳)

Salicaceae

Salix cortex

Favor and Qi: bitter, slightly acrid, astringent, cool

Channels entered: lung, liver

Actions: anti–inflammatory, febrifuge

Functions & Indications:

Clears heat and relieves pain. Willow bark is used for various painful conditions related to heat. Willow bark effectively clears heat from any source, i.e. replete heat or vacuity heat, to relieve pain. Willow bark is most commonly used to relieve pain in the joints and is an important herb in the treatment of impediment syndromes. Willow bark cools and drains heat with bitterness, while penetrating and gently moving with acridity. Acridity can penetrate heat-toxin or stagnated heat lodged in the joints. Willow bark can also be used in the treatment of other heat-associated pain such as heat lodged in the intestines with or without diarrhea, headache due to heat/fire rising, and heat-dampness pouring into the bladder.

Clears heat, cools the blood, and stops bleeding. Willow bark is used for blood in the stool, urine, or excessive menstrual bleeding. Willow bark can be used quite effectively for conditions where heat has damaged the network vessels leading to bleeding, but can also be used when there is fire toxin leading to blood moving frenetically out of the vessels. When heat enters the blood aspect, the blood can move frenetically. Willow bark is bitter and cool, upon entering the blood it is also slightly acrid, which helps to dissipate heat from the blood aspect, while draining with its bitterness and cool nature.

Cautions:

Large doses or prolonged usage of this herb can damage the stomach and spleen. Patients with allergies to salicylates should avoid its use.

Dosage and Preparation:

Decoction 3–10g; tincture 2–4ml

Major Combinations:

Combine with Figwort (either Western or Chinese) and *shēngdìhuáng* for yin vacuity wilting, which is yin vacuity fire damage to the sinews with stiffness, pain upon movement, and general weakness due to liver and kidney yin vacuity with fire.

Combine with *Angelica breweri* and *qiānghuó* for wind–damp–heat impediment with swollen, hot, painful joints.

Combine with *dàhuáng* for headache associated with constipation. Add *báizhĭ* for extreme cases where there is frontal headache that is piercing in nature.

Commentary:

Salix is a large part (~450 species) of the Salicaceae (Willow) family, comprising approximately one-third of the total species (~1210 species). The genus is found primarily in the Northern hemisphere and arctic regions and is quite variable, meaning that it is often difficult to distinguish what species you may be looking at. The primary species in this monograph is *S. alba*, a native of Europe, which has naturalized in many other regions of the world, including North America and parts of Asia. This happened primarily though human dissemination of the plant as a cultivated tree. The tree can grow up to 25 meters tall and is generally considered an attractive landscape plant, thus it is commonly found in cities and towns, often along waterways. The tree grows relatively fast, and the stems have long been used for other purposes, such as weaving baskets and producing other handicrafts.

Another species, *Salix nigra*, (*S. alba* was also used this way to a lesser extent) was used by many physicians in the 19th and early 20th century for all matters of sexual excess. I have never used this herb in this way but my guess is that it was used to clear kidney yin vacuity heat leading to excessive sexual desire. Although I cannot confirm the diagnosis of kidney yin vacuity in this specific use, it is worth noting because it may speak to how either species might be used to clear vacuity heat. In this regard, Culpeper (1653) said, "The leaves bruised and boiled in wine, stayeth the heat of lust in man or women, and quite extinguisheth it, if it be long used: The seed is also of the same effect." However, as noted in the cautions, this herb can damage the spleen/stomach with large dosage or prolonged use but, as with any cooling herb, it would never be used by itself without other herbs to balance it. And, since this medicinal is not nourishing yin, only clearing vacuity heat, it must be paired with herbs that nourish the yin humour. Thus, the first combination, or some variation thereof, may be efficacious in this pattern.

Parkinson (1640) lists 25 species of Willow in four categories, but lumps the uses into one monograph stating:

> "I thought fit to show you what particular property is in each of the Willows altogether, and not to make many places or repetitions. All of these in general are cooling, drying, thickening and binding: both the leaves and the bark, and the seed especially, are useful for any of those effects, as to staunch bleeding of wounds, and of the mouth or nose, and spitting of blood, as also all fluxes of blood in man or woman, and likewise to stay chasting, and the desire thereunto, if decocted in wine and drunk."

Willow is a well-researched herb with hundreds of studies showing its effectiveness. It has been shown to benefit a wide range of pain syndromes from osteoarthritis to migraine headache, and has significantly fewer adverse reactions than its pharmaceutical cousin, aspirin. Aspirin was originally synthesized from Willow bark's main constituent, salicin. Some studies comparing Willow to aspirin have shown similar benefits, with Willow having few to no adverse reports, as compared to aspirin's myriad adverse reports.

One such study showed that 39% of patients receiving a "high dose" of Willow were pain-free after 4 weeks of treatment, while 21% of those receiving a "low dose" were pain-free in the same time period; only 6% present of placebo users were pain-free. (High dose was defined as a standardized extract with 240mg salicin per day, while the low dose was the same extract with only 120mg of salicin per day.)[1]

Translation of Available Source Material:

Chinese medicine uses a number of *Salix* species in medicine, including *S. alba*, *S. babylonica*, *S. cheilophila*, *S. matsudana*, and *S. sinopurpurea*. The Chinese name for *S. alba*, or White Willow, is *báiliǔ* (白柳), which literally means "white willow;" the first character (白) means white and the second character (柳) is the Latin genus name *Salix* (in English, Willow). This medicinal grows, and is sometimes cultivated, below 3100 meters elevation in the provinces of Gansu, Qinghai, Inner Mongolia, Xinjiang, and Tibet, where it is also used for timber, weaving baskets and for nectar for beekeeping. As a medicinal, it is considered bitter and cold. It clears damp–heat and disperses wind–dampness. It is used for acute tonsillitis, upper respiratory tract infections, sore throat, pelvic inflammation, kidney inflammation, sores and boils. It is made into a decoction in a dose of 9–15g, or by pouring boiling water over it and allowing it to soak.

S. sinopurpurea shuǐyánggēn (水楊根) is considered bitter and neutral. It resolves toxin and disperses swelling and settles pain. It is used externally for mammary welling-abscess (acute mastitis) and incised wounds. *S. matsudana hànliǔ* (旱柳), of which the leaf and small branches are used, is considered bitter and cold. It clears heat and disinhibits dampness, dispels wind, and stops pain. It is used for jaundice, acute bladder inflammation, inhibited urination, arthritis, yellow water sores (impetigo), sore toxin, and toothache. It is used internally in decoction at 9–15g, or it can be pounded and applied externally. The stem of this medicinal is used in the following formula to treat arthritis with swelling: *hànliǔzhī* (旱柳枝) 15g, *jìshēng* (寄生) 9g, *sāngzhī* (桑枝) 9g, *tòugǔcǎo* (透骨草) (*Gaultheria yunnanensis*) 6–9g, *wǔjiāpí* (五加皮) 9g, taken as a decoction. (Note: see *Translation of Available Sources* under the Wintergreen heading (Garran 2008) for more information on *Gaultheria yunnanensis*, which also goes by the name of *tòugǔxiāng* (透骨香).

S. cheilophila shāliǔ (沙柳) is acrid, bitter, and slightly cold. It dispels wind and clears heat, dissipates stasis and stops pain. It is used for the onset of measles, maculopapular eruptions that have yet to outthrust, skin itching, furuncles and swollen welling-abscesses, and lumbar strain.

S. babylonica liǔzhī (柳枝) is bitter and cold, and enters the stomach and liver channels. It dispels wind and disinhibits dampness, resolves toxin and disperses swelling. It is used to treat wind–dampness impediment pain, urinary strangury–turbidity.

1. Chrubasik, Sigrun, et al. (2000). Treatment of Low Back Pain Exacerbations with Willow Bark Extract: A Randomized Double-Blind Study. *The American Journal of Medicine.* 109(1): pp. 9–14.

Vervain

Verbena officinalis L. and others
Verbenaceae
Verbenae herba
Chinese name: *mǎbiāncǎo* (馬鞭草)
Favor and Qi: bitter, acrid, slightly cold
Channels entered: liver, urinary bladder, gallbadder
Actions: diaphoretic, antispasmodic, antiinflammatory, diuretic

Functions & Indications:

Courses the liver, disperses stagnation, scatters stasis, and resolves constraint. Vervain enters the liver channel, opens the liver, rectifies qi and quickens blood for the treatment of binding constraint of the liver that has led to menstrual pain, menstrual block, rib–side pain, breast distention, or abdominal pain. Vervain is bitter, acrid, and slightly cold. The combination of bitter and acrid is commonly seen in medicinals that move qi and quicken the blood. Liver constraint, while primarily a qi stagnation issue, also frequently involves blood stasis; Vervain's acrid and bitter flavors are a perfect combination to treat this pattern. Because stasis and stagnation often lead to heat, and can also be caused by heat, Vervain's slightly cold nature is also important in the treatment of many conditions related to liver constraint.

Courses the exterior, scatters wind, and clears heat. Vervain is used for invasion of wind and heat, or wind–cold that has transformed to heat, with symptoms of fever or heat effusion, sore throat, dry mouth, red tongue with a yellow coat and floating rapid pulse. This herb can also be used in *shàoyáng* conditions.

Clears heat and disinhibits dampness. Vervain is used for damp–heat patterns in the liver, gallbladder, urinary bladder, and intestines with symptoms such as swelling and pain of the penis, gonads, or vagina; hemorrhoids; jaundice; scant painful urination; urinary stones; or bloody urination. Vervain is bitter, acrid, and slightly cold. The combination of the bitter flavor and slightly cold nature clears heat and drains downward to help move heat out through the urine. Its acrid nature helps to move the qi of the kidney/bladder system to facilitate the outward flow of urine and resolve stagnation of dampness in the lower burner.

Clears heat, dispels wind, and expels dampness. Vervain can be used for wind–damp–heat impediment with hot, painful, swollen joints. Vervain is bitter, acrid, and slightly cold. It enters the joints via the *tàiyáng* and *shàoyáng* channels to clear heat, dispel wind, and expel dampness. Vervain is not a primary medicinal in treating this disorder, but works as an excellent assistant to other medicinals used to treat this syndrome.

Cautions:

Use with caution for those with spleen and stomach vacuity cold. Also, due to its dispersing nature, this medicinal should be used with caution for yin vacuity.

Dosage and Preparation:

Decoction 3–9g, fresh plant tincture 2–4ml, dry plant tincture 3–5ml

Major Combinations:

Combine with *xiāngfù* and *yùjīn* for liver constraint menstrual pain. This combination can also be used for liver constraint pattern with abdominal or rib–side pain.

Combine with *zhǐshí* for liver constraint with fullness in the chest and vexation. Add Skullcap for anxiety associated with the same pattern.

Combine with *cháihú* and *huángqín* for *shàoyáng* patterns, especially when there is stronger heat effusion than chills.

Combine with Parsley root for inhibited urination and strangury with thick gravelly urine.

Commentary:

The genus *Verbena* has about 250 species of both annual and perennial herbs (some are woody), with the majority of these species being found in North America and Europe. The primary herb in this monograph is a well established weed from Europe and can be found in both North America and Asia.

This herb has a long history of use in the West, and also in China. Although not a major herb in China, it first appeared about 1400 years ago, and has appeared in many materia medicas since that time. This herb is found all along the Silk Road, and beyond, in China. Whether it came with early traders, as opposed to being native, is unclear. It easily could have come with early traders as a hitchhiker, rather than a purposeful delivery. It is, however, a worldwide temperate and tropical weed, and most sources attribute its native range to Europe.

One of Vervain's common names is "Simpler's Joy," owing to its many uses and wide applications. And, as we can see from its Latin binomial "*officinalis*," it is an important medicinal plant.

Gerard (1597) is the only primary source from the late 16th through early 18th Century that did not classify this medicinal as hot! Instead, he says: "...very dry, and do mainly bind and cool." This is of particular interest because it deviates significantly from the general ideas on classifying medicinal substances at that time, and is more in line with the Chinese interpretation of this medicinal. However, Gerard seems to only consider the external application of this medicinal. He says it is good for a variety of sores, headache, fever, and hemorrhoids, but only gives external applications for these ailments. Gerard gives us a bit of insight into what might be his bias about this herb with the following: "Many odd old wives bable are written of Vervain tending to witchcraft and sorcerie, which you may read elsewhere, for I am not willing to trouble your ears with such triffles, as honest ears abhorre to hear." And, to close the monograph, he states: "Most of the later physicians do give the juice or decoction hereof to them that have the plague; but these men are deceived, not only in that they look for some truth from the father of falsehood and leasings, but also because instead of a good and sure remedy they minister no remedy at all; for it is reported, that the devil did reveal it as a secret and divine medicine." This is quite damning, and may account for why Gerard considered this medicinal cool rather than hot (as did all his contempories), and why he only seems to use it as an external medicine.

Parkinson (1640) opens his monograh with: "Vervain is hot and dry, bitter and binding, and is an opener of obstructions, cleansing and healing, for it helps the yellow jaundice, the dropsy and gout, as also the defects of the reines [kidneys] and lungs, and generally all the inward pains and torments of the body [taken by decoction]." This is a very different approach to this medicinal than Gerard had just 43 years prior, and is also more in line with what the following authors wrote. Parkinson also states that Vervain is good for the plague or pestilence, as well as several types of fevers. And, in support of Vervain being known as

"Simpler's Joy," Parkinson included diseases of the liver, spleen, stomach, lungs, kidneys, and bladder as yielding to this medicinal, and actually names these organs specifically!

Culpeper (1653) considered this herb "hot and dry", and said it is "excellent for the womb to strengthen and remedy all the cold griefs of it, as Plantain doth the hot." He also said it opens "obstructions." The fact that Culpeper considered this medicinal to be hot is no surprise. He says, in his opening remarks about the qualities of herbs, that hot herbs come in four degrees. Hot in the first degree has three basic qualities and, for our purposes, the next three degrees are stronger versions of these."[1] To make the offending humours thin, that they may be expelled by sweat or perspiration.[2] By outward application to abate inflammations and fevers by opening the pores of the skin.[3] To help concoction, and keep the blood in its just temperature." (Note: The second degree and third degree hot herbs are said to cut "tough humours.") Thus, any herb that has the action to eliminate stagnation or stasis is considered "hot" to one degree or another. This is not parallel with the Chinese understanding of how hot herbs function. Thus, my disagreement with Culpeper here is really no matter, as we are not working within his paradigm; this must be clearly understood in order for us to use his work to our advantage. Also, Culpeper notes that this medicinal is useful for treating "yellow jaundice," "green wounds," "inflammations and deformities of the skin," and "it easeth the inveterate pains and ache of the head, and is good for those that are frantic," which all seem to be pointing at treating hot and/or toxic conditions.

Salmon (1710) agrees with Culpeper, but is more specific in saying, "Vervain is hot in the first degree and dry in the second." "It is drying, bitter and binding, an opener of obstructions, cleansing and healing. It cures the yellow jaundice, dropsy and gout, opens obstructions of the lungs, liver, spleen, reins [kidneys], mesentery and bladder; gives ease in the colick, and all inward pains and torments whatsoever." The seemingly opposing natures of "binding" and "opener of obstructions" might appear strange, but the bitter and, I suggest, acrid nature of this herb offers the answer. Bitter flavor is drying and draining, by nature, and the drying quality that stops or slows excretion of fluids (such as phlegm or dampness manifesting in the lung, spleen, or bladder) would be seen as "binding" by Salmon. It is clear from the rest of what he writes that this medicinal "opens obstructions." Salmon's description of this medicinal as "hot" is addressed above, with comments about Culpeper's similar description. Specific ailments mentioned by Salmon include: asthma; cough; colds; wheezing; hoarseness; bites from all manner of creatures; jaundice; dropsy; gout; strangury; obstructions of the kidneys and bladder; colic; pain in the bowels; worms; bleeding, both internally and externally; sores of the body, including the mouth and throat; skin diseases; and eye problems. Not a short list of ailments. There is no doubt that this was a very oft used medicinal plant at the beginning of the 18th Century.

Modern research supports much of the traditional literature although human trials are lacking. There is no surprise that Vervain's antiinflammatory properties are strongly supported in a number of studies including one based on the traditional use of the plant in Spain[1] and another study showing not only antiinflammatory but also analgesic activity based on the same tradition.[2] In a very interesting study done in China, aqueous extracts of Vervain showed neuroprotective activity on neurons and the researchers suggest that this could potentially be worth investigating in the field of Alzheimer's disease research.[3]

Translation of Available Source Material:

This herb first appeared in the *Míng Yī Bié Lù* (early 6th Century) but the entry simply states that it treats genital sores or hemorrhoids. The *Grand Dictionary of Chinese Medicinals* (2009) says it is bitter, acrid and slightly cold. It enters the liver and spleen channels. It clears heat and resolves toxin, quickens the blood and frees the menses, disinhibits water and disperses swelling, and interrupts malaria. It is used to try external invasion with heat effusion, throat swelling and pain, gum swelling and pain, damp-heat yellow jaundice, dysentery, malaria, strangury patterns, water swelling, inhibited urination, blood stasis menstrual block, painful menstruation, concretions/conglomerations/welling–abscess/sores, toxin swelling, external injuries due to knocks and falls.

The modern master Yán Zhèng–huá (2009) says that this herb is bitter and slightly cold and enters the liver and spleen channels, as well as the blood aspect. It quickens the blood and scatters stasis, cools the blood and frees the menses (concurrently disinhibiting water), interrupts malaria, and resolves toxin. He says it can be used for, among other things: concretions, conglomerations, accumulations, and gatherings; menstrual block and painful menstruation; injuries due to external trauma; blood stasis and painful swelling; and is important in the treatment of blood heat leading to stasis. For blood stagnation menstrual block or menstrual pain, he combines it with *dānshēn*, *zélán*, and *yìmǔcǎo*. For congretions, conglomerations, accumulations, and gatherings, he combines it with *sānléng*, *ézhú*, and *biējiǎ*. For injuries due to external trauma and blood stasis painful swelling he combines it with *hónghuā*, *táorén*, and *dāngguīwěi*.

1. Calvo, M.I., et al (1998). Anti–inflammatory activity of leaf extract of *Verbena officinalis* L. *Phytomedicine*. 5(6): pp 465–467.
2. Calvo, M.I. (2006). Anti–inflammatory and analgesic activity of the topical preparation of *Verbena officinalis* L. *Journal of Ethnopharmacology*. 107(3): pp 380–382.
3. Lai, Sau–Wan, et al. (2006). Novel neuroprotective effects of the aqueous extracts from Verbena officinalis Linn. *Neuropharmacology*. 50(6): pp 641–650.

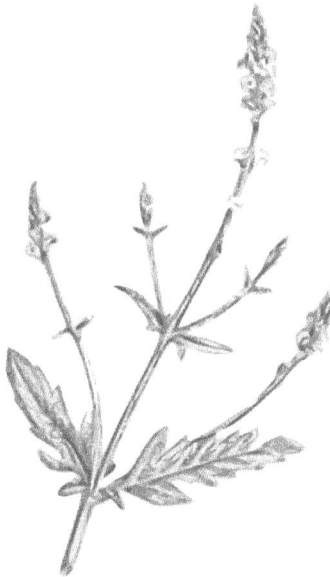

Medicinal	Nature	Flavor	Channels	Functions	Indications
Black Walnut	cold	bitter	stomach, large intestine	Clears heat, dries damp, and resolves toxicity; Clears heat and kills worms	purulent abscesses or wounds; anti-parasitic
Blessed Thistle	cool	bitter, acrid	liver, gallbladder, spleen	Courses the exterior, dissipates heat and abates fever; Clears heat, dries dampness, & downbears fire;	alternating heat effusion and chills, fullness in the chest and rib-side, bitter taste in the mouth, dry throat, slight dizziness; headache, red face, red eyes, vexation, dizziness, etc.
Chaparral	cool	bitter, acrid	lung, urinary bladder, large intestine	Clears heat, disinhibits dampness, and resolves toxin; Expels wind, clears heat, and resolves toxin; Clears heat, resolves toxin, generates flesh	scant, painful (burning), reddish (possibly) or yellow malodorous urine; fever, cough with think yellow sputum, sore throat, sinus congestion with purulent discharge, etc.; toxic-heat skin conditions
Willow bark	cool	bitter, slightly acrid, astringent	lung, liver	Clears heat and relieves pain; Clears heat, cools the blood, and stops bleeding	heat impediment; blood in the stool or urine, or excessive menstrual bleeding

Name	Temperature	Taste	Channels	Actions	Indications
Yellow Pond Lily	cold	bitter, slightly sweet, astringent	kidney, lung	Clears heat and dries dampness; Drains lung-heat and contains the yin	hot sloppy diarrhea, vaginal discharge with a strong odor, or hot, burning urination, with or without bleeding; cough, shortness of breath, difficulty breathing, and sweating
Vervain	slightly cold	bitter, acrid	liver, urinary bladder, gallbladder	Courses the liver, disperses stagnation, scatters stasis, and resolves constraint; Courses the exterior, scatters wind, and clears heat; Clears heat and dries dampness; Clears heat, dispels wind and expels dampness	menstrual pain, menstrual block, rib-side pain, breast distention, or abdominal pain; fever or heat effusion, sore throat, dry mouth, red tongue with a yellow coat and floating rapid pulse; swelling and pain of the penis, gonads, or vagina; hemorrhoids; jaundice; scant painful urination; urinary stones; bloody urination; hot, painful, swollen joints

祛風濕藥

Expel Wind and Dampness Medicinals

The expel wind and dampness category of medicinals is a group used to treat wind–dampness impediment patterns caused by invasion of pathogenic wind and dampness. These medicinals may be warm or cool in nature, but tend to be warm. Impediment patterns treated with this category of medicinals involve pathogenic factors that have penetrated the luò and affected the sinews and bones. Therefore, these medicinals expel wind and scatter cold, sooth the sinews and free the luò, dispel dampness and stop pain.

All of the medicinals in this category expel wind and dampness and are moving and activating in nature. There are several divisions often made within this broad category including: expel wind–cold–dampness medicinals, expel wind–dampness–heat medicinals, and expel wind dampness and strengthen the sinews and bones. Each of these sub–categories are represented in this materia medica. The first of the three listed above is represented by Yucca, the second by Bittersweet, and the third by Devil's Club.

This latter sub–category of medicinals is also known to supplement the liver and boost the kidney, and strengthen and invigorate the sinews and bones. Devil's Club represents this sub–category well, which in the standard Chinese medicine materia medica consist of medicinals such as *xùduàn* and *dùzhòng*.

This category of medicinals is traditionally prepared in alcohol in what Western herbalists would recognize as a tincture. These are generally taken in larger doses of around 0.5–2oz and formulas may consist of 5 to 25 medicinals. Part of reason for these preparations is that alcohol is known to be warm and activating to the channels and luo, thus the alcohol improves the function of the formula.

It is also important to recognize that these medicinals are often very drying and can damage the yin and blood. Because of this, it is important to be mindful when using these medicinals for patients with yin and or blood vacuity.

Yucca

Yucca sp. L.
Liliaceae
Radix Yuccae
Favor and Qi: acrid, bitter, hot, slightly toxic
Channels entered: liver, kidney, urinary bladder, small intestine
Actions: antiinflammatory, anti–arthritic, diuretic, laxative, antibacterial, antiprotozan

Functions & Indications:

Expels wind–damp–cold and courses the channels. Yucca is used for joint–running wind where wind–damp–cold has lodged in the joints causing acute pain, redness and swelling, with difficulty bending and stretching. May also be made into a paste and applied to the affected joints. Yucca is acrid and hot, and strongly dispels wind, dampness, and cold while coursing the channels to free the flow of qi and blood, thus reducing pain and clearing the stagnation associated with these pathogens.

Warms the yang and frees the bowels. Yucca is used for cold constipation with cold pain in the abdomen, desire for warmth over the abdomen and in the environment, and a swollen tongue with white fur. Yucca is acrid, bitter, and hot. Acrid moves, while bitter drains. Its hot nature warms yang and dispels cold pathogens, while its acridity helps to move qi. Its bitterness drains downward, assisting the bowels in moving stool.

Cautions:

Not for use in patients with yin vacuity heat. Use caution with very weak patients. Long term use can cause inflammation in the digestive tract and can reportedly slow absorption of fat soluble vitamins in the small intestine.

Dosage and Preparation:

Decoction 3–6g, tincture 0.5–2ml. The root of Yucca is gathered from late summer to early spring before it begins to put up its flowering stalk. The roots should be peeled and chopped for drying. The root is to be used dried only. It can be used as a tea, tincture, or powered herb (either a draft or in a capsule). Good quality is firm, white to tan, and without bark.

Major Combinations:

Combine in a bath with Yerba Mansa leaf for swollen painful hips, knees or ankles. This is a traditional Native American combination that was used by within the range of these two plants in the Southwestern United States and Northwestern Mexico. This combination was often used as a soak/bath.

Combine with Brewer's Angelica, Yerba Mansa, and California Figwort root for severe joint pain in the upper extremities with redness and swelling. Although this combination is overwhelmingly warming, most of the medicinals have an anti-inflammatory action, resulting in definitive action within 1-3 days of administration.

Commentary:

The Yucca genus is fairly small, with around 40 species. Since most can be used in medicine, I will give a general description of the genus rather than a description of a particular species. Yuccas range from a sub-shrub to tree-like, and some species die after they fruit. All species have rosetted leaves (either basal or elevated on the stalk) ranging from 2-15 cm in length, are linear, stiff, and sword-like, and armed with a spine on the tip. The base of the leaves is expanded and the edges curl upward. The inflorescence forms a dense panicle with whitish, drooping flowers ranging from 2-13 cm. The flower's perianth has six parts in two pedal-like whorls, with six stamens suspended on fleshy filaments. The ovary is superior, with a short, stalky style and a trebled stigma. Most of the species have capsules holding flat black seeds, two rows per chamber.

There are many species of Yucca, and many of them can be used interchangeably, to the best of my knowledge. It should be noted that one species of Yucca, the famous Joshua Tree (*Yucca brevifolia*) is protected in some areas. This plant is also quite large, and if the root is what you're after, cutting down a Joshua Tree is a poor choice. Based on the author's limited clinical experience with this medicinal, traditional usage, and modern research, he believes it deserves more investigation into its therapeutic usefulness. This plant has a long and wide history of use in shampoo and natural soaps because of its high saponin content. The genus is endemic to the Americas and most species are found in the Southwestern United States and Northwestern Mexico. Their pollinators are small moths that come in the night to lay their eggs in the ovary of the flower and unknowingly pollinate as they go.

Gerard (1597) was new to this plant, as it is not a native of Europe. He says that it comes from the Americas (though he does not use that word) and "in most of the islands of the canibals." He does not give uses for the plant but states that it is "hot and dry in the first degree." Gerard could not have had any significant experience using this plant therapeutically, and it is extremely unlikely that he had any reference point for its traditional use in its native habitat, but he had no problems suggesting its energetic, based on the little knowledge he did have.

Just over 100 years later, Salmon (1710) writes an extensive monograph on Yucca, naming three species. He says that it grows, and is used, from the southern tip of South America northward to New England, and had a primary use as a food substance by the Native peoples. He clearly has no clinical experience with the medicinal, but states that other authors have said that a vinegar or wine made from the peeled root "cools in fevers, and quenches thirst, and is admirable against malign and pestilential diseases." Also, when this preparation is made into a syrup with honey or sugar, it "cools singularly, any heat or inflammation or the viscera, opens obstructions of the lungs and causes free breathing." While we cannot rely on this information due to the lack of experience the author had with the plant, it does offer us an interesting look into how a new plant was integrated from a tradition from a foreign land.

There is little research into the use of Yucca as a medicine, but some work has been done on the anti–inflammatory saponins.[1,2] There also has been some, more recent, work on the phenolic compounds found in at least one species.[3] However, none of this work is conclusive, and we must rely more on historical usage and the experience of those currently using this medicinal.

1. Bingham R. "New and effective approaches to the prevention and treatment of arthritis", *J Appl Nutr* 28:38–47 (1976).
2. Bingham R, Bellow BA, Bellow JG., "Yucca plant saponin in the management of arthritis", *J Appl Nutr* , 27:45–51 (1975).
3. Olas B, Wachowicz B, Stochmal A, Oleszek W, "Inhibition of blood platelet adhesion and secretion by different phenolics from *Yucca schidigera* Roezl. Bark", *Nutrition* 21:199–206 (2005).

Bittersweet

Solanum dulcamara L.
Solanaceae
Solanum Dulcamarae stipites
Chinese name: *kǔqié* (苦茄)
Flavor and Qi: bitter, acrid, cool
Channels entered: urinary bladder, small intestine, liver
Actions: antirheumatic, anti–inflammatory

Functions and indications:

Expels wind, eliminates dampness, and stops pain. Bittersweet is used for wind–dampness impediment causing pain in the joints. When wind and dampness settle in the joints, qi stagnation occurs and dampness can accumulate. If left for a prolonged period of time, blood stasis and heat will also arise. Although this medicinal will clear heat, this is not its primary action. Instead, with acridity it expels wind, and with bitterness it eliminates dampness; by doing so, the qi can move, which, in turn, means the blood can move more freely and pain is relieved. This medicinal is particularly useful for chronic conditions with acute flare–ups of pain (e.g., gout), when the patient has clear signs of wind–dampness, but conflicting signs of heat and cold. Often, there may be heat in the joints or other areas, and yet the patient feels damp and cold. When dampness and cold settle into the body, the qi dynamic is impeded, blood can become static, and heat can arise; if it settles in the joints, both heat and pain will arise.

Courses the exterior and expels wind. Bittersweet is used for skin eruptions with dry, scaly skin. This herb effectively drains localized heat with bitterness, and courses the exterior and expels wind with acridity.

Cautions:

This herb is quite safe at appropriate doses, however overdose is possible and care should be taken to dose correctly. Like any other medicine, it should be kept out of reach of children. Use with caution with patients with spleen and stomach cold.

Dosage and preparation:
Tincture 2–4 ml (up to 6x/day for acute cases)

Major combinations:

I like to use this herb as a single–herb tincture or in combination with other herbs in tincture form because it is better suited to tinctures and much smaller dosages are needed. The primary reason that smaller doses are needed is that alcohol is a better solvent for some of the active constituents, thus a tincture contains higher amounts of those constituents.

This herb combines well with any of the Angelicas that are used for wind–damp, but my favorite combination is with *báizhǐ* in a 3:1 ratio in tincture.

Commentary:

This plant is native to Northern Europe and is also found on both the East and West coasts of North America, Russia, Southwestern China and Southeast Asia. It prefers water or wet areas, and is common along creeks, streams, and rivers.

It is part of the nightshade family (Solanaceae), and the nightshade genus (*Solanum*) as well. The name comes from either the Latin word *solare*, which means "to soothe", or *solamen*, meaning "a comfort." There are some 1500 species around the world, but most are concentrated in South America. Other plants in this genus include potato (*S. tuberosum*), eggplant (*S.melongena*), and tomato (*S. lycopersicum*), all of which are native to South America. There are at least 15 species used in medicine in China, and many others used around the world.

Many species within this genus, and indeed the entire family, are known to be toxic, or some parts of them are toxic. The berries of *S. dulcamara* are often thought to be toxic but, according to Collins & Hornfeldt (1990), it is only the unripe berries that show signs of being toxic in mice models, with no apparent signs of either gastrointestinal tissue changes, or changes in behavior suggesting solanine (a primary toxin found throughout the family) toxicity. This finding led the researchers to the following recommendation: "Aggressive treatment of children ingesting limited amounts of ripened *S. dulcamara* berries appears to be unnecessary."[1]

Gerard (1597) says: "The leaves and fruit of Bittersweet are in temperature hot, and dry, cleansing and wasting away." He also reports: "The decoction of the leaves is reported to remove the stoppings of the liver and gall: and to be drunk with good success against the yellow jaundice." And, "The juice is good for those that have fallen from high places, and thereby bruised, or dry beaten; for it is thought to dissolve blood congealed or cluttered any where in the entrails, and to heal the hurt places." And, while Gerard only seems to have experience with the leaves, he says that Hyeronimus Tragus (aka Hieronymus Bock, a mid–16th Century botanist and physician) "teaches to make a decoction of wine with the wood finely sliced and cut into small pieces, which he reports to purge gently both by urine and stool, those that have the dropsy and jaundice." While there is obvious correlation between what Gerard and Bock say and current usage, it is curious to see that while Gerard was only using the leaves, he tells of a similar use for the stems, but without comment. Furthermore, he prefers the decoction, presumably with water, but tells us the Bock makes a tincture, again without comment.

Parkinson (1640), gives a detailed description of Bock's preparation. This preparation is made by taking a pound of small–cut stems and three pints of white wine, and combining them in an earthen pot, which is then sealed. This mixture is boiled gently until two–thirds remain. It is then strained, and taken in the morning and evening. Parkinson does offer a warning from his own clinical experience. "It is held also effectual to open the obstructions of the liver and spleen, but so often as I have given it by appointment I have known it to purge very churlishly." Earlier in the monograph, in repeating what Gerard says, it seems as though he was using the leaves. This difference may account for why he found the "purge" [which is not meant in the downward draining sense of the word, but rather the purging humours by opening] to be rude or difficult, rather than smooth and easy, as many other authors (this one included) have reported.

Culpeper (1653) speaks of this herb with high regard. However, his use of the medicinal is dissimilar to that of my experience and other modern authors' experience. That being said, I believe his vast clinical experience is noteworthy. One thing we do agree on is the use of a tincture when applying this medicinal. He says, of the tincture, "you have a most excellent drink to open the obstructions of the liver and spleen, to help difficulty breathing, bruises and falls, and congealed blood in any part of the body; it help the yellow–jaundice, the dropsy and black jaundice, and to cleanse women newly brought to bed." This seems to suggest a direct action on the liver and blood, the two of which are inseparable in Chinese medicine. Of the symptoms he mentions, only dyspnea is not an obvious reference to either the liver or the blood, but binding constraint of liver qi could cause difficult breathing, especially if it were combined with other patterns, such as qi vacuity or phlegm.

Salmon (1710) says that the leaves and berries are hot and dry in the first degree, and essentially repeats what Culpeper said regarding the preparations of the juice and decoction. However, of the tincture he states, "It purges not, but very much strengthens the viscera, chiefly the liver and spleen, and represses vapors ascending from the stomach, and other parts, to the head and brain, causing vertigo, megrims [sudden depression], and distempers of the ventricle." (The meaning of the term "distempers of the ventricle" is not completely clear, however "distempers" is a term used to describe a derangement of the humors of the body and "ventricle" here is describing the head, or more precisely the cavity where the brain is found. Thus, this term has to do with a degrangement of the humors in the head.) Here, Salmon seems to be talking about what Chinese medicine might see as turbidity in the upper burner caused by liver fire or other similar patterns; there could even be liver wind involved, but it is very difficult to say for sure. Although I have no experience using this medicinal in this way, it may be worth considering and trying, when the appropriate case presents itself. The herb is cool, acrid, and bitter, which is an appropriate combination for this application.

Samuel Thomson (1825) used this medicinal in combination with Chamomile and Wormwood to prepare an ointment which could be applied externally for bruises, sprains, swellings, calluses, and corns.

Ellingwood (1919) said, "Dulcamara is a remedy for all conditions resulting from suppression of secretion, from exposure to cold and dampness." He continues on to state, "it assists in determining the eruption to the surface," which, when combined with the previous statement, shows that the Eclectic physicians had a similar way of thinking about diseases of the skin as does Chinese medicine, but with a different set of jargon. Chinese medicine says that exposure to cold and damp, when combined with wind (which the Eclectics didn't discuss), can enter the body and cause all manner of problems. In the case of skin diseases, pathogenic factors must be coursed from the exterior and expelled. As explained above, Bittersweet is cool in nature, but these problems, although originally caused by cold, have led to a condition of localized heat and congestion.

Felter & Lloyd (1905) state that Bittersweet is best for "scaly cutaneous" skin diseases and suggests it be combined with Yellow Dock and *Guaiacum officinale*. Yellow Dock is a bitter cold herb (see Garran 2008 pp. 86–88.) and *Guaiacum officinale* is a warming and acrid, resinous wood similar to *chénxiāng* or the resins *mòyào* and *rŭxiāng*. Although *Guaiacum officinale* is no longer available as a medicine due to its endangered status and listing with CITES, *chénxiāng* is available and this may be a reasonable substitute. Currently there is some concern with both *mòyào* and *rŭxiāng* due to ecological and social/political issues in their native ranges.

Translation of available sources material:

Found in the south-west of China, this plant is considered bitter, acrid, and cold. It expels wind and eliminates dampness, and clears heat and resolves toxin. It is used to treat wind-dampness pain, lockjaw, swollen welling-abscess, malign sores and other sores, external injury with bleeding. Internally, it is used as a decoction in 15–30g dosages. Externally, either the leaf or the whole herb is ground to a powder and applied as a paste. It is also commonly prepared as a tincture (see above).

1. Hornfeldt, Carl S. & Collins, James E. (1990). Toxicity of Nightshade Berries (*Solanum dulcamara*) in Mice. *Clinical Toxicology*. 28: pp 185–192.

Devil's Club

Opolopanax horrididum (Sm.) Miq.
Araliaceae
Opolopanax horrididi cortex
Favor and Qi: acrid, bitter, slightly sweet, warm
Channels entered: liver, kidney
Actions: anti-arthritic, antitussive, diaphoretic

Functions & Indications:

Expels wind and dampness and boosts qi. Devil's Club is used for the treatment of chronic wind–damp–cold taxation with symptoms of joint pain, muscle aches (especially those that get better with mild exercise but worse with excessive exercise), fatigue, and sluggishness of speech/thought. Devil's Club is warm and acrid and dispels wind and dampness strongly. However, it is also warm and sweet, so it can boost the qi, particularly of the spleen, thus assisting in the movement or elimination of dampness in the body.

Expels wind, transforms phlegm and rheum, boosts qi, and stops cough. Devil's Club is used for the treatment of chronic taxation cough with accumulation of phlegm and/or rheum. This herb can also be used for acute coughs, especially when there is concurrent qi vacuity. Devil's Club is bitter, acrid, and warm and can strongly dispel wind, and penetrate the lung to transform phlegm or rheum, while also assisting the lung to stop cough. This is assisted by its warm and slightly sweet nature and flavor, which boosts qi and helps to recover from illness.

Courses the exterior, expels wind, and supplements vacuity. Devil's Club is used for external contraction of wind–cold with concurrent qi vacuity. Devil's Club courses the exterior and expels wind with bitter acridity, while supplementing qi with its slightly sweet flavor. Although this herb has supplementing properties, I, as well as some other herbalists, do not consider it a strong supplementing herb, although definite in action. However, some herbalists do consider it a strong supplementing herb, so there is some debate about this.

This herb has also been used in a biomedical sense to treat diabetes and sub-clinical blood sugar problems. This function may be related to its traditional value as a tonic. Gottesfeld and Anderson report, "Regular chewing of the fresh devil's club *inner bark* [emphasis added] is believed to maintain good health. Good health and vigor among older people has been attributed to regular use of devil's club. An infusion of the fresh bark is a tonic and "energizer."[1]

Cautions:

Not for use with yin vacuity heat. Use caution with repletion heat patterns.

Dosage and Preparation:

Decoction or infusion 3–10g; fresh plant tincture 1–3ml; dry plant tincture 2–4ml.

Major Combinations:

Added to *Dú Huó Jì Shēng Tāng*, it strengthens the two primary actions of the formula, which are to dispel wind–dampness and strengthen the liver and kidney.

Added to *Jīng Fáng Bài Dú Sǎn* to strengthen the formula and boost the qi to help the person overcome the pathogen. Also, when taking a decoction of this formula, the dosage of *dúhuó* and *qiānghuó* may be reduced to facilitate palatability of the formula for the patient while retaining effective clinical action. This is something I have done numerous times (in fact, I have eliminated the herbs several times with good success) because *dúhuó* and *qiānghuó* are so difficult for many patients to stomach, because of their very strong acrid flavor. The addition of 10g of Devil's Club compensates for the reduction in, or elimination of, these two medicinals. Also, any of the Angelicas discussed in Garran (2008) can be substituted for either *dúhuó* or *qiānghuó*.

Combine with Yellow Pond Lily and *shāshēn* for cough and/or panting, possibly with chest pain, due to phlegm or rheum lodged in the lungs.

Commentary:

Devil's Club is a member of the Ginseng family (Araliaceae), a family that is comprised of primarily tropical and subtropical plants; the family is otherwise not well represented in North America. A native of the

Pacific Northwest of North America, this deep forest dweller is an extremely well-guarded plant with spines on the stem as well as the leaves, and was likely one of the most important medicinal plants for the native peoples within its region. Gottesfeld (1992) states, "Devil's Club branches and inner bark are the most important medicinal bark preparations in the Northwest Coast region."[2] And, Turner (1971) states, "This plant was used by almost every Indian tribe from Oregon to Alaska..."[3] As for many other plants of Western North America, our ethnobotanical records for this medicinal are scant, and our history of use since Europeans and Asians entered the continent is also not particularly well documented, as compared to medicinal plants from the Eastern part of North America. However, due to the importance placed on this plant, there are quite a few references. Dan Moerman's Ethnobotanical Database shows the following uses: of 152 entries, 31 (>20%) are for pain (mostly for arthritic pain, but some are for other types of pain), 20 (>13%) entries are for gastrointestinal disorders, 18 (>11%) are for dermatological ailments, 16 (>10%) are for lung diseases, and 15 (>9%) are for colds and influenza. If we combine lung diseases with colds and influenza (noting that many lung diseases start with what might be categorized as a "cold," and that most lung diseases in Chinese medicine are said to originate from invasions of external pathogens) we come up with 31 (>20%), the same amount as for pain; together, pain and lung diseases make up more than 40% of all the uses for this plant (not shown in chart) throughout its native range.

This illustrates how modern herbalists and Native Peoples have come to very similar conclusions. The two other categories, dermatological and gastrointestinal diseases, are not found in the monograph above, but account for a combined 25% of the total uses for this plant found in the literature. Many of the dermatological uses for this plant were for external application, for which we have a plethora of other plants that might be useful. Nevertheless, considering the importance of this plant within its range (and also the plant family Araliaceae), studying this plant for these types of ailments seems like a worthwhile endeavor.

Traditional extracts of medicinal plants (in pre–European invasion North America) were almost exclusively made with water, either by infusion or decoction. These are, naturally, different than those made with alcohol, which is a common sovlent in modern Western herbal medicine. One attribute of medicinal plants is that resins and similar compounds from various plant parts are more soluble in alcohol than in water. These compounds often come from roots/rhizomes (e.g., *Angelica, Ligusticum, Notoptyrigium,* etc.) or stems/barks such as Devil's Club. Gottesfeld and Anderson (1988) report, "Regular chewing [as opposed to an infusion or decoction] of (preferably fresh) Devil's Club bark is reported to be helpful in treating rheumatism or stiffness of the joints." They add "The chewed bark is swallowed by the user."[4] This suggests that a water extraction does not liberate the necessary chemical constituents from the bark, which further suggests that a tincture may be the best extraction technique for this medicinal when employing it for joint pain and other pain syndromes. When chewing a plant, the enzymes in our mouth and the mechanical chewing process will help to break it down and facilitate the ingestion of compounds that may not otherwise be consumed in a standard decoction. A similar example of this is a *draft* in Chinese medicine (also used in traditional Western herbal medicine). By grinding the medicinals, pouring water over them, then consuming the entirety of the beverage, this allows one to ingest the whole plant and allows the body to digest and utilize compounds that otherwise would not be available in a simple water extraction, i.e. decoction.

Some research into the chemistry of Devil's Club supports traditional usage. Extracts of the inner bark have been reported to be active against a number of different bacteria and fungi, including *Mycobacterium tuberculosis* and *M. avium* (two species that commonly cause tuberculosis),[5] as well as having some antiviral activity.[6,7,8,9,10]

Translation of Available Source Material:

There is at least one species of Oplopanax used in Chinese medicine, *O. elatus* Nakai *cìrénshēn* (刺人参). The *Grand Dictionary of Chinese Medicinals* says it is sweet, slightly bitter and warm. It supplements qi and reinforces yang, stops cough, and frees the network vessels. It is used to treat qi vacuity with body weakness, neurasthenia, impotence, weakened body with enduring cough, and wind–cold with enduring impediment. Although the author has no experience with this medicinal, botanical relationships suggest potential similar uses and the literature seems to support this.

1. *Journal of Ethnobiology* 8(1): pp 13–33. 1988.

2. Gottesfeld, Leslie M. Johnson, (1992). *Economic Botany* 46(2): pp 148–157.

3. *Economic Botany* 25(1): pp 63–104. 1971.

4. *Journal of Ethnobiology* 8(1): pp 13–33. 1988.

5. McCutcheon, AR, et al. (1997). *International Journal of Pharmacognosy*, (35)2: pp 77–83.

6. McCutcheon, AR, et al. (1992). *Journal of Ethnophrmacology*, 37: pp 213–223.

7. McCutcheon, AR, et al. (1995). *Journal of Ethnopharmocology*, 49: pp 101–110.

8. Kobaisy, Mozaina, et al. (1997). *Journal of Natural Products.* 60: pp 1210–1213.

9. Bloxton, James D. (2002). *Economic Botany*, 56(3) pp 285–289.

10. Calway, T. et al, (2012). *Journal of Natural Medicines*, 66(2) pp 249–256.

Medicinal	Nature	Flavor	Channels	Functions	Indications
Bittersweet	cool	bitter, acrid	urinary bladder, small intestine, liver	Expels wind, eliminates dampness, and stops pain; Courses the exterior and expels wind	Joint pain; skin eruptions with dry, scaly skin
Devil's Club	warm	acrid, bitter, slightly sweet	liver, kidney	Epels wind and dampness and boosts qi; Expels wind, transforms phlegm and rheum, boosts qi, and stops cough; Courses the exterior, expels wind, and supplements vacuity	joint pain, muscle aches, fatigue, and sluggishness of speech/thought; chronic taxation cough with accumulation of phlegm and/or rheum; wind-cold with concurrent qi vacuity
Chaparral	cool	bitter, acrid	lung, urinary bladder, large intestine	Clears heat, disinhibits dampness, and resolves toxin; Expels wind, clears heat, and resolves toxin; Clears heat, resolves toxin, generates flesh	scant, painful (burning), reddish (possibly) or yellow malodorous urine; fever, cough with think yellow sputum, sore throat, sinus congestion with purulent discharge, etc.; toxic-heat skin conditions
Willow bark	cool	bitter, slightly acrid, astringent	lung, liver	Clears heat and relieves pain; Clears heat, cools the blood, and stops bleeding	heat impediment; blood in the stool or urine, or excessive menstrual bleeding

芳香化濕藥

Aromatic Transform Dampness Medicinals

The aromatic transform dampness category is a small but specific group of aromatic, warm, and drying medicinals. These medicinals are used to transform dampness and move the spleen for patterns when dampness is obstructing the middle burner. These herbs are used to awaken the spleen and transform dampness in other patterns such as summerheat dampness, as well to repel foulness accumulated in the middle and lower burners. When dampness obstructs the middle burner symptoms such as nausea, vomiting, sloppy diarrhea, low appetite with no thought of drinking, sweet taste in the mouth with excessive salivation, and a white greasy tongue coating may be present.

In this materia medica Bee Balm is well-suited for summerheat dampness pattern as it both transforms dampness in the middle and resolves the exterior. Juniper is a premiere medicinal to repel foulness in the middle and lower burner (and even the upper burner to a lessor extent). The third medicinal here is Sage Brush when strongly repels foulness and treats dampness obstructing the spleen.

Although these medicinals are warm in nature, with appropriate formula they can be, and are commonly, used to treat damp-heat and summerheat patterns. These medicinals are drying in nature and are generally only used for short term therapy in acute conditions. When using these medicinals for any length of time care should be taken when administering them to patients with yin or blood vacuity due to their drying nature and for patients with qi vacuity due to their scattering nature. It is also important to note that, because of their aromatic nature, these medicinals should not be cooked for long periods of time and work very well as alcoholic extracts.

Juniper

Juniperus communis L., *J. californica* Carr.

Cupressaceae

Fructus Juniperi Communis

Favor and Qi: acrid, bitter, aromatic, warm, slightly toxic

Channels entered: spleen, kidney, triple burner

Actions: diuretic, antiseptic, carminative, antiinflammatory

Functions & Indications:

Aromatically transforms dampness, drains damp turbidity, and moves qi. Juniper is used for chronic damp conditions with symptoms of oppression in the chest, pain and distention in the abdomen, strangury, nausea, and loss of appetite. Juniper is aromatic, acrid, bitter, and warm. With warm acridity, Juniper utilizes its aroma to transform dampness, and its bitter flavor to move turbidity downward and drain it out. Owing to its warm acrid nature, Juniper is very effective for moving qi and transforming dampness and turbidity, making this medicinal very useful when stagnation of dampness has led to stagnation of qi, or vice versa. Although Juniper is warm in nature, it is frequently combined with other herbs such as *huángbāi*, *huángqín*, *huánglián*, or Oregon grape root for heat conditions.

Dispels dampness and expels cold. Juniper is used for wind–damp–cold impediment with dampness being the predominant pathogenic mechanism. Symptoms include heaviness of the limbs and fixed pain in the joints. Juniper has a long history of use for "arthritic" conditions but seems to have the best effect on joints in the lower part of the body. This may be because Juniper is very good for moving dampness, and dampness tends to settle downward into the lower extremities.

Warms the kidneys and transforms phlegm. Juniper is used for phlegm-dampness lumbar pain with a cold, heavy, dragging sensation in the lower back. Phlegm is often a product of the kidneys, which are the root of phlegm. This can be due to either yin vacuity fire steaming dampness into phlegm, or kidney yang vacuity unable to assist the spleen in transforming fluids, which will lead to phlegm. The latter of these is where Juniper is best administered. Although it can be used in kidney yin vacuity patterns, it must be done with caution because of its warming and moving qualities. Juniper warms the yang, which is then able to assist the spleen in transformation of fluids and removal of phlegm.

Cautions:

Due to mild toxicity, this herb should not be used for long periods of time, nor should it be given to those with overt kidney damage.

Dosage and Preparation:

Light decoction 2–6g; tincture 0.5–2ml. The oil is prepared as an external salve for the treatment of a variety of skin ailments. This is not something I have experience with, but is noted in the literature.

Major Combinations:

Combine with Parsley root and *fúlíng* for damp-heat in the lower burner. Add *huángbǎi* for scanty, painful urination. If the heat is very strong or there is fire, add *shānzhīzǐ*, Echinacea, and/or Usnea. If there is bleeding, add *báimáogēn*. If there are nodules, add Cleavers, Red Root, and/or *liánqiáo*.

Combine with *Liù Jūn Zǐ Tāng* for spleen qi vacuity and damp encumberance where the urination output is low due to cold dampness obstructing the qi mechanism of the bladder.

Combine with *yìyǐrén* added to *Juān Bì Tāng* for damp impediment.

Commentary:

Juniper is a member of the Cypress family (Cupressaceae), a family with noted importance throughout the world. In the Western US we find the related Western Red Cedar (*Thuja plicata*), the most widely used plant in Western North America, and the Cypress called Port Orford Cedar (*Cupressus lawsoniana*), a revered wood by fine woodworkers around the world, especially Japan. The main plant discussed in this monograph is the "Common" Juniper (*J. communis*), a circumboreal plant. Juniper grows throughout many parts of the Northern Hemisphere, preferring rocky, well-draining soils and lots of sun.

Juniper is a small often spreading shrub, generally staying under 1 meter (but can grow up to 10 meters tall), with thin, peeling red-brown bark and needle-like leaves spreading in whorls of three. Juniper generally requires both a male and female plant to produce fruit or seed cone. The resinous seed cone is 5-8mm, ripening from red to a blue or black; these, like the Yews, appear more like a fruit than a cone.

The seed cones are gathered in the spring and early summer when ripe and sticky. The cones can either been tinctured fresh, or dried and reserved for future use. Good quality is blue to black and sticky. The cones should not be brittle and broken.

Dioscoridies (2000 *trans.*) states, "[the berries are] round and fragrant, sweet, and a little bitter to chew. [They are] mildly warming and astringent, good for the stomach, good taken in drink for infirmities of the chest, coughs, gaseousness, griping, and poisons of venomous creatures. [They are] also diuretic; as a result [they are] good for convulsions and hernia, and those who have congested or blocked wombs." The first set of ailments listed by Dioscoridies is in line with how this herb has been used continuously since his time (1st Century C.E.). However, the author has no experience with the use of this herb for the treatment of chest complaints such as cough, and, as this is a much lesser known application of this herb today, these indications have been left out.

Gerard (1597) says: "Juniper is hot and dry, and that in the third degree, as Galen teaches; The berries are also hot, but not altogether so dry." Thus, we can gather that, at least since Galen's time (2nd Century), Juniper has been used and classified in much the same. He continues his monograph by saying: "The fruit of the Juniper tree clenses the liver and kidney, [also attributing this to Galen]. It also makes thin, clamy and gross humours." The "clamy and gross humours" are likely what we term "turbid dampness" (sometimes termed "damp–turbidity") in Chinese medicine, and could also be related to some forms of phlegm. Like other medicinals in this category in the Chinese materia medica (i.e. *hòupò, cāngzhú*), Juniper is used when dampness becomes turbid and inhibits the functions of the various organ systems that move fluid in the body.

Parkinson (1640) repeats much of what Gerard and Galen have said. However, his monograph is extensive and includes information from other Greek and German authors who, he says, use a "condensed juice of the berries...in all diseases, almost." He says that it is "profitable against strangury and stoppings of urine" and "powerful against dropsy." All of this is more or less in concert with other writers of that era. However, he seems to support my claims regarding this medicinal as a kidney yang warming medicine to treat turbid dampness and phlegm when he says: "The berry are very comfortable to the brain and strengthen the memory and sight, and all the senses and the heart also." Most chronic phlegmatic conditions are due to vacuity, either kidney yang or yin. Although the turbid dampness or phlegm may be excess in nature, the cause is often either the waning of kidney yang or kidney yin vacuity causing fluids to "condense." Thus, it is critical to warm kidney yang and supplement the kidney qi/yang in order to treat diseases associated with these pathogens, especially if they rise to the chest or head and cause problems with the senses or heart.

Culpeper (1653) says of Juniper: "The berries are hot in the third degree, and dry but in the first..." Here, Culpeper states that the medicinal is very hot, but not overly drying, at least not in a way that will damage the body unless taken in excessive doses. He also says, "...they provoke urine exceedingly, and therefore are very available to dysuries and stranguaries." This remains, probably, the most common use of this medicinal today. As noted in the monograph above, Juniper is a very good medicinal for the treatment of turbid dampness in various parts of the body, but is likely most known for treating urinary problems. Culpeper also notes, "[the berries] break the stone." In another part of his monograph he says, "... [Juniper] strengthens the stomach exceedingly, and expels wind; indeed there is scarce a better remedy for wind in any part of the body, or the colic, than the chemical oil drawn from the berries." Also, it "procure appetite when lost". While I have not used the oil, I can say that the berries serve this function quite well. It is important to note that the "wind" of Culpeper's writing is not the same as that of Chinese medicine. Culpeper was talking about "gas" in the body as evidenced by burping, flatulence, and abdominal fullness.

He also makes a number of references to its possible connection to the treatment of turbid dampness or phlegm with statements such as, "the berries stay all fluxes," "are excellent good for all palsies, and falling sickness," "strengthen the brain exceedingly, help the memory...help the gout....are excellent in all sorts of agues...and strengthen all the limbs of the body." Although these statements alone are difficult to evaluate and understand in terms of turbid dampness or phlegm from the Chinese Medicine point of view, when looking at these statements and the rest of the medicinal's uses, one can see that there is a strong connection between Culpepper's and Chinese Medicine's understanding of these pathologies.

Translation of available literature:

There are two species of Juniper listed in the *Grand Dictionary of Chinese Medicinals* (2009). *Juniperus rigida* Sieb. Et Zucc. *dùsōng* (杜松) uses the strobili (aka berry) as is used in *Juniperus communis* and *J. californicum*. It was first listed in the *Guó Yào De Yào Lǐ Xué* (1952), although it was likely used long before that time. It is native to the north central and northeast part of China. It is considered sweet, bitter, and neutral, although other sources list it as cool. It dispels wind, settles pain, expels dampness, and disinhibits urination. It is used to treat wind–damp joint pain, painful wind, kidney inflammation, water swelling, and urinary tract infections.

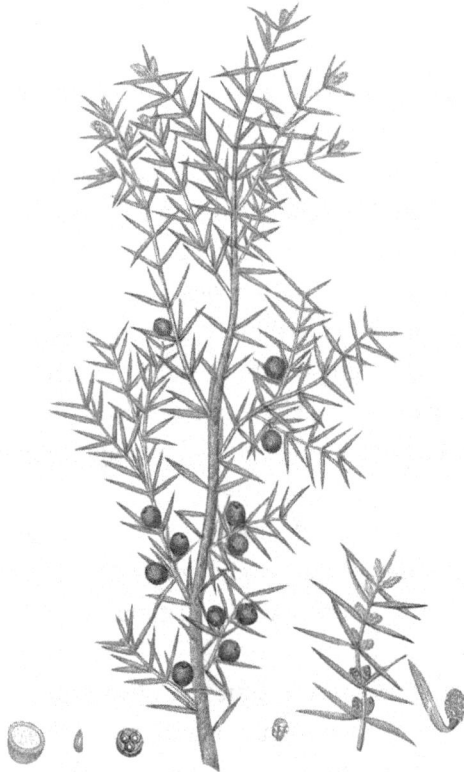

Beebalm

Monarda sp. L.

Lameaceae

Monardae herba

Favor and Qi: aromatic, acrid, bitter, warm

Channels entered: spleen, stomach, urinary bladder

Actions: diaphoretic, anti–inflammatory, antimicrobial, antispasmodic

Functions & Indications:

Aromatically transforms dampness. Beebalm is used for middle burner dampness obstruction with symptoms of fullness in the abdomen and chest, with or without nausea or vomiting. Beebalm warms the spleen and aromatically transforms dampness with its warm nature and aromatic, acrid, and bitter flavors. Its warm, aromatic, acrid, and bitter actions also help to dry and revive the spleen when it has been damaged by dampness and cold. This herb can be used for acute conditions like food poisoning, while also being valuable for more chronic conditions such as damp–cold invasion hampering the action of the spleen, or spleen vacuity leading to damp-obstruction in the middle burner. In this way, Beebalm is similar to *zǐsūyè* and *huòxiāng*.

Courses wind, resolves the exterior, and dispels cold. Bee Balm is used for external invasion of wind–cold with symptoms of chills, no sweating, feeling (or fear of) cold or wind, and nasal congestion. Beebalm is very good for coursing and resolving the exterior, and can be thought of as similar to *jīngjiè* of Chinese medicine. It is able to dispel wind, and also course the exterior.

Cautions:

None noted. However, due to this medicinal's strong scattering nature it should be used with caution for those with qi vacuity.

Dosage and Preparation:

Strong infusion 3–10g; fresh plant tincture 2–4ml

Major Combinations:

Combine with *shēngjiāng*, *hòupò*, and *huánglián* for acute middle burner obstruction due to food poisoning or other external causes, with symptoms of nausea, vomiting, headache, etc.

Combine with *cāngzhú* and *báizhú* for dampness obstructing the middle burner causing symptoms of pain, fullness, nausea, loss of appetite, diarrhea, etc. Add *gānjiāng* for combined coldness with symptoms of chilly feeling, especially in the abdomen, sloppy diarrhea, and desire for warm foods and drinks.

Combine with Osha and Echinacea for wind–cold external invasions with chills, fear of cold and/or wind, slight fever, and a tight, floating pulse.

Commentary:

Beebalm is a member of the Lamiaceae (Mint) family, and is a common name for a collection of plants in the *Monarda* genus. The genus is comprised of 16 species and is only found in North America. Some species are prized cultivars and may be found outside of their native range, including *M. didyma* (Scarlet Beebalm) and, to a lessor extent, *M. fistulosa* (Wild Bergamot), the latter of which is the most widespread species growing throughout most of North America. The author has experience with four of these species, including the two mentioned above, as well as *M. citriodora* (Lemon Beebalm) and *M. punctata* (Spotted Beebalm). Although they are mostly similar, there are some slight differences. Other than saying that Scarlet Beebalm is likely the "weakest" of these medicinals for the purposes set forth above, my experience is not rich enough with all four species to be able to give definitive differentiation.

Cook (1869) states of *M. punctata*: "This herb is diffusively stimulating and relaxant, of the distinctly carminative nervine and antispasmodic order. It makes a grateful and useful addition to diaphoretic drinks in the treatment of recent colds, catarrhal and typhus fevers, and measles." Here, Cook primarily discusses this medicinal's action to resolve the exterior and aromatically transform dampness in the middle burner. While his mention of measles is likely an exterior resolving action, the author has never used this medicinal for any skin conditions. Cook also believes that *M. punctata* is superior to *M. fistulosa*.

Felter & Llody (1905) state, of *M. punctata*: "Horsemint [an old name for Beebalm] is stimulant, carminative, sudorific, diuretic, and anti–emetic. The infusion or essence is used in *flatulence, nausea, vomiting*, and as a diuretic in *suppression of the urine*, and other urinary disorders." While Felter & Lloyd mention Beebalm's action as a diaphoretic, the focus of their monograph is on Beebalm's action on the middle and lower burners, especially the middle burner. They only give a few symptoms (shown above), but there seems to be a relatively clear link between these symptoms and the medicinal category of Aromatically Transforming Dampness in this text. Felter & Lloyd also note that both *M. fistulosa* and *M. didyma* can be used as substitutes for *M. punctata*.

There are some ethnobotanical records for most of these species. Mostly, they echo what has been said above, but the records are scant and sketchy, thus are not very dependable. However, a more recent publication states that another species, which is reported in the paper as *M. austromontana* (but is actually a subspecies of *M. citriodora*), is considered a highly valued medicinal by the Tarahumara of Northeast Mexico. They state that the: "leafy stems of napá [the Tarahumara name] are brewed into a tea (along or in mixture) to treat sore throats, colds, and gastrointestinal ailments; it is considered a general medicinal tea."[1]

There is a small amount of other modern research, mostly on the essential oils of a number of species. Both *M. didyma*[2] and *M. citriodora*[3] have shown antifungal properties. Unfortunately, the latter of those studies used the oil on agricultural pathogens, so we have no indication whether this species has antifungal properties against human pathogenic fungal species.

1. Bye, Robert A., (1986). Medicinal Plants of the Sierra Madre: Comparative Study of Tarahumara and Mexican Market Plants. *Economic Botany*. 40(1): pp. 103–124.
2. Fraternale, Daniele, et al., (2006). Chemical Composition, Antifungal and In Vitro Antioxidant Properties of *Monarda didyma* L. Essential Oil. *Journal of Essential Oil Research*. 18(5): pp. 581–585.
3. Bishop, Chris D. & Thornton, Ian B., (1997). Evaluation of the Antifungal Activity of the Essential Oils of *Monarda citriodora* var. *citriodora* and *Melaleuca alternifolia* on Post-Harvest Pathogens. *Journal of Essential Oil Research*. 9(1): pp. 77–82.

Sage Brush

Artemisia tridentata Nutt.
Asteraceae
Artemisiae tridentatae herba
Favor and Qi: bitter, acrid, aromatic, warm
Channels entered: lung, large intestine, spleen
Actions: antibacterial, antiviral, antifugal

Functions & Indications:

Transforms dampness and resolves toxin. Sage Brush is used for dampness accumulation with resulting toxicity. It transforms dampness with warm, acrid aroma, and resolves toxin with bitterness and warmth. This is particularly important in patients with acute heat–toxin impeding the small intestine's function of separating the pure and impure which can cause an accumulation of dampness with symptoms of fullness, diarrhea that does not offer much relief, cramping, and pain. Although this medicinal is warm, it uses bitterness, acridity, and aroma to effectively resolve toxicity, and when it is combined with appropriate cooling herbs, is exceptionally effective for treating these types of bowel complaints.

Resolves the exterior and scatters cold. Sage Brush is used for externally contracted wind–cold, especially when complicated by constitutional dampness. A symptom complex of feelings of chilliness, sore achy muscles, loss of appetite, and runny nose and nasal congestion is common with a swollen tongue and thick coating. Sage Brush resolves the exterior with warm acridity, while addressing constitutional dampness that can complicate this pattern with both its warm–bitter (draining) and warm–acrid (moving) nature-flavor combination.

Disperses wind and resolves dampness. Sage Brush is used for external application to wind–damp (either heat or cold) skin diseases with itching, suppuration, pus, or other damp qualities. Sage Brush is warm, acrid, and aromatic; a combination that effectively disperses wind and resolves dampness. Externally, this medicinal works as an effective wash, alone or in combination, to help resolve many skin conditions associated with these pathologies.

Cautions:
Sage Brush is a strong aromatic medicinal; large doses could cause nausea. Use caution with internal application for children and the very weak. There is no known toxicity. This medicinal should not be used during pregnancy or nursing.

Dosage and Preparation:
Tincture 0.5–2 ml; decoction or strong infusion 2–5g; external wash or use of tincture is exceptionally effective against fungal infections.

Major Combinations:
Combine with Goldenseal, *dàhuáng*, and *huángqín* for acute heat toxin in the intestines with fever, sweating, pain, bloating, with or without diarrhea (when there is diarrhea, the *dàhuáng* should be cooked for at least 20 minutes). Add *mùxiāng* and Yarrow for cramping pain. Dicentra may also be used for severe pain, added to this combination as a simple to be taken in 5–10 drop dosages every 15–20 minutes until the pain in relieved.

Combine with Yerba Mansa, *kǔshēn*, and Oregon Grape root, as a powder for external application to damp–heat skin infections (often fungal), such as athlete's foot.

Combine with Chenopodium and Black Walnut for worm infestation of the intestines with bloating and pain.

Commentary:
Sage brush is one of the most common plants (if not the most common) in the Great Basin area, and of most of the rest of the high desert area in the Western United States. Its common name, Sage Brush, is erroneous since it is not a true sage. Sages are part of the Laminaceae family "Mint," but Sage Brush is an Asteraceae family plant, and thus is more closely related to the common daisy or the Chrysanthemum (*júhuā*). It has long been a popular "smudge", which is prepared by tying together a collection of stems to form a thick "stick" (about 3–6cm diameter) which is burned for its purification qualities. In a number of Native American traditions, this was a popular use for this plant, which was used in ceremony, when people were ill, or to purify a room or home after someone had either been sick or died.[1]

Moore (2003) states of Sage Brush: "The cold infusion is suprisingly useful for impaired digestion, with poor gum health, coated tongue and chronic bad breath in the mornings. It is NOT appropriate for indigestion with excess salivation and a red–tipped tongue." While it is a bit difficult to understand this pattern from a Chinese medicine perspective, it seems to be some mechanism associated with the stomach and/or small intestine, and that complex being over–whelmed by dampness.

Sage Brush was also used by many Native American groups, both internally and externally, for various infections such as athlete's foot. The plant has shown 'good' to 'very good' results when used to treat a number of common pathogenic fungi, particularly *Microsporum cookerii* and *Microsporum gypseum.*[2]

For unknown reasons, this plant has been more or less overlooked as a medicine by herbalists in the 19th and 20th Centuries. There is essentially no modern literature on this plant other than a mention in Michael Moore's work from the 1990's. The plant covers an enormous amount of land in the Great Basin region of the Western United States, and there are few ecological concerns from overharvesting at the moment. This plant is worth a second look, perhaps leading to a place in our materia medica.

1. Shemluck, Melvin (1982). Medicinal and Other Uses of the Compositae by Indians in the United States and Canada. *Journal of Ethnopharmacology.* 5; pp 303–358.
2 McCutcheon, A.R., Ellis, S.M., Hancock, R.E.W., Towers, G.H.N. (1994). Antifungal screening of medicinal plants of British Columbian native peoples. *Journal of Ethnopharmacology.* 44: pp 157–169.

Medicinal	Nature	Flavor	Channels	Functions	Indications
Juniper	warm	acrid, bitter, aromatic	spleen, kidney, triple burner	Aromatically transforms dampness, drains damp turbidity, and moves qi; Dispels dampness and expels cold for wind–damp–cold impediment; Warms the kidneys and transforms phlegm	oppression in the chest, pain and distention in the abdomen, strangury, nausea, and loss of appetite; heaviness of the limbs and fixed pain in the joints; lumbar pain with cold, heavy, dragging sensation in the lower back
Beebalm	warm	aromatic, acrid, bitter	spleen, stomach, urinary bladder	Aromatically transforms dampness; Courses wind, resolves the exterior, and dispels cold	fullness in the abdomen and chest, with or without nausea or vomiting; wind–cold with symptoms of chills, no sweating, feeling of (or fear of) cold or wind, and nasal congestion
Sage Brush	warm	bitter, acrid	lung, large intestine, spleen	Resolves the exterior and scatters cold; Resolves toxin and transforms dampness; Disperses wind and resolves dampness	feeling of chilliness, sore achy muscles, loss of appetite, runny nose and nasal congestion; fullness, diarrhea that does not offer much relief, cramping and pain; itching, suppuration, pus

利水滲濕藥

Disinhibit Water Percolate Dampness Medicinals

The disinhibit water percolate dampness category of medicinals is a large and often used group of both warm and cool nature medicinals. These medicinals are used to free and disinhibit the water pathways and percolate and drain water–dampness. This category of medicinals is primarily used for patterns where water-dampness is collecting internally. This can manifest in a number of patterns and medicinals in this category are often divided into three sub-categories; disinhibit water and disperse swelling, disinhibit urination and free strangury, and disinhibit dampness and abate yellow (jaundice). Common symptoms of these patterns are inhibited urination, water swelling, diarrhea, phlegm-rheum, strangury pattern, yellow jaundice, dampness sores, and vaginal discharge.

The medicinals in this materia medica cover many of the patterns and symptoms mentioned above. Goldenrod is likely the most familiar to the readers and likely the most versatile of the group. Bidens is a very important medicinal in this category but I believe much underutilized by many Western herbalists. The last, Parsley root, has a long history of use in the West, but has fallen out of favor in recent years.

Because the medicinals in this category affect the bodily fluids care should be used when patients have yin depletion with scant liquids (thinner fluids), kidney vacuity with loss of essence, and with caution during pregnancy.

Goldenrod

Solidago canadensis L. and others
Asteraceae
Solidagi herba
Chinese Name: *yīzhīhuánghuā* (一枝黄花)
Favor and Qi: acrid, bitter, slightly sweet, cool
Channels entered: kidney, bladder, lung
Actions: diuretic, diaphoretic, anti-inflammatory, antimicrobial

Functions & Indications:

Clears heat, disinhibits dampness, relieves pain, and stops bleeding. Goldenrod is used for damp-heat strangury and other damp-heat conditions in the lower burner with scant, dark-yellow urine (with or without blood present), and pain in the lower back (anatomical kidney area). Although this medicinal is cool in nature, its acrid flavor moves the qi, while its bitter flavor drains. The combination of these actions will clears heat not only by its bitter flavor and cool nature, but also by resolving damp stagnation. When combined with other medicinals that clear heat in the lower burner, the heat-clearing action can be greatly enhanced.

Diffuses the lung and courses the exterior. Goldenrod is used for external contraction of wind-heat or wind-cold congesting the lung channel, with symptoms such as sinus congestion, cough, sore throat, and heat effusion with a floating and rapid or floating and tight pulse. This medicinal is both cooling and slightly nourishing, so it can be particularly beneficial in cases of external contraction of wind evils in deficient patients, particularly those with yin vacuity. This medicinal is bitter and acrid. Goldenrod uses cool bitterness to drain the lung and help clear lodged congestion in the lung channel; with cool acridity, it courses the exterior and diffuses the lung, bringing the lung's depurative function into harmony.

Quickens the blood, reduces swelling, and stops pain. Goldenrod is used for both internal and external application to bruises, trauma, sores, and tissue damage whenever there is blood stasis, swelling, and pain. Goldenrod has long been noted as an excellent medicinal for wounds with swelling and pain. Goldenrod quickens the blood with cool acridity, thus reducing swelling and stopping pain, while its bitter flavor is particularly useful (combined with its cool nature) when there is heat or toxin associated with these traumas.

Nourishes the kidney, clears heat, and disinhibits strangury. Goldenrod is used for kidney yin vacuity, or damp–heat brewing in the lower burner damaging yin humors, leading to scanty dark urine, lower back pain, painful urination, night sweating, etc. Goldenrod is cool, bitter, acrid and slightly sweet. Goldenrod drains heat and disinhibits dampness with cool bitterness, and with cool acridity it assists the qi dynamic of the kidney to disinhibit dampness. However, it is also slightly sweet, and this cool sweetness gently nourishes kidney yin, making it an important herb for conditions where the kidney yin humors are damaged in combination with strangury patterns.

Cautions:

This herb is diuretic and should be used with caution if the patient is taking another diuretic. Patients who have pollen allergies could possibly react to this medicinal with an allergy, however this is uncommon.

Dosage and Preparation:

Decoction or infusion 3–10g; fresh plant tincture 2–4ml

Major Combinations:

Combine with *niúxī* and Dandelion for damp–heat in the lower burner with painful strangury accompanied by scant dark urine and lower back pain. Add *báimáogēn* for the presence of blood, detected either by lab tests or visual confirmation of reddish urine. Add Marshmallow root for heat damage to yin humors.

Combine with Ambrosia and *xīnyíhuā* for allergic rhinitis, add *báizhǐ* for associated facial pain.

Combine with *shègān* and Echinacea for wind–heat invasion fettering the lung with swollen sore throat. Add Grindelia for cough.

Combine with *báizhǐ* and Elecampane for wind–cold congesting the lung with sinus congestion and coughing of thin, clear or white sputum.

Combine with Calendula and *hónghuā* for external or internal use, to quicken the blood and stop pain due to trauma. These three herbs

(Goldenrod, Calendula, and *hónghuā*), combined with St. John's Wort and Cayenne, and infused into olive, sesame, or sweet almond oil, are an excellent external application for pain due to traumatic injury with redness and swelling, or after a bruise has developed, to hasten the healing time.

Combine with *yíncháihú* and *shēngdìhuáng* for kidney yin vacuity with scant, difficult urination, night sweats, and a rapid floating pulse.

Commentary:

Solidago is a member of the Asteraceae (Sunflower) family in a genus (*Solidago*) of about 120 species with a center of biological diversity in North America. There are a handful of species in Mexico, South America, and Europe, but only three species native to China. All three species are, or have been, used in medicine with similar indications (see below for translations).

Although the center of biological diversity may be in North America, review of the literature clearly shows that across the globe, wherever there is a species of *Solidago*, there is some record of medicinal use. And, what's more, the continuum of usage across the genus is striking. There are no less than 10 species (probably a lot more) from four continents used in medicine, and the overwhelming majority of the usages for these species are the same or similar. Kovaleva and Batyuk (1985) state: "Thus, free flavonols and their biosides have been detected in *S. canadensis* [North America] and *S. virgaurea* [Europe/Asia]. The flavonoid compositions of the species of Goldenrod studies are similar to one another; differing only by the ratios of the individual components."[1] The importance of this statement is not so much in the recognition that these two plants have the same or similar usage and chemical components, but that, despite their geographical disparity, other plants within the genus, having similar documented usage, might also have similar chemistry. It is noteworthy that the major species mentioned in Chinese medicine (*S. decurrens*) is also native to a number of surrounding countries, including Russia, where there appears to be a significant amount of research available. Since 2011, I have been using this species as a local (to Beijing) substitute and find that it fits the description in the monograph above.

Gerard (1597) states: "Goldenrod is hot and dry in the second degree; it clenses with a certain astriction or binding quality." That Gerard classifies this medicinal as hot and dry is not strange when considering that it promotes urination (hot) and stops bleeding (drying). He further states: "Goldenrod provokes urine, wastes away stones in the kidneys, and expels them; and withall brings down tough and raw phlegmatic humors sticking in the urine vessels, which now and then do hinder the coming away of the stones..." Although it is impossible to be sure what, specifically, Gerard was talking about here, it is likely related to the kidney, urinary bladder and, possibly, prostate enlargement. It is entirely possible that the "tough and raw phlegmatic humors" are simply turbid dampness or phlegm in the lower burner, and not true stones coming from the kidneys or urinary bladder. However, stones may also have been present in some of these cases, but correct diagnosis of the problem may not have been true stones. Dampness can congeal into phlegm via scorching of the fluids from excessive heat or yin vacuity. It can also congeal into phlegm because of kidney yang vacuity unable to warm and move fluids (through its action both directly on the fluids and humor and also its support of the spleen and trible burner). In the lower burner, the cause of turbid dampness or phlegm is often yin vacuity (see discussion in *Commentary* section of Juniper). This can lead to inhibited urination.

Parkinson (1640) puts a slightly different spin on the above quote that may help us to understand it better. He says: "...provokes urine in abundance, whereby the gravel and stone engendered in the uritory parts, by raw and tough phlegmatic humours, may be wasted down into the bladder, from growing into a stone in those parts, and thence my be voided with the urine." This seems to suggest that Goldenrod disinhibits damp–turbidity so that stones are not formed, or that if stones do form, then Goldenrod will thin damp–turbidity and disinhibit dampness to allow for stones to pass more easily.

Of the decoction, Parkinson states that either the fresh herb or dried is "very effectual" for bruises, being taken both internally and externally. He also says of the decoction: "...helps to fasten the teeth that are loose in the gums." This latter comment may support the author's idea that Goldenrod nourishes the kidney.

Culpeper (1653) says of this herb, "...provokes urine in abundance, whereby also all the gravel and stone may be voided." This is one of the most common uses of this plant; in fact, Culpeper is actually quoting another source. Later, he states, "It is a sovereign wound herb, inferior to none, both for inward and outward hurts; green wounds, old sores and ulcers, are quickly cured therewith." Although Goldenrod has fallen out of favor, to some extent, as a medicinal for traumatic injuries and wounds, there is abundant traditional literature to support this use. In fact, Salmon (1710), who treated two English/European species and one American species (presumably *S. canadensis*) as the same, states: "It is one of the most noble wound–herbs, curing wounds and ulcers in an admirable manner." Later in the monograph, he states: "...for the curing of wounds inward and outward, it do as much as any other can: green wounds, it quickly cures them; and old sores and ulcers, it digests, cleanses, dries, and speedily induces their healing; drying up, stopping, or removing that moisture and flux of humors which hinders their cure."

A related plant, *S. chilensis*, which is native to South America, is sometimes called Brazilian Arnica, owing to both its resemblance to the European Arnica and to its traditional use similar to that of Arnica.[2] Bocek describes *S. californica* being decocted and used for both bruises and burns by the Costanoan Indians of Central California.[3]

Based on the above references, it appears that there is much room for cross–genus usage within *Solidago* species, which warrants further investigation into the understanding and usage of many species within the genus.

Also worthy of note is that although Goldenrod is often blamed for seasonal allergies, the pollen of this genus are too heavy to become airborne in any significant amount, thus this plant *is not* a cause of seasonal allergies despite common folklore to the contrary.[4]

Translation of Available Source Material:

There are several species of *Solidago* listed in the *Grand Dictionary of Chinese Medicinals* (2009), but there are three main entries. *S. decurrens* (yīzhīhuánghuā, 一枝黄花) appears to be the primary of the three. It is distributed from east to west, through central and southern China, as well as Shanxi Province. It is considered acrid, bitter, and cool (two other sources say "neutral", and one of those adds "sweet" but omits "acrid"). The functions are to course wind and clear heat, and resolve toxin and disperse swelling. Three other sources list a direct action on the blood, one suggesting it breaks blood, while the others are a bit more moderate, suggesting it quickens blood and stops pain. Furthermore, one source says that this medicinal frees and opens the orifices. It is indicated for wind–heat common cold, throat swelling and pain, lung heat cough, jaundice, heat-strangury, welling–abscess swelling with sores, poisonous snake bite, and knocks and falls.

S. pacifica cháoxiǎnyīzhīhuánghuā (朝鮮一枝黃花) is known in the Chang Bai Shan region in the northeast, which is most famous for its Ginseng. This medicinal is considered acrid, bitter, and cool and has the functions of clearing heat and resolving toxin, transforming phlegm and calming panting, stopping bleeding and dispersing swelling. It is indicated for common cold with heat effusion, swollen and painful throat, bronchitis, panting, lung inflammation, pulmonary tuberculosis with expectoration of blood [Note: The Chinese term for pulmonary tuberculosis is *fèijiéhé* (肺結核), which literally translates as "lung bind kernel (or pit)" suggesting that there is something bound like a kernel inside the lung], chronic kidney inflammation, blood in the urine, and uterine bleeding. Externally, it is used for welling–abscess and carbuncles with toxin, mastitis, and bites from poisonous snakes.

The third species is *S. virgaurea, xīnjiāngyīzhīhuánghuā* (新疆一枝黃花) which, as the name indicates, grows in Xinjiang Province in the northwest part of China and is the major species used throughout Europe and Central Asia. This medicinal is bitter, slightly acrid, and cool. Its functions are to course wind and clear heat, resolve toxin and disperse swelling, disinhibit water, and disperse swelling, and stop pain. It is indicated for wind–heat common cold, throat swelling with pain, kidney and bladder inflammation, welling–abscess and carbuncles with toxin, and knocks and falls. Note: This is the same species discussed by all the European authors above.

1. V. S. Batyuk and S. N. Kovaleva (1985). Flavonoids of *Solidago canadensis* and *S. virgaurea. Chemistry of Natural Compounds.* 21(4): pp. 533–534.

2. Mercandeli, Angélica A., et al. (2012) Evidence for the Safe Use of the Extract from the Brazilian Arnica, *Solidago chilensis* Meyen, in Primary Health Care. *Chinese Medicine.* 3: pp. 4–8. Published online in March, 2012 http://www.SciRP.org/journal/cm.

3. Bocek, Barbara R., (1984). Ethnobotany of Costanoan Indians, California, based on collections by John P. Harrington. *Economic Botany.* 38(2): pp. 240–255.

4. Abrahamson, Warren and Paul Heinrich, *The Solidago Eurosta Gall Homepage: A Resource for Teaching and Research.* (http://www.facstaff. bucknell.edu/abrahmsn/solidago/main.html)

Parsley Root

Petroselinum crispum (Mill.) Fuss
Apiaceae
Petroselini Crispi radix
Chinese name: ōuqíngēn (歐芹跟)
Favor and Qi: sweet, bitter, slightly acrid, cool
Channels entered: spleen, urinary bladder, kidney
Actions: potassium-sparing diuretic, anti-inflammatory

Functions & Indications:

Disinhibits dampness and clears heat for damp-heat accumulations. Parsley root is used for damp-heat accumulation where dampness is predominate, particularly in the lower part of the body. It is used to treat damp-heat patterns including urinary bladder damp-heat, liver/gallbladder damp-heat, spleen/stomach damp-heat, damp-heat jaundice, etc. Parsley root disinhibits dampness with bitter acridity, while clearing heat with coolness. Parsley's sweet flavor can benefit the middle qi and thus support the main function of this medicinal.

Opens the stomach and strengthens the spleen. Parsley root is used for food stagnation with accumulation of food and dampness causing symptoms of fullness, lack of appetite, foul breath, constipation or diarrhea, etc. Parsley downbears the stomach and opens with bitter acridity, while strengthening the spleen with sweetness.

Cautions:
This herb should be used with caution in damp-cold conditions.

Dosage and Preparation:
Decoction 3-10g; wine stir-fried strengthens its function to open the stomach

Major Combinations:

Combine with *huángbái* and *shānzhīzi* for damp-heat in the lower burner with dark yellow and possibly bloody urination, hemorrhoids, or sores in the genital area.

Combine with Dandelion and Gentian (or *lóngdǎncǎo*) for damp-heat in the liver/gallbladder with a red tongue and thick greasy yellow coating.

Combine with *cāngzhú* and *huíxiāngzǐ* for food stagnation and damp accumulation with sloppy diarrhea, painful distended abdomen, and foul breath. Add oil of Peppermint for serious cramping pains. If the tongue coating is yellow and thick, add *dàhuáng*, cooking for at least 20 minutes (longer cooking times will *decrease* the laxative action of this medicinal).

Commentary:

Parsley root is a common, safe, but too often forgotten medicinal plant. It is a member of the Apiaceae family, which is sometime called "the Parsley family." This family is well known for both its medicinal, spice, and food plants. Medicinals include species in the genera of *Ligusticum*, *Angelica*, *Notopterygium*, *Bupleurum*, *Osmorrhiza*, etc.; spices such as coriander, cumin, caraway, etc.; and foods such as carrot, celery, and parsnip. The family is made up of 300 genera and about 3000 species worldwide, primarily in temperate zones. There are several toxic members of this family, including *Conium maculatum* (Poison Hemlock), which is the plant that Socrates ingested in 399 BCE after being condemned to death; and *Cicuta maculata* (Water Hemlock), which is known as the most poisonous of all native species in North America.

Parsley has been used since antiquity with mentions in the literature as early as Pliny (23–79 CE). The leaf is also used in medicine, with similar actions, but drains dampness more strongly. The leaf is an important ingredient or garnish in many Western dishes and offers exception nutritional value as well.

Parsley root clears heat but not strongly, thus is always combined with heat–clearing herbs that are most appropriate for the pattern being treated. However, while it is not a strong heat–clearing herb, it generally is not used for cold conditions. It has a definite dampness–draining effect, while also being somewhat strengthening to the spleen, thus it will assist the spleen in resolving dampness while disinhibiting urine.

The seeds are also used in medicine and are acrid, bitter, and warm. They move qi and open the stomach. They can be used for bloating, gas, abdominal swelling with pain, various menstrual disorders, and have also been used to kill lice by external application.

The essential oil of this herb, found throughout the plant but most highly concentrated in the fruits (seeds), has been used for many years. Felter & Lloyd (1905) state: "It is highly recommended as a substitute for quinine in *intermittent fevers*, and has proved very efficient. It has likewise been found valuable in *menstrual derangements*; as *fetid menstruation*, *neuralgic dysmenorrhea, neuralgic uterine colic, amenorrhea*, etc.; also in the *night-sweats of consumption.*" Although the monograph in this text is concerned with the root only, some of the oil found in the roots.

The concentration of Apiole (a major constituent) is between 30–86% depending on the variety, the time of year the seeds are sown, and when the plant is harvested. Interestingly, later planting and harvesting yield a higher concentration of this constituent, as well as Myristicin.[1] This helps explain some of its ability to move qi and clear heat; although it also hints toward quickening the blood, I don't believe this to be a feature of the root, only the seed or oil.

Parsley leaf is a potassium-sparing diuretic,[2] which makes it an important herb for some situations. Parley leaf assists the body in eliminating sodium along with water through the urine, while allowing for the re-absorption of potassium into the blood. This is especially important when treating patients with high blood pressure, kidney disease, and heart disease, since potassium is a key electrolyte associated with these disease processes. There is no research to support the use of the root for this action, but because the chemistry is similar, there is a high likelihood that the root also offers this benefit.

In Turkey, Parsley leaf is commonly used for diabetes and liver toxicity. There are several animal studies that support this use. In one study, the serum ALP (which indicates bone and liver disease) and ALT (which reflects damage to the liver and underlying liver disease) activities were decreased, and findings showed statistically significant improvement over controls. This study also showed significant reduction or absence of hepatocytes in diabetic rats treated with parsley.[3] In another study, the extract of Parsley leaf showed a decrease in blood glucose levels in rats.[4]

Gerard (1597) speaks of the root, leaf, and seeds, more or less counting them as the same medicine, but to different degrees. He says that the root, specifically, is moderately hot (in the second degree), causes diuresis, and is agreeable to the stomach.

Parkinson (1640) states: "...the root moves the belly downwards and is one of the five opening roots, but also binds the body as Dioscorides says, and hereby also is profitable for the yellow jaundice and dropsy." He also says that while most say the seed is the most effectual part of the plant, others say it is the root that is most effective. The term "five opening roots," is not readily found elsewhere in the literature, so it is unclear what the other four roots are. Parkinson also gives us the following formula from Bock, the famous German botanist and physician, which is used for the treatment of "jaundice and falling sickness, the dropsy, and stone in the kidneys and urinary bladder":

Seeds of: (an ounce of each)
Parsley, Fennel, Annise, and Carraways
Roots of: (an ounce and a half of each)
Parley, Burnet, Saxifrage and Carraways

This is made into a tincture by first bruising the seeds and cutting the roots small. The medicinals are allowed to steep in a bottle of white wine overnight, then the mixture is transferred to an earthen vessel and cooked "until a third part more be wasted, then straining and clarified. This is then taken in 4 oz. doses first thing in the morning and last thing in the evening, while abstaining from drink for three hours after. Of the uses of this preparation he says that this "openeth obstructions of the liver and spleen, and expelleth the dropsy or jaundice by urine." This formula is repeated by Culpeper, without crediting Bock for the recipe.

Culpeper (1653) states of the root: "it is very comfortable to the stomach; helpeth to provoke urine and women's courses (menstruation), to break wind both in the stomach and bowels, and doth a little open the body, but the root much more. It openeth obstructions both of the liver and spleen, and is therefore accounted one of the five opening roots." This statement shows a clear connection between this root (and the herb to some extent) and its use for both digestive problems (food stagnation) and dampness accumulation.

Salmon (1710) also calls Parsley "one of the five opening roots" and further states, "therefore the juice thereof must be profitable against all diseases proceeding from obstructions." Salmon also states that Parsley root should be combined with herbs that either gently or strongly "move the belly downward." Salmon echoes much of what Culpeper wrote half a century earlier, but his monograph is more extensive and discusses the leaf, root, and seed. He states that the leaf is the weakest and the seed is the strongest. The leaf and root are considered hot and dry in the second degree, while the seed is hot and dry in the third degree. This is most likely due to the difference in volume of essential oil present in the seeds, which generally yields a more pronounced and clinically visible effect on the body of both warming and drying.

Translation of Available Source Material:

Material available in Chinese language is either translation of English language material or based on a few current research studies. The author was unable to find any literature supporting a Chinese medical approach to using this plant.

1. Petropouus, S.A., Daferera, D., Akouminanakis, C.A., Passam, H.C., and Polissiou, M.G. (2004). The effect of sowing date and growth stage on the essential oil composition of three types of parsley (*Petroselinum crispum*). *J Sci Food Agric*. 84, pp. 1606–1610.

2. Kreydiyyeh, Sawsan Ibrahim & Usta, Julnar, (2002). Diuretic effect and mechanism of action of parsley. *Journal of Ethnopharacology*. 79(3): pp. 353–357.

3. S. Bolkent, R. Yanardag, O. Ozsoy-sacan and O. Karabulut-Bulan. (2004). Effects of Parsley (*Petroselinum crispum*) on the Liver of Diabetic Rats: a Morphological and Biochemical Study. *Phytother. Res.* 18: pp. 996–999.

4. Tunali T, Yarat A, Yanardag R et al. (1999). Effect of parsley (*Petroselinum crispum*) on the skin of STZ induced diabetic rats. *Phytother Res* 13: pp. 138–141.

Bidens

Bidens pilosa L. and others
Asteraceae
Bidens herba
Chinese Name: *guǐzhēncǎo* (鬼針草) or *mángchángcǎo* (盲腸草)
Other Names: Spanish Needles, Beggar's Tick
Favor and Qi: sweet, slightly bitter, cool
Channels entered: kidney, liver, spleen, urinary bladder, small intestine
Actions: anti-inflammatory, diuretic, antitumor, antibacterial, antiparasitic

Functions & Indications:

Clears heat and disinhibits dampness. Bidens is used for damp-heat stagnating in various parts of the body including the throat, groin area, and urinary bladder. The *Shī Wēn Lùn* (circa 1735) states, "[When] dampness pathogen stays in the *yángmíng* and/or *tàiyīn* for an extended period of time, heat will be generated. Extreme heat leads to 'lesser fire' (少火), which in turn becomes vigorous fire." Dampness can both lead to heat and combine with heat generated from another source. This can lead to fire, and fire can congeal pathogenic dampness and form nodules, which can become red and hot and cause pain. Bidens effectively clears heat and disinhibits dampness with cool bitterness, while harmonizing the spleen/stomach with sweetness.

Abates vacuity heat. Bidens is used for heat associated with either yin or qi vacuity. While yin vacuity and qi vacuity (see Commentary for more on qi vacuity heat) are two separate patterns, Bidens can be used equally well with both (although it needs to be used with some caution when treating yin vacuity because of its disinhibiting dampness action). However, when symptoms such as night sweats, spontaneous sweating, scant yellow urination, and anxiety/irritability are associated with these patterns, Bidens gently abates heat (and disinhibits dampness) without causing further depletion of the source yin or qi.

Cautions:

None noted, but because this medicinal is draining by nature, caution is advised when fluids are damaged.

Dosage and Preparation:

Decoction 6–15g; fresh plant tincture 3–6ml

Major Combinations:

Combine with Oregon Grape Root and Dandelion for damp–heat pouring into the urinary bladder with symptoms of scant, dark yellow, malodorous urine. For pain, add Kava. For blood in the urine, add *báimáogēn*.

Combine with *báizhú* and *zhìhuángqí* for qi vacuity heat with symptoms of lethargy, heat effusion, low appetite, scant dark urination, and a weak slippery pulse.

Add to *Bǔ Zhōng Yì Qì Tāng* to strengthen its draining action, particularly when the formula is indicated but there is yellow urination.

Commentary:

Bidens is a large genus within the Asteraceae (Sunflower) family of mostly tropical and semitropical plants. Many plants within the *Bidens* genus are used throughout the tropical and semitropical parts of the world. *B. pilosa*, the primary medicinal in this monograph, is a pan-tropical weed traditionally used in medicine in North & South America, Africa, Asia, and the South Pacific. Although it is considered "tropical", the author has found it growing well into the temperate zone to approximately the 45th parallel both in North America and Asia. It is commonly found near water, such as the edges of slow moving creeks and streams, as well as along ponds and lakes. It can also be found growing in disturbed areas, such as along roadsides and vacant lots.

In Brazil, *B. pilosa* is traditionally used for a variety of ailments, including malaria and liver diseases. Modern research done in Brazil shows significant support for its use in the treatment of malaria.[1,2] Bidens' use for liver ailments can be found traditionally throughout its native range and there has been a fair bit of research to support its use for both direct influence on the liver[3] and as an immunomodulatory and anti–inflammatory medicinal that can be used for hepatitis.[4] Bidens is also well-known for its use for type–2 diabetes. Modern research supports this use, which is common throughout its native habitat, which works by enhancing insulin secretion and possibly islet protection;[5] the research also suggests that Bidens could help prevent type–2 diabetes through T–cell modulation.[6]

Qi vacuity heat is a pattern often overlooked by practitioners because qi is a part of yang, and therefore many practitioners find the concept hard to understand. However, this pattern is often encountered in the clinic due to Westerners' propensity for damaged spleen/stomach from inappropriate eating and drinking habits. There are two causes of qi vacuity heat: 1) internal damage to the spleen/stomach or spleen/lung leading to spleen/stomach or spleen/lung qi vacuity, and 2) summerheat dampness pattern damaging the qi. The former is a relatively common pattern and is what Lǐ Dōng-yuán frequently discussed in his *Pí Wèi Lùn*. The *Zhèng Zhì Huì Bǔ* (1687) states, "[When there is] qi vacuity heat, use sweet and warm [medicinals] to eliminate the heat." Although this medicinal is neither warming nor supplementing, it is sweet and, when combined with warm qi supplementing medicinals, offers an excellent combination to treat this pattern. The latter pattern may be less frequently encountered, but should be considered when there is qi vacuity heat. The *Sù Wèn* says, "[When there is] qi vacuity and the body is warm, it is due to summerheat damage." Summer-heat pathogens consume the qi and damage the bodily fluids; the body becomes warm and the pulse is vacuous. The appropriate course of action is to clear summerheat, supplement qi, and engender fluids. The primary formula for this pattern is Lǐ Dōng-yuán's *Qīng Shǔ Yì Qì Tāng*, which has only sweet and bland *zéxiè* as a dampness draining medicinal. Bidens may be added to this formula only if there is more dampness associated with the pattern, but it is important to be aware not to further damage the bodily fluids.

Translation of Available Source Material:

There are at least six species of *Bidens* used in Chinese medicine. The *Grand Dictionary of Chinese Medicinals* (2009) lists *B. pilosa*, *mángchángcǎo* (盲 腸草) as sweet, slightly bitter, and cool, which are the same classifications that the author arrived at independently, and are offered above. Functions are listed as clearing heat, resolving toxin, disinhibiting urination, and strengthening the spleen. The *Gui Zhou Collection of Herbal Folk Remedies* (1978) lists *B. pilosa* as a medicinal that clears heat and resolves toxin, and is used to treat liver inflammation, abdominal water, high fever, clove sore, ejections of blood, and intestinal welling-abscess.

1. Brandao, M.G.L., Krettli, A.U., Soares, L.S.R., Nery, C.G.C., Marinuzzi, H.C. (1997). Antimalarial activity of extracts and fractions from *Bidens pilosa* and other *Bidens* species (Asteraceae) correlated with the presence of acetylene and flavonoid compounds. *Journal of Ethnopharmacology*. 57; pp 131–138.

2. Andrade–Neto, V.F., et al (2004). Antimalarial activity of *Bidens pilosa* L. (Asteraceae) ethanol extracts from wild plants collected in various localities or plants cultivated in humus soil. *Phytotherapy Research*. 18; pp. 634–639.

3. Yuan, Li–Ping, et al. (2008). Protective effects of total flavonoids of *Bidens pilosa* L. (TFB) on animal liver injury and liver fibrosis. *Journal of Ethnopharmacology*. 116(4); pp 539–546.

4. Abajo, Celia, et al (2004). In vitro study of the antioxidant and immunomodulatory activity of aqueous infusion of *Bidens pilosa*. *Journal of Ethnopharmacology*. 93(3); pp 319–323.

5. Hsu, Yi–Jou, et al. (2009). Anti–hyperglycemic effects and mechanism of *Bidens pilosa* water extract. *Journal of Ethnopharmacology*. 122(3); pp 379–383.

6 Chiang, Yi–Ming, et al. (2007). Cytopiloyne, a novel polyacetylenic glucoside from *Bidens pilosa*, functions as a T helper cell modulator. *Journal of Ethnopharmacology*. 110(4); pp 532–538.

Medicinal	Nature	Flavor	Channels	Functions	Indications
Parsley root	cool	sweet, bitter, slightly acrid	Kidney, urinary bladder	Drains dampness and clears heat; Opens the stomach and strengthens the spleen;	urinary bladder damp-heat, liver/gallbladder damp-heat, spleen/stomach damp-heat, damp-heat jaundice; fullness, lack of appetite, foul breath, constipation or diarrhea
Bidens	cool	sweet, slightly bitter	kidney, liver, spleen, urinary bladder, small intestine	Clears heat and drains dampness; Drains vacuity heat and is used for heat associated with either yin or qi vacuity	damp-heat stagnating in various parts of the body including the throat, groin area, and urinary bladder; night sweats, spontaneous sweating, scant yellow urination, and anxiety/irritability
Goldenrod	cool	acrid, bitter, slightly sweet	kidney, lung, urinary bladder	Clears heat, drains damp, relieves pain, and stops bleeding; Diffuses the lung and courses the exterior; Nourishes the kidney, clears heat, and disinhibits strangury	damp-heat strangury and other damp-heat conditions in the lower burner with scant, dark-yellow urine (with or without blood present), and pain in the lower back; sinus congestion, cough, sore throat, and heat effusion with a floating and rapid or floating and tight pulse; bruises, trauma, sores, and tissue damage whenever there is blood stasis, swelling, and pain; kidney yin vacuity, or damp-heat brewing in the lower burner leading to scanty dark urine, lower back pain, painful urination, night sweating, etc.

化痰止咳藥

Transform Phlegm and Stop Cough Medicinals

T he transform phlegm stop cough category of medicinals is a very important category used to expel or disperse phlegm; this is known as transforming phlegm in Chinese medicine. This category is also important to mitigate or check coughing (and even calm panting) and thus called stop coughing. Medicinals in this category may be either warming or cooling in nature and tend to have bitter and acrid flavors.

This category is divided into three subcategories; warm and transform cold phlegm, clear heat and transform phlegm medicinals, and stop cough and calm panting medicinals. In this materia medica all of the medicinals discussed are cooling in nature; for a discussion of some Western medicinals in this category with a warm nature I would encourage you to see Garran (2008) where I discuss warming medicinals in this category including Yerba Santa and Elecampane (although the latter was put in the Supplementing category, it is clearly a very good medicinal for treating phlegm). Mullein and Eucalyptus are very important medicinals in the Western materia medica for the treatment of phlegm and are covered here. Horehound, Wild Cherry bark, and Wild Lettuce stand out as some of the most important medicinals in the Western materia medica for the treatment of cough, particularly the first two.

Phlegm can appear in other places in the body, but medicinals in this category are most commonly used for phlegm in the lungs (and its channel). The medicinals in this materia medica are primarily used for this common therapeutic action. When treating phlegm, medicinals from two other categories are often used in formulas. The first is medicinals that strengthen the spleen because the spleen is the origin of phlegm and by strengthening the spleen we can stop the phlegm before it is generated. The second category frequently combined with the medicinals in this category is medicinals that move the qi. By moving the qi, phlegm is more easily dispersed and thus adding qi moving medicinals to a formula for transforming phlegm will bring about resolution more swiftly.

Mullein Leaf

Verbascum thapsus L. and others
Scrophulariaceae
Verbasci folium
Chinese Name: 毛蕊花 (*máoruǐhuā*) or 大毛叶 (*dàmáoyè*)
Favor and Qi: bitter, slightly acrid, cool
Channels entered: lung, triple burner, kidney
Actions: demulcent, diuretic, expectorant, sedative

Functions & Indications:

Clears heat, transforms phlegm, and stops cough. Mullein leaf is used for phlegm–heat in the lungs with yellow or green phlegm and coughing. Mullein leaf drains heat with bitterness, and with bitterness and acridity helps to restore the depurative downbearing action of the lungs. However, Mullein also has a fluid–nourishing action, making it an effective herb for treating heat in the lungs. The lungs are "the delicate viscus" and are easily damaged by dryness or heat. Mullein has a mild but definite action to moisten the lungs and mediate damage due to heat pathogens invading the lungs.

Clears heat and promotes urination. Mullein leaf is used for heat–dampness accumulation, particularly when the lung's ability to control water in the body has been disturbed. Although this herb has a major action on the lungs, it is also very important in the treatment of heat strangury. It clears heat in the bladder while also helping to restore the lung's depurative downbearing action to assist the elimination of dampness in the body. When the urine is inhibited or scanty due to heat, Mullein clears heat and facilitates the flow of urine. Mullein leaf is bitter, slightly acrid, and cool. Cool bitterness can clear heat and drain dampness from the urinary bladder, while the cool and slightly acrid nature of this medicinal can act on the lung to restore its depurative downbearing action. The combination of these make Mullein leaf an effective medicinal for the treatment of heat–dampness in the lower burner.

Clears vacuity heat, nourishes fluids, and transforms phlegm. Mullein leaf is used for "scrophula" (*luǒlì*瘰疬) due to lung and kidney yin vacuity. This disease pattern arises from yin vacuity heat in the kidney and lung (or other internal heat) scorching the fluids and transforming them into phlegm; it can also arise with chronic liver constraint or contraction of wind–fire–toxin. Mullein leaf clears heat with cool bitterness, while utilizing its acrid–cool nature to transform lodged phlegm. Mullein's gentle moistening action nourishes fluids without being cloying, thus serving a particularly important function when treating this ailment.

Clears heat, transforms toxin, reduces swelling, and stops pain. Mullein leaf is used for heat–toxin swellings such as sores (including bed–sores), ulcerations, and other hot–swellings. This is for external application where the leaf is sometimes applied directly to the affected area. Mullein leaf clears heat and transforms toxin with cool bitterness, while also reducing swelling. Its acrid flavor helps to move qi and relieve pain and, combined with its cool nature, helps to reduce swelling. This herb has also been used externally for hemorrhoids, swollen glands, and traumatic injury. The internal application of this herb is also indicated for these complaints.

Cautions:
See note in *Dosage and Preparation* below.

Dosage and Preparation:
Decoction or strong infusion 3–10g, tincture 2–4ml. Note: Care should be taken to strain a tea through a fine cloth or coffee filter, as the hairs found on the leaves could cause irritation of the throat when swallowed.

Major Combinations:
Combine with Grindelia and *yúxīngcǎo* for cough with thick green phlegm that is difficult to expectorate.

Combine with *huángqín* and *tiānhuāfěn* for cough due to prolonged heat lodged in the lungs damaging the humors and fluids of the lungs, with sticky yellow sputum that is difficult to expectorate.

Combine with *màiméndōng* and American Ginseng for a yin vacuity cough with weakness and sticky yellow sputum that is difficult to expectorate.

Combine with Marshmallow and *kuǎndōnghuā* for dry cough due to wind–dryness pathogen invading the lung. This combination can also be used for other types of dry coughing without severe damage to lung yin. Honey mix-fried *kuǎndōnghuā* should be used in this combination.

Combine with Yerba Santa for cough with difficult to expectorate sputum. This combination can be further modified for heat patterns with *huángqín* and *tiānhuāfěn*, or with Elecampane and *bànxià* for cold patterns with abundant or watery phlegm.

Combine with Figwort, Red Root, and *zhèbèi* for "scrophula" (瘰疬), also known as lymphatic swellings or phlegm nodulation, in the neck, armpits, or groin. This basic combination can be modified by adding Echinacea for red, hot, and potentially infected swellings, or by adding Ocatillo for swellings in the groin area. Cleavers should be added in damp–heat patterns.

Commentary:

Mullein is a Scrophulariacea (Figwort) family member of the *Verbascum* genus, which is biogeographically centered in Turkey and surrounding areas. It is a relatively large genus consisting of about 228 species, many of which are used medicinally by local cultures in their native habitat. The species primarily noted in this monograph has naturalized throughout much of Europe and North America. It is very easy to grow and has even become weedy in some areas. It will grow in a wide range of ecosystems and elevations, but tends to prefer open disturbed areas.

Mullein is a biennial, which means that it blooms in the second year, after which it dies. The leaves are large and soft because of the abundant soft hairs. They hold a significant amount of water, which is important to note if you want to harvest them, because drying too slowly will produce a darker color due to oxidation. However, if you find yourself in the woods with no toilet paper and can't make it home, Mullein leaves do provide a very good substitute! Many people have asked if the leaf hairs can lead to irritation of the mouth or throat. Although I have never know this to be a problem, it might be wise to take care when straining any tea made with Mullein.

Mullein is a stately plant. The flowering stalk can reach over two meters and is covered in yellow flowers, which are also medicinal (see below). The leaves should be gathered in the summer and early autumn of the first year, or early spring of the second year. Once the plant begins to flower, the medicinal properties of the leaf diminish, and it should be left to flower and fruit. Mullein is a weed in many parts of the world, but it is not terribly difficult to manage, so it generally doesn't garner much attention from native plant enthusiasts who are out to eliminate alien species.

The leaves are best prepared as a strong infusion or, preferably, a decoction. The tincture is definitely effective, although it is stronger for dealing with cough and moving fluids than it is with nourishing dryness. Interestingly, decoctions have shown the best antibacterial activity against the most common bacteria involved in lung and kidney infections.[1] Decoction is the best all–around preparation, so this is an herb that easily fits into standard Chinese medical practice and should be incorporated. In some parts of India, the leaves of this plant are smoked as a sedative and also applied externally to wounds.[2]

Most of the modern research on this plant does not yield clinically useful information that is not already well understood by herbalists using Mullein. Mullein is one of the first medicinal plants that many Western herbalists learn, and is a primary botanical medicine for treatment of many lung conditions.

The lung being the "tender yin organ" in Chinese medicine means that qi transformation within the lung, as well as humors and fluids of the lung, are easily damaged by pathogenic influences such heat, cold, wind, dryness, etc. These pathogens can disrupt the qi dynamic within the lung and lead to cough, shortness of breath, and other breathing problems. Although Mullein is not truly a "lung yin supplementing" medicinal, I can safely say that it nourishes the fluids and humors of the lung (and kidney). Therefore, although it can address some of the symptoms associated with lung yin vacuity, and also nourishes the fluids and humors, it does not possess the depth of nourishment needed in these cases and must be combined with other medicinals that specifically nourish lung yin. Medicinals that nourish yin in the Western material medica include Marshmallow and American Ginseng; in the Chinese materia medica, *màiméndōng*, *shāshēn*, and *bǎihé* are most frequently used, while herbs such as *tiānhuāfěn* are used to nourish the fluids and humors of the lung.

Mullein leaf affects fluid movement of the body, so, in addition to its more obvious effects on the lung, it also works to mildly transform or move dampness. Mullein does not transform dampness in the spleen, but it has an action of moving and transforming dampness when dampness has accumulated in a particular area. This suggests an action on the triple burner, i.e. damp–heat lodged in the triple burner with oppression in the chest and short voidings of urine, or any manifestation of the triple burner qi not transforming fluids, which then can accumulate in a particular area of the body. Many organ systems are involved with the transformation and movement of water (lung, spleen, kidney, bladder, small intestine, stomach, and large intestine) but these functions all coalesce in the triple burner. Clavey (2004) states:

> "San Jiao [triple burner] is the pathway for the body's yang qi to ascend and descend, and is thus the source of all qi transformation; it is also the pathway for fluids to be moved about the body by the qi. Any treatment of damp–heat disease must necessarily open San Jiao, so that yang qi flows smoothly and qi transformation occurs normally, after which the fluid metabolism will be regular and harmonious, and pathogenic damp will have no place to exist. With no damp to hold it in, any heat will disperse as it is formed."

Mullein's action on two of the most prominent of those organ systems (lung and kidney) plays a key role in its ability to affect the triple burner, but Mullein also seems to have a direct action on the triple burner channel, making it an important medicinal in the treatment of impaired movement of fluid in many different scenarios.

Parkinson (1640) discusses Mullein at length, describing how Dioscorides and other well-known Greek physicians used this medicinal since at least the beginning of the Common Era (CE). In his discussion of the plant, he mentions uses for the root, flowers, seeds, and leaves (see the monograph on Mullein flowers for more of what Parkinson said about using them).

Parkinson says of the leaves, "A decoction of the leaves hereof, and of Sage, Marjoram, and Chamomile flowers, can be used to bath areas of the body where veins or sinews are stiff with cold, or with cramps, to bring much ease and comfort." Later he says, "A decoction of the root, and also the leaves, is of great effect to dissolve the tumors or swellings, as well as inflammations of the throat."

Parkinson does not state this plant's nature, but these two quotes illustrate two contrasting natures. On one hand, it is combined with Sage (warm), Marjoram (warm), and Chamomile (cool) to be applied for cold conditions, while on the other hand, he says that it can "dissolve tumors" and treat "inflammations of the throat." Although both warming and cooling herbs can be used to treat tumors and swellings, cooling herbs are generally used to treat throat inflammation (a notable exception discussed in my first book is *Ligusticum grayi* and *L. porter*). I propose this herb to be cooling.

Salmon (1710) is much more specific in regards to the above combination, which may help to shed a little light on this preparation. "Take leaves of Mullein two parts, Chamomile flowers, Marjoram, and Sage, of each one part, decoct all these together in wine. With this bathe morning and night where the veins are swollen, or the nerves are contracted, or where the cramp commonly afflicts, it gives relief, ease, and comfort." The combination seems to be more or less neutral in nature and yet is used to treat a cold condition. However, what Parkinson calls "stiff with cold" is not necessarily without inflammation, e.g. heat.

Salmon states that this medicinal is "temperate" (meaning its nature is "neutral") and drying in the first degree, which may help us to understand Parkinson's indications. Salmon also states that Mullein is specific for "coughs, colds, obstructions of the lungs, asthma, diarrhea, strangury, intermittent fever and chills, hemorrhoids, and relieves pain of gout." He states that the juice, taken in 1-3 spoonful doses with wine, "cures diarrhea, dysentery...catarrh, and abundant rheum in the lungs...And being drunk morning and night for 30 days together, it cures the gout." Salmon states that the tincture of the leaves in 3.5–10.5ml doses "cures a vehement pain of the stomach, and is profitable against convulsions, faintings and swooning fits [loss of consciousness], palpitation of the heart, sickness at the heart [possibly heart vexation], and vomiting, a vehement diarrhea with bloody discharge." This is a relatively large dose, but certainly not excessive by many standards. This is the only time I have seen Mullein referenced for use in treating the heart.

Translation of Available Source Material:

This medicinal was first recorded in China in *Selected Medicinals from Yunnan* in 1970. Thus, many of the indications are biomedically oriented. Chinese medicine recognized the entire plant (leaves, stem, root, etc.) as one herb and recommend it used as a decoction in 10-15g dosages. The *Grand Dictionary of Chinese Medicnials* (2009) calls it acrid, bitter, cool, with mild toxicity. It ascribes to Mullein the functions of clearing heat and resolving toxin, dispersing constraint and staunching bleeding, while recommending it for lung inflammation, chronic appendix inflammation, toxin of sores, knocks and falls (traumatic injury), and damage by sores with bleeding."

Selected Medicinals from Yunnan (1971) calls it bitter and cold, and lists the functions of dispersing inflammation, staunching bleeding, and drawing out toxin. The book recommends the herb for the treatment of sore toxin, knife and gun wounds, and knocks and falls.

Frequently Used Chinese Medicinals of Tibet (1971) calls is cool and bitter, and ascribes the functions of clearing heat and resolving toxin, and staunching bleeding. The book recommends it for the treatment of lung inflammation, "damage by sores with bleeding," joint sprains, sore toxin, etc.

Case Study

Male, 32 years old

Primary complaint: hot, red, swollen lymph nodes in groin.

Other symptoms: scant dark yellow urine, slightly dry irregular bowel movements, dry sore throat, hemorrhoids, lack of energy, difficulty sleeping.

Tongue: red, dry, cracked, thin yellow coat (thicker in the back)

Pulse: thin, floating, rapid

Diagnosis: kidney and lung yin vacuity with internal heat scorching the fluids and transforming them into phlegm.

Treatment strategy: clear heat, transform phlegm, nourish fluids

Herbs:

Echinacea 4pts, Mullein 3pts, Figwort 3pts, *zhèbèi* 3pts, Ocotillo 2pts, Red Root 2pts, California Coffee Berry bark 2pts, Licorice 1pt

The formula was give as a tincture and the patient was told to take 4ml every 3 hours for the first three days, every 4 hours for the following two days, then after each meal for the final two days before returning in a week's time. The patient was instructed to contact me via phone if there was no positive change within 48 hours, or if the condition worsened during that time.

These herbs were given as a tincture because the patient did not want a tea or decoction, and because I wanted him to start taking the herbs immediately. The primary function of this formula is to clear heat, although it also transforms phlegm and nourishes fluids. This formula was given for one week, at which point most of the primary symptoms were significantly improved. At that time, the Echinacea and the California Coffee Berry bark were removed, and I was able to convince the patient to take a powdered extract tea. I gave him a powdered extract of *Zhī Bǎi Dì Huáng* formula to be taken in 4 gram dosages, twice daily, 20–30 minutes prior to eating. He also continued to take a tincture formula of Mullein 3pts, Figwort 3 pts, Ocatillo 2 pts, and Red Root 2 pts for another 10 days. After one week of this subsequent treatment, the patient reported that his swellings were gone and all other symptoms were either resolved or nearly so. He continued the treatment, as far as I know, but did not come for a return visit.

Explanation of formula:

Echinacea is a primary herb for clearing heat and resolving toxin. It is used for nearly all cases of lodged heat in the body, whether from excess or vacuity. All pathogenic heat, no matter the origin, is still an excess and, when lodged like this, is generally classified as heat-toxin. The primary combination of Mullein, Figwort, and *zhèbèi* is employed here to resolve the swellings by clearing heat, transforming phlegm, and nourishing fluids. Red Root is a primary herb for the treatment of congestion and swellings (瘰疬) and, when combined with Ocotillo, works very well for problems in the groin and lower body in general. California Coffee berry was chosen in this case to drain heat from the bowels by gently moving the stool. Rhubarb could have been chosen here, but my affinity for this native California plant won out. Licorice was added to harmonize the formula, as well as clear heat and nourish fluids.

1. Turker A.U, Camper N.D, (2002). Biological activity of common mullein, a medicinal plant. *Journal of Ethnopharmacolgy* 82(2–3): 117–125.
2. Author unknown, (2009). *Ethnobotanical Leaflets* 13: 1240–56.

Horehound

Marrubium officinalis L.
Lamiaceae
Marrubii herba
Favor and Qi: bitter, acrid, slightly cold
Channels entered: lung, liver, spleen, stomach
Actions: antispasmodic, antihypertensive, anti–inflammatory, analgesic, antimicrobial

Functions & Indications:

Transforms phlegm, clears heat, downbears qi, and stops cough. Horehound is used for phlegm–heat congesting the lung and obstructing the depurative downbearing function of the lung. Horehound is profoundly bitter and strongly downbears qi with bitterness; its acrid flavor helps to move the qi, enabling the lung qi to return to its natural downward motion. Its strong bitterness makes it a difficult medicinal to drink. It is cold in nature and, with bitter cold, effectively clears heat, while its acrid–coldness helps to transform phlegm–heat.

Courses the liver, clears heat, and harmonizes the middle. Horehound is used for Wood–Earth disharmonies when constrained liver qi invades and plunders the spleen or stomach. Symptoms of these disharmonies include headache, bitter taste in the mouth, feeling of stuffiness or oppression in the chest, rib–side fullness or pain, glomus, fullness after eating (liver–spleen) or stomach–duct pain ("heartburn"), regurgitating stomach acid, lack of appetite, fullness and distention in the abdomen, rib–side pain, and inappropriate anger (liver–stomach). Horehound is slightly cold, bitter, and acrid and effectively courses the liver to resolve constrained qi while clearing the heat associated with constraint. Its slightly cold bitterness helps to move upsurging qi (manifesting as stomach-duct pain, fullness in the chest, inappropriate anger, etc.) downward, while it's acridity helps to harmonize the middle and reorder the spleen and stomach.

Cautions:

Although Horehound is used for Wood–Earth disharmonies, it can damage the spleen and stomach in patients who exhibit spleen/stomach qi vacuity or vacuity cold, and should be avoided or used cautiously in these cases. However, due to the relatively short duration of use, this should rarely be an issue.

Dosage and Preparation:

Light decoction or infusion 2–6g, fresh or dry plant tincture 1–3ml.

Major Combinations:

Combine with Mullein, *chuānbèimǔ*, and *tiānhuāfěn* for cough with sticky, yellow, difficult-to-expectorate phlegm due to phlegm–heat lodged in the lungs. I generally add *huángqín* to the combination for heat effusion.

Combine with Grindelia and Wild Yam for spasmodic cough due to external pathogens. Add Pleurisy Root when this cough is dry or has sticky, difficult-to-expectorate phlegm. Add Elecampane and Yerba Santa when this cough is wet due to wind–cold invasion.

Combine with *xuánfùhuā* and *jiāngbànxià* for copious frothy sputum with a choking sensation, difficult expectoration, and possible vomiting.

Combine with Elecampane and Hyssop for chronic cough due to spleen–lung dual vacuity. This combination requires the honey mix–fried version of Elecampane, and should always be combined with other herbs to strengthen the spleen and lung qi.

Combine with Wild Yam and *Sì Nì Sǎn* for liver qi invading the stomach with symptoms of stomach–duct pain, regurgitating stomach acid, lack of appetite, fullness and distention in the abdomen, and rib–side pain.

Combine with Wild Yam and *Tòng Xiè Yào Fāng* for liver qi invading the spleen with symptoms of feeling of stuffiness or oppression in the chest, rib–side fullness or pain, glomus, and fullness after eating.

Commentary:

Horehound is a member of the Lamiaceae "Mint" family in the genus *Marrubium*. *Marrubium* comes from the Hebrew word meaning "bitter juice", and it is commonly believed that a plant from this genus, perhaps *M. vulgare*, was one of the bitter herbs discussed in the Bible. The genus has 30 species, all native to Eurasia (mostly in the Mediterranean region), many of which are used in medicine, though several are reported as toxic.

Its crinkled, gray–blue leaves and bur–like sepals are an obvious indicator of the species. Horehound is a noxious weed in many locations, but struggles in extreme cold environments, especially with wet clay soil.

Horehound is an extremely bitter medicinal and is also acrid. This can make the use of Horehound a bit challenging, even for those accustomed to taking Chinese decoctions. Although I don't see this medicinal used as commonly as I once did, it is an important medicinal for phlegm-heat in the lung, and for coughing. It is particularly useful for more acute conditions, as its acridity will help to dispel wind-heat. Thus, it is often used for acute conditions rather than chronic conditions. However, this medicinal is also very useful in chronic coughs, particularly difficult, painful, hot coughs, with or without expectoration. This type of cough is often associated with other signs and symptoms such as tightness in the chest, spasmodic coughing fits, constipation, headache, and the tongue is usually red to scarlet and is often cracked. Modern research literature has shown that Horehound effectively treats many of these symptoms. A group in Spain has published two separate papers showing both the analgesic[1] and antispasmodic[2] actions of this medicinal.

Gerard (1597) says that: "Galen teaches [Horehound] is hot in the second degree, and dry in the third, and of a bitter taste." Those are words that Salmon echos over 100 years later (see below). Gerard introduces four species of Horehound, but in his monograph only mentions the species discussed above. He states: "Common Horehound boiled in water and drunk, opens the liver and spleen, clenses the breast and lungs, and prevails greatly against an old cough, pain of the side, spitting of blood, the consumption, and ulcerations of the lungs." Gerard speaks of Horehound with great zeal when it comes to the fresh herb being processed into a syrup, stating: "[It] is a most singular remedy against the cough, and wheezing of the lungs." He also says: "The same syrup doth wonderfully and above credit, ease such as have been long sick of any consumption of the lungs, as hath been often proved by the learned physicians of our London College." This syrup is a common product and is still made today. The syrup is also cooked into hard candy and sold as lozenges. In modern times, this is generally compounded into a formula incorporating other medicinals such as Wild Cherry bark, Mullein, Elecampane, etc. I have used such a syrup of the following formula to great advantage:

Cough Syrup

Horehound	3pts
Elecampane	3pts
Yerba Santa	3pts
Wild Cherry bark	2pts (*xìngrén* may be substituted)
zhèbèimǔ	2pts
Echinacea	2pts
Mullein	2pts
jiégěng	1pt
gāncǎo	1pt

The medicinals (except the Wild Cherry bark/*xìngrén*, either of which is prepared as a cold water infusion the night before) are combined and simmered with water and alcohol (70:30) for one hour. After the decoction has cooled to handling temperature, it is strained and filtered. To this filtered liquid, add sugar in a 1:2 ratio (sugar:decoction) and bring to a boil. Right before boiling, add the cold infusion of Wild Cherry bark or *xìngrén*. Boil briefly, about 2 minutes, remove from heat and allow to cool for 10 minutes, stirring occasionally. Transfer to bottles to reserve for later use. Do not cap tightly until syrup is cooled to room temperature. I have changed the recipe a number of times over the years and there is room to play with it depending on the patient's needs. More warming, more cooling, stronger phlegm–resolving action, etc. can all be achieved by modifying this formula. Even essential oils, such Eucalyptus, may be added at the end. The final product is about 25–30% alcohol, sweet enough for kids to take easily, yet effective. Total time, depending on volume, is about 3–4 hours. (Note: Due to recent developments in cGMP regulations and enforcement, selling this *could* get you in a bit of hot water with the FDA.)

Parkinson (1640) quotes Dioscorides as saying, "a decoction of the dried herb with the seed, or the juice of the green herb taken with honey, is a remedy for those that are pursie [meaning unknown to author, possibly a reference to pleurisy], and short winded, for those that have a cough, and for such as by long sickness, or thin distillations of rheum upon the lungs are wasted and fallen into consumption" Parkinson is expanding on what Gerard said, rather than simply repeating or rewording it.

Culpeper (1653) wrote about Horehound extensively. He modifies what Parkinson said regarding Iris or Orris. Parkinson states that this combination "brings down womens curses [menstruation]" but Culpeper uses the combination for "tough phlegm in the chest," which is sensible. (Note: Iris and Orris, though not often used in modern herbalism, were common medicinals in the past and have a similar action to that of medicinals that "sweep phlegm", such as *tiānnánxíng*, or strong phlegm-resolving medicinals such as *bànxià*.)

"A decoction of the dried herb, with the seed, is a remedy for those that are short-winded, have a cough, or are fallen into a consumption, either through long sickness, or this distillations of rheum upon the lungs. It helpeth to expectorate tough phlegm from the chest, being taken with the roots of Iris or Orris." "The leaves used with honey, purgeth foul ulcers, stays running or creeping sores, and the growing of the flesh over the nails; it also helpeth pains of the sides. The juice thereof with wine and honey, helpeth to clear the eye sight; and snuffed up into the nostrils, purgeth away the yellow jaundice." "Galen saith, it openeth obstructions both of the liver and spleen, and purgeth the breast and lungs of phlegm."

Finally, in a rare nod to the medical profession, he says: "There is a syrup made of Horehound to be had at the apothecaries, very good for old coughs, to rid phlegm; as also to void cold rheums from the lungs of old folks, and for those that are asthmatic or short-winded."

Gerard, Parkinson, and Culpeper thought of this medicinal as a cooling herb, or at least used it to treat many hot, toxic conditions. The exception to this is when Culpeper says, "to void cold rheums from the lungs of old folks." However, what he called "cold" is likely to have been manifesting as a heat condition, as we would describe it in Chinese medicine. He considered ALL phlegm to be cold and moist (no matter how thick or thin it was) owing to its apparent congealed nature ("cold congeals, heat thins" was a common axiom of the time). He also considered pus to be a type of phlegm, as did Chinese doctors of that period. Although Culpeper considered phlegm to be cold in nature, it is very likely that the above description is of a heat condition, judging by symptomology such as "foul ulcers," "running and creeping sores," etc. Furthermore, if the phlegm was thick (more congealed), this would have been a sign of cold rather than heat, according to the energetics of Culpeper's time. This is the opposite of how we generally view congealed phlegm in Chinese medicine, since it is heat that congeals phlegm. Although these authors treat this medicinal as "hot", this classification is entirely based on their understanding of health and disease in the body. It is important to note that although I disagree with this classification of Horehound as cold, my view is based on the Chinese medicine idea of health and disease in the body. Each viewpoint has classified the use of Horehound to treat the opposite manifestation of phlegm; authors of the late Middle Ages say phlegm is cold, therefore treat it with hot medicinals, while Chinese medicine says phlegm (here we are talking about congealed phlegm that is obviously associated with heat patterns) is hot, therefore treat it with cold herbs.

This and other species figure prominently in the literature. There is promising research to support the traditional use of this medicinal as an external application. Horehound out–performed Walnut (see Black Walnut monograph) at both preventing formation and adherence of biofilms of Methicillin–resistant *Staphylococcus aureus* in both low and high concentrations.[3] This study used alcoholic extracts made with denatured alcohol (which is toxic to humans), but concentrations of the extract were only 1:10 (standard tinctures are usually 1:5, often more concentrated). Although the use of denatured alcohol might affect the clinical results as compared to ethanol, the more concentrated preparations used by herbalists might be even more effective. Futhermore, many herbalists use this medicinal as a fresh plant tincture, which is also likely to improve outcomes due to increased amount of essential oils present in fresh, versus dried, material.

1. de Souza, M.M, et al., (1998). Analgesic profile of hydroalcoholic extract obtained from *Marrubium vulgare*. *Phytomedicine*. 5(2): pp. 103–107.
2. Schlemper, V. et al., (1996). Antispasmodic effects of hydroalcoholic extract of *Marrubium vulgare* on isolated tissues. *Phytomedicine*. 3(2): pp. 211–216.
3. Quave, Cassandra L. et al., (2008). Effects of extracts from Italian medicinal plants on planktonic growth, biofilm formation and adherence of methicillin–resistant *Staphylococcus aureus*. *Journal of Ethnopharmacology*. 118(3): pp. 418–428.

Wild Cherry Bark

Prunus virginiana L., and others
Rosaceae
Pruni virginianae cortex
Favor and Qi: acrid, bitter, cool
Channels entered: lung, stomach
Actions: antitussive, antispasmodic, sedative

Functions & Indications:

Stops cough and settles panting. Wild Cherry bark is commonly used for all types of coughing and panting—replete and vacuous, acute and chronic, as well as for adults and children—but is particularly good for spasmodic coughs associated with heat. Although this medicinal is cool it can be added to any formula to treat coughing and/or panting. However, this medicinal excels in heat patterns, particularly in vacuity heat conditions. Wild Cherry bark is acrid, bitter, and cool, and with cool acridity it moves qi and assists with impaired diffusion and depuration of the lung qi. Wild Cherry bark clears heat and unblocks qi stagnation. It moves downward with cool bitterness, again assisting the lung, but in this case it is more closely related to its depurative downbearing function.

Harmonizes the middle, and courses and downbears qi. Wild Cherry bark is used for retching, belching, swallowing of upflowing acid, distention and pain in the stomach duct, with a red tongue, and a string-like pulse. Wild Cherry bark treats liver invading the middle, but its action is stronger on the spleen/stomach than the liver. Wild Cherry bark is bitter and acrid, effectively downbearing counterflow qi in the middle with bitterness, and moving stagnant qi. It works as an assistant to medicinals such as Horehound, or formulas such as *Sì Nì Sǎn* or *Chái Hú Shū Gān Sǎn*. In small doses, it is both appropriate and easy (it doesn't taste nasty!) for children.

Cautions:

Although this medicinal is very safe, large doses could cause stupor in small children, animals, and possibly adults.

Dosage and Preparation:

This medicinal is best prepared as a cold infusion (2–6g). If used in a decoction (4–10g), it must be added at the end. Tincture is useful (1–3ml), but the cold infusion is the superior product.

Major Combinations:

Combine with Mullein and *tiānhuāfěn* for dry, spasmodic cough with difficult expectoration, or expectoration of thick phlegm.

Combine with *zhǐshí* and *guālóupí* for spasmodic cough with chest pain and fullness.

Combine with *mùxiāng* and *huánglián* for retching and swallowing of upflowing stomach acid.

Commentary:

Prunus is a member of the Rosaceae "Rose" family and is an extremely valuable genus to humans for its food, ornamental value, timber, and medicine, and likewise for a multitude of animals and birds for food and protection. The foods produced by this genus are known as "stone fruits" and include cherries, apricots, nectarines, plums, and almonds. The cherry tree (*Prunus serotina*) is prized for it hard, attractive, deep reddish–colored wood, and has been used for furniture making and other applications for centuries. Ornamental species and their varieties generally flower before the leaves emerge, often drawing large crowds at city parks throughout China, Korea, and Japan. The exact number of species is unclear, but sources place the number from 30 to 450, with a large number of cultivars. *P. virginiana*, the species of this monograph, is native to the eastern part of North America and is known as Choke Cherry. It is widely cultivated for its fruit and is one of the most common small trees or shrubs within its native habitat.[1] Unfortunately, a disease known as X-disease is causing enough economic damage to draw the attention of bioengineers, who are now creating genetically modified varieties of this species.[2] How this will affect the native species is unknown, and we can only hope that the results will not be permanently damaging.

The well-known Chinese medicinal *xìngrén* is closely related to Wild Cherry bark, and is produced from the common apricot kernel (*P. armeniaca*) or several closely related species in the sub-genus *Armeniaca*. These two genera (*Prunus* and *Armeniaca*) are very closely related and there has been much "lumping and splitting" of the two genera for many years. The origin of Apricot is controversial, with many scholars placing it in Armenia (hence the species name "armeniaca") while others argue that it originated in China. This plant has been grown in China for centuries, with references going back to at least the time of Zhuāngzǐ in the 4th Century BCE, and the medicinal appearing the *Bēn Cǎo Jīng*.

The primary connection between the species in this monograph and xìngrén, other than botanical, is the presence of compounds known as cyanogenic glycosides. These compounds are present in the kernel, bark, and leaves of many species of *Prunus*, and these parts of the plant have been used in medicine around the world for all of written history, and likely much longer. They can be fatal in large doses, but are perfectly safe when used in reasonable medicinal dosages. Their sweet almond smell likely attracted humans, and the development of their use as medicinal agents followed.

Cook (1869) states: "It is chiefly valued for the soothing influence which accompanies its tonic action; for while it gently improves appetite, digestion, and the general strength, it quiets nervous irritability and arterial excitement." He also says that it is good for chronic gastritis with indigestion, irritable nervousness, "and will be received by the stomach when most other tonics are objectionable, and improve the strength without inducing feverishness." His observation closely resembles what Chinese medicine classifies as Wood–Earth disharmony. In referencing Wild Cherry bark's action on the lungs, he states "The lungs are much acted on by it; and it is a superior article for irritable coughs, whether acute or chronic." When Cook uses the term "irritable cough" in other places in his text, he mentions either dryness or an inflammatory disease, or both. So, it seems that an irritable cough is a heat condition, likely of a chronic nature.

Scudder (1898) wrote "used in advantage in cases of dyspepsia; especially when connected with an irritable state of the stomach, or when attended with general irritability of the nervous system, over which it exerts a manifestly sedative influence." Scudder is discussing this medicinal's ability to harmonize the stomach and downbear qi. In the last part, he mentions that it has a sedative effect on the nervous system, a use not often employed by modern herbalists. However, this may be a partial physiological explanation for how this medicinal works to downbear qi.

Felter and Llody (1905) state "Its chief property is its power of relieving irritation of the mucous surfaces, making it an admirable remedy in many *gastro-intestinal, pulmonic,* and *urinary troubles.* Like lycopus [Bugleweed], it lessens vascular excitement, though it does not control hemorrhages like that agent. It is best adapted to chronic troubles." They also say "[It is specific for] rapid, weak, circulation; continual irritative cough, with profuse muco-purulent expectoration; cardiac palpitation, from debility; dyspnea; loss of appetite; and cardiac pain." This montage of symptoms relates strongly to what is described in this monograph. The authors are describing heat in most of the patterns they trace, and there is even a hint of heat from vacuity in phrases like, "rapid, weak, circulation [pulse]", which we can safely assume is yin vacuity, although it may also be qi vacuity heat.

Modern literature on this medicinal is scant, but ethnobotanical literature is overflowing with references. Nearly every native society within its range in North America used this plant. There are 337 references in Moerman's database (see bibliography) and while there are reported uses for everything from strengthening the hair to helping nursing mothers, the vast majority of the reports are either for gastrointestinal disorders or pulmonary complaints. It appears to be safe for both adults and children alike.

Translation of Available Source Material:

There are two native species of *Prunus* used in China, *P. salicina*, *yángméihérén* (楊梅核仁) and *P. simonii, jīxuělǐ* (雞血李). Not surprisingly both species are used in a similar way to Wild Cherry bark. *P. salicina* is found primarily in the north and northwestern part of the country (although it is found in most provinces) and is used in a number of different preparations; the root, root bark, stem, leaf, flower, and seed are all used. Because the functions and indications are similar for all the parts, I only provide the translation for the root bark. The root bark is called *lǐgēnpí* (李根皮) and the *Grand Dictionary of Chinese Medicinals* (2009) says that it is bitter, salty, and cold. It enters the liver channel. Its functions are to clear heat, downbear qi, and resolve toxin. It is used to treat qi counterflow running piglet,* damp-heat dysentery, red and white vaginal discharge, diabetes, foot qi, cinnabar toxin, and sores. It is used in 3–9g dosages in decoction, and also externally. The other species, *P. simonii* is reported in the *Grand Dictionary of Chinese Medicinals* (2009) to be bitter and cold. Its functions are to clear heat and eliminate vexation, disinhibit water and free strangury, and stop bleeding and dissipate stasis. It is used to treat diabetes, heart vexation, white turbidity, water swelling, spitting blood, flooding and leaking [menstrual], menstrual block, and blunt force trauma.

*Running piglet is a traditional disease name originating in the *Jīn Guì Yào Lüè*, which Wiseman & Ye (1998) define as "A disease characterized by a sensation of upsurge from the lower abdomen to the chest and throat, accompanied by gripping abdominal pain, oppression in the chest, rapid breathing, dizziness, heart palpitation, and heart vexation." The term sounds strange in both English and Chinese, but the characters do not offer much wriggle room for a different translation. The characterization is that the sensation is similar to a feeling as if there were very small pigs running up from your abdomen to your chest. Strange as it may sound, you can imagine if that happened, you might exhibit similar symptomology.

1. Dai, Wenhao, et al., (2004). Plant Regeneration of Chokecherry (*Prunus viginiana* L.) from *in vitro* Leaf Tissues. *Journal of Environmental Horticulture.* 22(4): pp. 225–228.
2. ibid

Wild Lettuce

Lactuca virosa L. and others
Asteraceae
Lactucae herba
Favor and Qi: bitter, cool
Channels entered: lung, stomach
Actions: anodyne, antitussive

Functions & Indications:

Downbears lung qi, clears lung heat, and stops cough. Wild Lettuce is used for spasmodic coughing due to replete heat in the lungs, especially when heat has dried yin fluids. This medicinal is also frequently employed for cough at night with difficulty sleeping, especially in children. Although this medicinal can be used in phlegmatic conditions, it is probably best for coughs that are dry or mostly dry. Wild Lettuce is bitter and cool; with bitterness, it downbears, and with coolness, it clears lung heat.

Clears stomach and intestinal heat, and stops pain. Wild Lettuce is used for replete heat in the stomach and intestines with cramping pain. This is especially good for children who, due to improperly regulated food intake, often have replete heat in the stomach and intestines associated with food stagnation. This is not a strong pain relieving substance, yet it is very effective within its reaches as a therapeutic agent.

Cautions:

This herb should be used with caution for those with cold in the middle, although it is only used for a short time and, therefore, unlikely to cause any harm.

Dosage and Preparation:

Fresh plant tincture with 10% vinegar 2–4 ml, dry plant tincture with 10% vinegar 3–6 ml, 3–6g decoction or infusion

Major Combinations:

Combine with Grindelia for stubborn spasmodic cough. Add Lobelia for intense spasmodic coughing that does not yield to therapy.

Combine with Catnip for spasmodic cough in young children. Add Lemon Balm for coughs that are keeping a child awake.

Combine with Chamomile and Lemon Balm for stomach pain in children due to overeating. This combination is also effective for children with nighttime crying and difficulty sleeping due to over-indulgence in sweet and/or oily foods.

Commentary:

Wild Lettuce is a member of the *Lactuca* genus of the Asteraceae "Sunflower" family. The genus has around 70 species, which are found throughout most of the northern temperate areas of the world. China and North America have 12 and 10 species respectively, while the remainder of the genus is found throughout Central America (including Mexico), Europe, West Asia, and northern Africa.

I have classified this medicinal as "cool", and although I can't go so far as to say it is cold, it might be better understood as "very cool" or "slightly cold," but this is not a common designation and so I have left the main heading as "cool." As I noted earlier in the book, these designations are somewhat arbitrary, and largely the opinion of any author.

Although this monograph is about Wild Lettuce, the domesticated versions most likely derive from one or more of the wild species that are still used in medicine. The cultivation of lettuce is thought to have originated in the Kurdistan–Mesopotamia area, then migrated to Egypt, where it is depicted in paintings found in temples and tombs from as early as 2500 BCE.[1] The common lettuce of today, of which there are many varieties, are all derived from *L. serriola*, and/or perhaps another species.[2] In Asia, lettuce is primarily grown for its edible stem rather than its leaves, as is most common throughout the rest of the world. The leaves are largely discarded and the stem is peeled and prepared in a wide variety of both hot and cold dishes.

There are many species of Wild Lettuce, and it is unclear whether there is a significant difference within the genus in regards to their medicinal quality. The domesticated species has been bred to reduce the bitterness and, thus, the amount of latex or sap in the plant, which is the primary medicinal portion, and from where it derives its bitter flavor. The bitter quality of the plant is what makes it medicinal, therefore the domesticated varieties are not good for medicine.

Based on the literature, one can see that there is a lot of variation in the usage of this plant from region to region, which, as noted above, may be due to differences within the genus. Most people use the plant for some sort of pain, and they all seem to consider it a cooling medicinal. How it was applied varies somewhat, due to cultural context within each region. It is also possible that there is enough difference between species to warrant some differences in usage.

Gerard (1597) calls the medicinal cold and moist, but not in an extreme degree. In his discussion he mentions six different kinds of lettuce, noting that some are cultivated while others are wild, yet does not distinguish between the two in his medicinal uses. It is likely that even the garden varieties of that time were quite bitter. He says: "Lettuce cools a hot stomach, called heart burning; and helps it when it is troubled with choler; it quenches thirst, causes sleep, makes plenty of milk in nurses, who through heat and dryness do grow barraine and dry of milk; for it breeds milk by tempering the dryness and heat. But in bodies that be naturally cold, it does not engender milk at all, but is rather an hinderance thereunto." I have included this entire quote primarily to show Gerard's thinking with respect to hot and cold, and how medicinals and the bodies' reaction to them were viewed in late 16th Century England. Gerard states that a cold medicinal will cool heat, but also that, if given to a person who is cold, it will have the opposite effect, actually damaging the person's ability to perform otherwise normal functions.

Parkinson (1640) separates the wild from the garden lettuces, telling us that the wild is more bitter. Explaining the connection between the bitterness and coldness of the medicinal, he states: "The Wild Lettuce is near the same property of cooling that the Garden kind is, although the bitterness therein makes it more opening, but not heating even as it is in Succary, Poppy, Opium and the like, whose bitterness doth rather open a way for the qualities to work the better, no cold quality being powerful of it felt and therefore...it is more available to procure sleep than the garden kind."

Culpeper (1653) says that lettuce both cools and moistens, and "it helpeth to lossen the belly; it helpeth digestion, quencheth thirst, increaseth milk in nurses, easeth griping pains in the stomach and bowels that come of choler." He also says, "the use of Lettuce is chiefly forbidden to those that are short–winded, or have any imperfections of the lungs, or spit blood." This last statement suggests that this medicinal should only be used for replete conditions. Although he is not specific about the cause of the spitting of blood, it is likely that he is referring to "consumption" (i.e., tuberculosis), which is generally considered to be a constitutional vacuity with replete pathogenic factors such as phlegm and heat. Also, the entirety of the monograph suggests that this caution refers to vacuity causes, considering that he said lettuce is cooling and moistening. I am not entirely sure why it would be contraindicated for "spitting blood," except in cases of vacuity where cooling medicinals need to be used more carefully.

Salmon (1710) writes that garden lettuce is "cold and moist in the second degree: anodyne, digestive, emollient, relaxive, and galectoguge . . . It allays inflammations, gives ease in the strangury, induces sleep, and represses bodily lust." In his writings on Wild Lettuce he says;

> "Wild Lettuce is cold in the end of the second degree, and moist in the end of the first. It has nearly the same properties of cooling, which the Garden Kind has; but the bitterness of this makes it the more aperitive [opening obstructions of the visera]; and yet it is more somniferous than the mature sorts, and comes up, as it is thought by some, almost to the degree of Opium; but this opinion I can never assent to, my experience having proved the contrary."

Much of what Salmon says is similar to what Culpeper wrote half a century earlier, but it is interesting to note that Salmon calls this herb an "aperitive," which he defines as "a medicinal that opens obstructions of the viscera." However, he also states that aperitives are "all hot at least in the second degree, for the most part in the third, and many times in the forth." Yet Salmon classifies Garden Lettuce as cold in the second degree and Wild Lettuce as cold "at the end of the second degree." This nature designation of cooling is contrary to his statement of aperitives in general and is especially interesting since he made such an absolute statement on the nature of this class of medicinals. Contrarily, Culpeper seems to consider this more of a relaxing medicine, which helps to explain some of its functions, and while Salmon also calls it a "relaxive," he also (likely due to its bitterness) sees it as an "aperitive." Salmon calls this medicinal "somniferous," but is quick to note that it is not as strong as Opium. I have heard some suggest that, while not as strong, Wild Lettuce can be used similarly to Opium. This may be true to a certain extent, but one must remember that there are no opiates in Wild Lettuce and the action of Wild

Lettuce with regard to relieving pain or inducing sleep is but a very small fraction of the strength of Opium, so much so that it is perfectly safe to administer to children.

Translation of Available Source Material:

The monograph on Wild Lettuce was mostly written for the first edition, and is now being finished. I now have much more access to Chinese literature, and can present several species of Wild Lettuce from these sources. My opinion differs from the source literature primarily in terms of indications, rather than in method of use. This could be due to differences in cultural context, chemical composition of the species, growing conditions, or the types of diseases seen currently versus those in the past.

L. sativa is first mentioned in the *Dietary Therapy Materia Medica* (8th Century), but only as a food, in combination with other species used in cooking. The *Grand Dictionary of Chinese Medicinals* (2009) says it is bitter, sweet, and cool, and enters the stomach and small intestine channels. It disinhibits urine, frees breast milk, and clears heat and resolves toxin. It is used to treat inhibited urination, blood in the urine, breast milk not free-flowing, insect and snake bites, and toxic swelling associated with chigger bites. It is used in 30-60g dosages in decoction and applied externally (pound and apply). It is contraindicated in spleen/stomach vacuity weakness.

L. raddeana Maxim. *shānkǔcài* (山苦菜) was first mentioned in the *Guì Zhōu Materia Medica*, a modern regional materia medica. This species is common throughout Eastern Asia and is listed in the *Flora of China* as *máomàichìguǒjú* (毛脉翅果菊). This plant is not a well-established plant in Chinese medicine, although it has probably been used in the folk tradition. There are no entries available about its qi or nature, nor the channels entered. The *Grand Dictionary of Chinese Medicinals* says the herb clears heat and resolves toxin, dispels wind and eliminate dampness and is used to treat wind-damp impediment pain, heat-stroke with abdominal pain, sores, boils and swellings, and snake bites. Use 15-30g in decoction, or 1.5-3ml tincture. For external use, the leaf is made into a paste or liniment.

L. formosana Maxim. *kǔdīng* (苦丁) was first found in the *Annals of Sichuan Chinese Medicinals* (1960), where it was listed as cold, bitter, and non-toxic, and the seed is said to regulate the channels. The *Grand*

Dictionary of Chinese Medicinals (2009) says it is bitter and cold, clears heat and resolves toxin, dispels wind–dampness, and quickens the blood. It is used to treat cinnabar welling–abscess and swelling, breast pain, intestinal sores, swelling and pain in the throat, boils, snake bites, painful wind-dampness impediment, and knocks and falls. Either the root or the whole plant is used. It is used internally in 15–30g doses (or 45–90g when used fresh), and it is prepared as a tincture. It can also be applied externally, either pounded or boiled first.

L. indica L. *shānwōjù* (山萵苣) was first listed in *Materia Medica to Help Relieve Famine* (1406), where it is said to be slightly bitter. The *Grand Dictionary of Chinese Medicinals* (2009) says it is bitter and cold. It clears heat and resolves toxin, quickens the blood and stops bleeding. It is used for throat swelling and pain, intestinal sores, cervical inflammation, postpartum blood stasis and pain, flooding and spotting, swollen and toxic sores and boils, warts and tumors, and bleeding hemorrhoids. It is used in 9–15g dosages in decoction, or pounded and applied externally.

L. tatarica C.A. Mey. *kǔǎo* (苦芺) was first listed in *Collected Commentaries of the Classic of Materia Medica* (5th Century). The *Grand Dictionary of Chinese Medicinals* (2009) says it is bitter and slightly cold, clears heat and resolves toxin, cools the blood and stops bleeding. It is used for summerheat with vexation and oppression, cinnabar toxin, swollen sores, hemorrhoids, external bleeding due to injury, and knocks and fall. It is used in 15–30g dosages in decoction, or chewed fresh. Externally, it is pounded and applied, or boiled and then applied.

1. de Vries, I.M. Origin and Domestication of *Lactuca sativa* L. *Genetic Resources and Crop Evolution* 44(2) pp. 165–174, 1997.
2. Lindqvist, K. 1960. On the Cultivation of Lettuce, *Hereditas* 46 pp 319–350.

Eucalyptus

Eucalyptus globulus Labill.
Myrtaceae
Eucalypti folium seu oleum
Favor and Qi: acrid, bitter, aromatic, cool
Channels entered: lung, stomach, spleen, liver*
Actions: antibacterial, antiviral, antiparasitic, anti–inflammatory

Functions & Indications:

Courses the exterior, expels wind, and opens the orifice of the nose. Eucalyptus is used for external wind invasion patterns, particularly when wind combines with a warm/heat pathogen with symptoms of sinus congestion, headache, facial pain due to congestion, and painful itchy eyes. This medicinal is cool, acrid, and light so it can penetrate the orifices of the nose and open them, clearing heat and loosening lodged phlegm, thus allowing for easy expulsion. The combination of acridity and bitterness courses the exterior and expels wind and, combined with its cool nature, makes it very well suited for wind–warmth, warm pestilence, and other contagious external diseases that manifest in the upper burner.

Courses wind and resolves the exterior. Eucalyptus is used for external wind invasions with symptoms of high fever with headache, as well as lung heat with cough. Also used for pain due to wind and dampness, and whooping cough. Eucalyptus is an acrid, bitter, and aromatic herb with a cooling nature. With cool acridity, it courses wind and resolves the exterior, opening the pores and forcing the pathogen out from whence it came; with cool bitterness, it clears heat and reduces fever.

Clears heat and resolves toxin. Eucalyptus is used for damp–heat toxin with symptoms of diarrhea and dysentery, pain and distension in the stomach duct and abdomen, swollen welling-abscess toxin, eczema with scab and lichen, and malaria. Eucalyptus is cool in nature, thus it clears heat and can resolve toxin. Damp–heat toxin is often difficult to treat and requires a combination of cool/cold medicinals with bitter and acrid medicinals to drain dampness and resolve toxin, while moving qi to restore a poorly functioning qi dynamic. Eucalyptus does this, and its aroma aromatically transforms dampness and relieves pain.

Kills parasites and stops itching for ancylostonmiasis and filariasis. This is primarily for external application and is a traditional use of the herb and its essential oil.

Cautions:

Use caution for those with yin vacuity, dryness patterns.

Dosage and Preparation:

Decoction (added at the end) or simple infusion 6–10g. It can also be ground to a powder and taken in 1g dosages up to 4 times a day. Externally, it can be applied in several ways, but I consider the essential oil to be the best way to employ this medicinal externally. The essential oil is relatively safe and can be used as a steam, inhalant, or directly on the skin with a carrier oil. The essential oil can also be used internally, but this requires special training.

Major Combinations:

Combine with Yerba Mansa, Ambrosia, and *huángqín* for sinus congestion with purulent yellow/green phlegm that is difficult to discharge. This combination also can be added to formulas like *Bí Yán Piàn* and *Cāng'ěr Zǐ Sān*.

Combine with *báizhì*, *huángqín*, and Goldenrod for thick yellow congested phlegm in the sinuses with facial pain.

Commentary:

Eucalyptus is a genus of about 700 species within the Mytaceae family that is native to Australia and surrounding island nations. There are only nine species of Eucalyptus that do not grow in Australia, and an additional six that grow both within and outside of Australia. This means that, of the 700 species of Eucalyptus, 685 are endemic to Australia, or nearly 98%, an exceptional feature for such a large genus.

The leaves are aromatic and have been used in medicine by Australian native peoples for probably as long as people have been there. Unfortunately, there is no written record of these uses, so we have little knowledge of traditional uses beyond what has been established since the period of colonization. However, since that time, Eucalyptus has found a solid place in medicine, and its essential oil is one of the most famously used on the planet (although this may be, at least in part, due to its relatively inexpensive price tag). Eucalyptus trees are the most common plantation tree around the world, now found on every continent.

The essential oil is what is primarily used in medicine and, although the leaves can be used, the essential oil is what I have the most experience using. That said, my early days as an herbalist were in Santa Cruz, California where Eucalyptus is found abundantly, I have used both the leaves (as tea) and the tincture. I find the leaf prepared as a tea is tolerated by most people, even children, although others find it rather offensive. This medicinal is cool, acrid, and light. The *Treaties on Warm Heat* (1746) states, "The lung governs qi, it is connected to the skin and body hair, that's why it is said to be on the exterior. [When the pathogen is] at the exterior first use acrid, cool, light medicinals." Eucalypus is acrid, cool, and light and is an excellent medicinal for treating the initial invasion of warm–heat pathogens.

The aroma, when used for upper burner conditions, also makes a profitable steam that can be breathed in when cooking the tea for an extra benefit, or primer, to ingesting the tea. By doing this, the phlegm of the sinuses and lungs can be loosened to some degree, which improves the results from drinking the tea. As a pure steam using the essential oil alone, this is an exceptional remedy for exceedingly difficult cases of sinus congestion. For this, 1–3 drops of essential oil can be added to a small pot of boiled water; a towel is draped over the person's head to help keep the steam focused, and the Eucalyptus oil steam is breathed in. As the steam passes through the nasal cavities, the congestion begins to loosen, and after a few minutes, the congestion is dramatically reduced. This is mostly a temporary effect, but nevertheless offers the patient some relief, and helps the performance of the internal application of herbs. A note of caution when doing a steam: inhaling steam, especially with essential oils can cause a choking sensation, burning of the sinuses and/or throat, and tearing eyes. To avoid these, start by only inhaling a very gentle short breath. Let your breathing passages get accustomed to the heat of the steam and the oil. Breathing will become slightly easier as the person gets used to it, and the sinuses will start to open. There is no need to force this process, go slowly and get as much as possible without causing these problems. If they occur, stop and try again once they disappear. None of these are serious, but if one inhales a large amount of the essential oils directly into the lungs, it could cause more serious problems. DO NOT exceed the recommended dosage.

The constituent eucalyptol, taken from the essential oil, is found in a wide range of external products, from creams to lip balms and mouth washes. It is a primary ingredient in the famous Vicks Vapor Rub that is still produced today with a combination of plant essential oil constituents, such as eucalyptol, thymol, and menthol, in a petroleum jelly base.

Translation of Available Source Material:

The information available in Chinese on this medicinal is based on Western use and does not show any clear Chinese Medicine thought process, so I have not included it here.

*The designations in sections marked in this monograph come from the *Grand Dictionary of Chinese Medicinals* (2009).

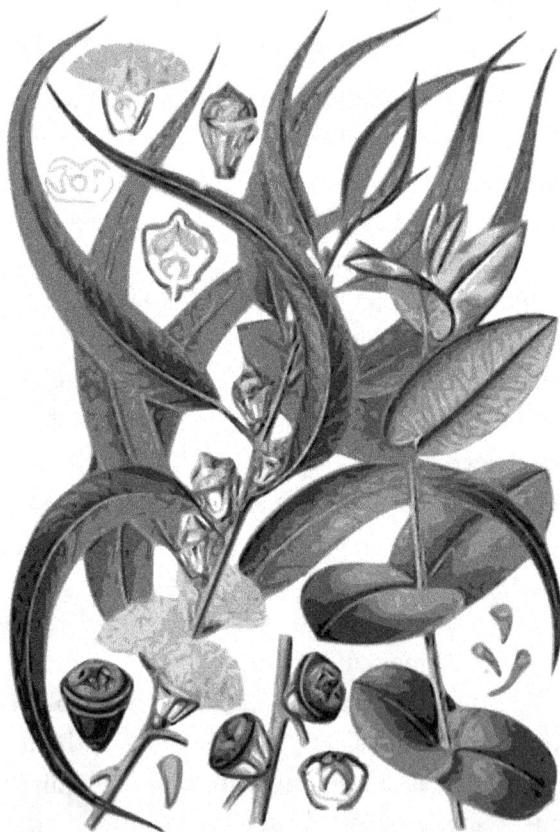

Eucalyptus Cross Leaflets

Medicinal	Nature	Flavor	Channels	Functions	Indications
Mullein Leaf	cool	bitter, slightly acrid	lung, triple burner, kidney	Clears heat, transforms phlegm, & stops cough; Clears heat & promotes urination; Clears vacuity heat, nourishes fluids, & transforms phlegm; Clears heat, transforms toxin, reduces swelling, & stops pain	phlegm-heat in the lungs with yellow or green phlegm and coughing; heat strangury; scrophula; heat-toxin swellings such as sores (bed-sores), ulcerations, and other hot-swellings
Horehound	slightly cold	bitter, acrid	lung, liver	Transforms phlegm, clears heat, downbears qi, and stops cough	phlegm-heat congesting the lung
Wild Cherry Bark	cool	acrid, bitter	lung, stomach	Stops cough and settles panting; Harmonizes the stomach and downbears qi	coughing and panting; retching, belching, swallowing of upflowing acid, distention in the stomach duct, with a pale tongue and white coat; retching, belching, swallowing of upflowing acid, distention in the stomach duct
Wild Lettuce	cool	bitter	lung, stomach	Downbears lung qi, clears lung heat and stops cough; Clears stomach and intestinal heat and stops pain	spasmodic coughing, difficulty sleeping due to cough; stomach and intestinal cramping

Medicinal	Nature	Flavor	Channels	Functions	Indications
Eucalyptus	cool	acrid, bitter, aromatic	lung, stomach, spleen, liver	Courses wind and resolves the exterior; Courses the exterior, expels wind, and opens the orifice of the nose; Clears heat and resolve toxin for damp-heat toxin; Kills parasites and stops itching	Headache, cough; sinus congestion, headache, facial pain due to congestion, and painful itchy eyes; diarrhea and dysentery, pain and distension in the stomach duct and abdomen, swollen welling-abscess toxin, eczema with scab and lichen, and malaria; ancylostonmiasis and filariasis

理
氣
藥

Rectify Qi Medicinals

The rectifying qi category of medicinals is, perhaps, one of the most unique categories in the Chinese materia medica. This category is used to course and rectify the qi for patterns of qi stagnation and qi reversal (qi going in a direction other than its normal healthy flow). Although many of the medicinals in this category are warm in nature, there are also many cooling medicinals. In this materia medica Wild Yam is the sole cooling medicinal. Because acrid flavor tends to move, most medicinals found in this category are acrid in nature; in this materia medica they are all acrid.

When qi stagnates pain arises, so many of the medicinals in this category are used to relieve pain. Medicinals that have functions such as regulate qi and strengthen the spleen, course the liver and resolve constraint, regulate qi and loosen the chest, and break qi and disperse binding.

There are three primary divisions, treating a broad range of patterns within this large and important category. The first, spleen/stomach qi stagnation is very common and well-known in other systems of botanical medicine and are similar to carminatives in Western herbal medicine. These medicinals treat symptoms such as fullness in the abdomen, sour belching, vomiting, and irregular bowel movements. This group is represented in this materia medica by European Angelica and Dill Seed. The second pattern is liver constraint qi stagnation. Common symptoms associated with this pattern include abdominal and rib-side pain, emotional constraint without happiness, irregular menses, breast distention and pain, and lumps and bindings. European Angelica, Wild Yam, and Beth Root represent much of this sub-category in this materia medica. The third pattern is lung congestion qi stagnation. Common symptoms associated with this pattern are impeded breathing, chest oppression and chest pain, and coughing and panting. Wild Yam and European Angelica both address symptoms within this sub-category.

European Angelica

Angelica archangelica L.

Apiaceae

Angelicae Archangelicae radix

Favor and Qi: acrid, bitter, warm

Channels entered: stomach, spleen, liver

Actions: carminative, diaphoretic, anodyne

Functions & Indications:

Moves qi, warms the middle, and opens the stomach. European Angelica
is used for abdominal pain with accumulation of cold and damp, with
associated qi stagnation. This pattern is often associated with a
disharmony between the liver and spleen or stomach. European
Angelica is an important medicinal in the treatment of cold and
dampness (and phlegm) in the middle and lower burners. The spleen
and stomach can be damaged by inappropriate eating of cold and damp
foods. On the other hand, the spleen and stomach can become weak,
causing accumulation of cold and dampness. European Angelica is
warm, acrid, and bitter. With warm acridity, it effectively treats cold
stagnation by both warming and dispersing, and with warm bitterness,
it effectively drains. When there is concurrent spleen/stomach qi
vacuity, prepare this medicinal prior to use by stir-frying in honey.

Resolves liver constraint and stops pain. European Angelica is used for
constraint patterns with pain in the rib-sides and lesser abdomen due
to constraint of liver qi. This medicinal has a long history of use for
menstrual disorders (similar to *dāngguī*). However, it moves qi much
more strongly than blood. It can be added to formulas to help resolve
menstrual pain with a combination of qi stagnation and blood stasis,
but should be combined with medicinals which more strongly move the
blood. This medicinal is warm and acrid, moves qi and disperses
stagnation, and its bitterness helps to drain accumulation.

Warms the lungs and transforms phlegm-cold. European Angelica is
used for abundant clear or white phlegm. When cold and dampness
accumulate in the middle and transform into phlegm, the lungs will
become the storage house for the phlegm. European Angelica's warm
and acrid nature warms the spleen and stomach to stop phlegm

production at the source. It also effectively warms the lungs. With acridity, it disperses, and with bitterness, it drains. The combination of warmth, acridity, and bitterness, accompanied by its action on both the spleen/stomach and the lungs, makes this medicinal an effective herb for resolving phlegm–cold in the lung.

Courses the channels, expels wind, and dispels cold and damp. European Angelica is used for the treatment of wind–cold–damp impediment pain with evils lodged in the channels. This medicinal can also be used for wind entering the *tàiyáng* channels in acute illness where wind can be combined with cold, damp, or even heat. With warm acridity, European Angelica is penetrating and effectively courses and frees the channels, helping to restore the flow of qi and blood, thus relieving pain. This warm acridity also effectively expels wind and eliminates cold and damp from the body. Because of this, it can also be used for acute external attacks of wind–cold. This herb can also be used to treat heat conditions when combined with the appropriate medicinals.

Cautions:
European Angelica is warm and acrid and should be used with caution with those with yin vacuity, especially stomach yin vacuity.

Dosage and Preparation:
Decoction 3–9g, dry plant tincture 1–3ml, fresh plant tincture 0.5–2ml

Major Combinations:
Combine with Elecampane for accumulation of cold and dampness in the middle and upper burner, especially where dampness is the predominant factor. This combination is also good for phlegm accumulation in either the lung or intestine. In this *duìyào* combination, when treating phlegm in the lung, the Elecampane is used raw while the Angelica is honey stir-fried. When using this *duìyào* for digestive problems, both medicinals are honey stir-fried in order to warm and dry, while also harmonizing the spleen and stomach. However, if a strong qi moving action is desired, the raw/unprepared European Angelica can be used.

Combine with *chuānxiōng* for any type of blood stasis that has either been caused by qi stagnation or has led to qi stagnation. While *chuānxiōng* is considered a very important medicinal for quickening the blood, it is said to act on the qi within the blood. Likewise, European Angelica does the same thing, but has a much stronger effect on the qi dynamic while having a weaker effect on the blood. The combination of the two medicines is an important *duìyào* for liver constraint patterns without heat. If treating heat patterns, this combination must be combined with heat-clearing herbs such as *shānzhīzǐ*.

Add to *Chái Hú Shū Gān Sǎn* to strengthen the effects of the formula's principal function to rectify qi function, while assisting *chuānxiōng* to move the qi within the blood. Because of its action on the stomach, it will also strengthen the effect of *chénpí* in rectifying qi and opening the stomach.

Combine honey mixed-fried European Angelica with *Sì Jūn Zǐ Tāng* for spleen vacuity leading to accumulation of phlegm-dampness, especially when there is a liver-spleen disharmony.

Commentary:

European Angelica, also known as Garden Angelica, is a member of the genus *Angelica*, which is made up of over 90 species (approximately half are found in China), and is part of the Apiaceae (Parsley) family. This is a plant that I did not immediately love. When I first started studying and practicing, I was living in Northern California and there were a number of species of *Angelica* both in the coastal area and in the Sierra Nevada that I was learning to use (not to mention several Chinese species). But as time passed, I found this plant to have an important place in the materia medica. While the genus of *Angelica* is widely known for its actions on the blood, (as is this species), I believe that *A. archangelica* has a much stronger action on the qi dynamic.

The genus has some 60 to 90 species, depending on the source consulted. There is a lot of ambiguity in the botanical literature, and some species from closely related genera may move to or away from the *Angelica* genus once a complete overhaul of the botany is performed. The center for the genus is in China, with roughly 32 endemic species and ~45 present. North America has 22 native species with all but 3 found in the West, and one, *A. lucida*, which is a bi-coastal species. In an interesting note on the biogeography of the genus in North America, there is a complete absence of the genus throughout the plains of both Canada and the United States.

European Angelica is especially useful when there is a disharmony between the liver and spleen, as well as liver and stomach disharmony. European Angelica courses the liver with acrid warmth and acts on the spleen with warmth to assist its transformative functions, while using warm–acridity to dry any dampness accumulated from untransformed fluids. Likewise, in liver–stomach disharmony it has the same action on the liver, utilizing acridity to open, and bitterness to help downbear stomach counterflow caused by the disharmony between the liver and stomach.

Furthermore, this medicinal has a strong action to resolve dampness and transform phlegm. This is important because dampness and phlegm are two common results of qi stagnation. As noted above, if the liver qi becomes constrained, this will often cause a disharmony between it and the stomach or spleen. This will result in poor functioning of the either the spleen, stomach, or both, which can (especially in the case of the spleen) cause the accumulation of dampness. Disharmony with the stomach is more likely to cause accumulation of food, which can then cause accumulation of dampness. Although there is no equivalent syndrome/pattern in Western herbal medicine with which to compare food stagnation, I have successfully used European Angelica for food stagnation patterns on a number of occasions.

Gerard (1597) speaks of two species of *Angelica*, the species of this monograph and another "Wild Angelica," known as *A. sylvestris*. (This latter plant is well-known and grows in Northern Europe, Greenland and Northeastern North America.) Gerard says that although they possess the same virtures, the Garden Angelica is stronger and better used in medicine. He calls the Garden Angelica "hot and dry in the third degree, therefore it opens, attenuates, or makes thin [that which is thick], [assists] digestion, and procures sweat." He also recommends the fresh root to "extenuate and make thin, gross and tough phlegm." This latter quote speaks to my assertion that this medicinal for the treatment of phlegm.

Parkinson (1640) tells us that a distilled preparation of either a water extraction or wine extraction "doth ease all pains and torments that come of cold and wind, so as the body be not bound." Here we seem to have direct reference to cold (and perhaps wind) in the channels causing pain and a stagnation of qi (bound sensation). He also states, of the decoction: "it helps digestion in the stomach, and is a remedy for surfet." Surfet is now spelled 'surfeit', and is an ailment or sensation caused by overindulgence of food and drink. So, Parkinson is telling us that this medicinal is good for food stagnation.

Culpeper (1653) had much to say about this herb, including;

> *"They [roots and seeds] are likewise serviceable in all cold flatulent complaints, and seldom fail of removing the ague.."*

and

> *"[it] easeth all pains and torments coming of cold and wind, so that the body be not bound..."*

and

> *"[it] helpeth the pleurisy, as also all other diseases of the lungs and breast, as coughs, phyisick, and shortness of breath; and syrup of the stalks doth the like. It helps pains of the cholic, the stranguary and stoppage of the urine, procureth woman's course, and expelleth the after-birth, openeth the stoppings of the liver and spleen, and briefly easeth and discusseth all windiness and inward swellings."*

Culpepper addressed four primary organ systems here: the stomach and spleen, the lungs, the liver, and the urinary bladder. There appears to be a focus on the *tàiyáng* and *yángmíng*. It is clear that Culpeper used this medicinal quite extensively and thought highly of it. In my experience, most of what he discusses continues to be appropriate today.

Salmon (1710) says the root is hot and dry in the second degree, and the candied root "...is good against coughs, hoarsness; and strengthens, heals and comforts a cold and weak stomach." This supports the notion that, when treating coldness and vacuity of the spleen/stomach this medicinal should be used in its honey mixed–fried form. Excessive cold and dampness invading the interior and affecting the spleen/stomach can be treated with this preparation. I frequently use the tincture in these cases to good effect, and the seed tincture is a very nice, more gentle way of using this medicinal in preparations that also expel cold and dry dampness in the middle.

Another species native to the British Isles and naturalized in Eastern Canada and Northeastern US is *Angelica sylvestris*. This plant was used much less, or so it appears, than the common Angelica of this monograph. However, Allen and Hatfield (2004) tell us that it was used similarly for lung and chest complaints, rheumatism, and as a "spring tonic."

While this species has abundant historical literature, there is surprisingly little modern research on the plant outside of the cataloging of its chemical constituents. One such study shows its antimicrobial activity.[1] However, there are two studies that investigated less obvious, and perhaps more interesting, features. The first showed Garden Angelica's antitumor effects[2] and strong potential for future research. This study was done on mice, using breast tumor cells, and showed that nearly 90% of the mice did not progress to larger tumor size when the *leaf* extract was administered. Although the leaf is not commonly used in medicine, the chemisty of the leaf and the root is similar. The other outstanding study was done with the essential oil produced from the root of Garden Angelica. This study showed a significant anticonvulsive activity,[3] which suggests that the alcohol extract could possibly be used in a similar way (alcohol is a better solvent for the essential oils of plants, while water extracts are generally quite poor). However, larger dosages might be needed, which may cause problems due to other chemisty in the root. The plant is also known to cause contact dermatitis[4] when encountered in the wild. The author's experience with this issue is that children and fair skinned individuals are most likely affected, but anyone could have this reaction. The condition is self–limiting and generally mild unless there is significant exposure. This reaction is caused by the oils in the leaves and also roots, therefore, care should be taken when harvesting and preparing the fresh plant. The dried plant is not likely to cause this reaction.

There are also a number of species of *Angelica* native to North America (particularly in the West) and used in medicine (see Garran, 2008).

Translation of Available Source Material:

There is scant Chinese language information on the internet about this medicinal, and it is merely translations from English to Chinese. It is named ōubáizhǐ (歐白芷), the "ōu" refers to Europe, ōuzhōu (歐洲) and of course *báizhǐ* comes from the commonly used Chinese herb (*Angelica dahurica*). These two medicinals are not all that similar, *báizhǐ* being a unique medicinal with no other *Angelica* species that compares to it, definitely not European Angelica.

1. Ojala, Tiina, et al, (200). Antimicrobial activity of some coumarin containing herbal plants growing in Finland. *Journal of Ethnopharmacology*. 73(2): pp 299–305.
2. Sigurdsson, Steinthor, et al, (2005). Antitumour Activity of *Angelica archangelica* Leaf Extract. *In vivo*. 19: pp 191–194.

3. Pathak, Shalini, et al, (2010). Evaluation of Antiseisure Activity of Essential Oil from Roots of *Angelica archangelica* Linn. in Mice. *Indian Journal of Pharmaceutical Science.* 72(3): pp 371–375.

4. Knapp, Charles F. & Elston, Dirk M., (2009). Botanical Briefs: Garden Angelica (*Angelica archangelica*). *Close Encounters with the Environment.* 84: pp 189–190.

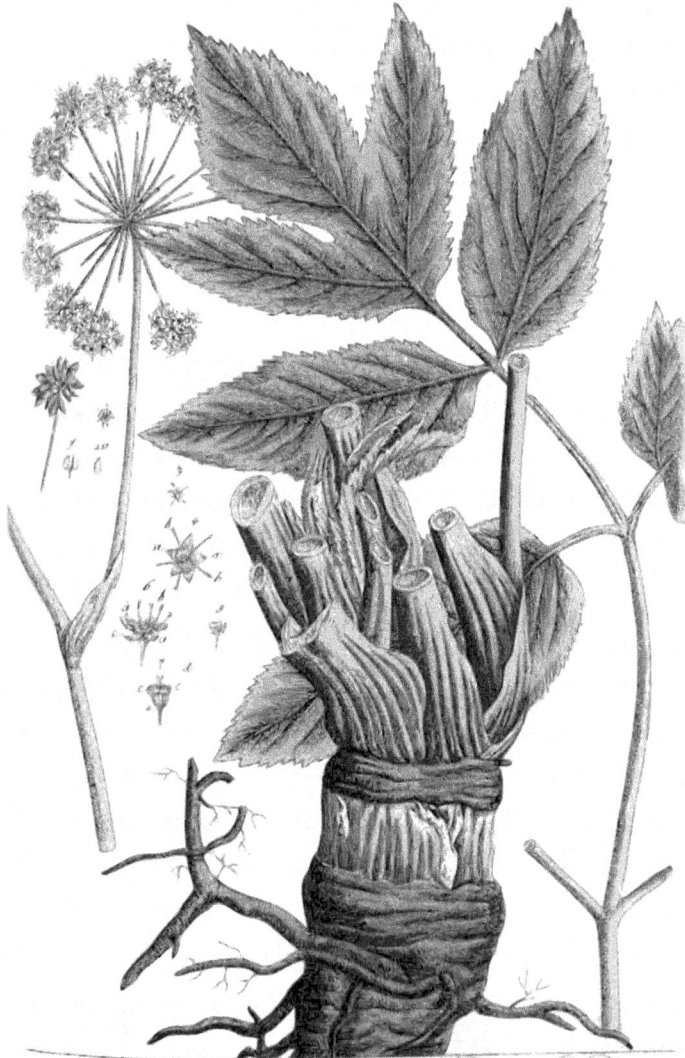

Angelica   Angelit-Wurk:

Wild Yam

Dioscorea villosa L.
Dioscoraceae
Dioscoreae villosae rhizoma
Favor and Qi: acrid, bitter, cool
Channels entered: liver, lung, small intestine
Actions: antispasmodic, diaphoretic

Functions & Indications:

Transforms stagnation and relieves pain. Wild Yam is used for liver constraint qi stagnation leading to menstrual and abdominal spasms and pain, as well as pain due to any pattern associated with liver qi constraint. Shěn Jīn-áo (1774) said: "[In] all qi constraint, the first [treatment] is always to transform stagnation." Wild Yam very powerfully transforms stagnation and relieves pain without damaging right qi. It is acrid, bitter, and cool. Acridity can move qi, while bitterness can drain it. Wild Yam very effectively utilizes these flavors to strongly move qi and transform stagnation, while its cool nature gently clears heat accumulation from stagnation. This latter function is not strong, but assists Wild Yam's primary function to move qi and transform stagnation.

Diffuses and downbears qi, stops cough, and calms panting. Wild Yam is used for coughing and panting due to non-diffusion and counter-flow of the lung qi. When the lung loses its depurative downbearing function, lung qi will run counterflow, and coughing and panting will result. This can happen either from contraction of external pathogens or internal damage. Wild Yam is generally most effective for "spasmodic" coughing, which is most frequently found in patterns of contraction of external pathogens. Wild Yam's acrid flavor acts on the lung to restore its normal depurative function, and its cool bitterness assists in returning the lung qi to its normal downward motion.

Cautions:

None noted.

Dosage and Preparation:

Decoction 3–10g; dried plant tincture 1–4ml

Major Combinations:

Combine with fresh Ginger and European Angelica for lower abdominal pain and diarrhea associated with liver overacting on the spleen. (See *Major Combinations* in the Horehound monograph)

Combine with fresh Ginger and Peppermint for abdominal pain with nausea (and vomiting) associated with liver overacting on the stomach. (See *Major Combinations* in the Horehound monograph)

Combine with *Guì Zhī Fú Líng Tāng* for the treatment of abdominal masses with abnormal bleeding, lower abdominal pain, excessive menstrual bleeding, and spasms. When combining Wild Yam with this formula, use *chìsháo* instead of *báisháo* because the Wild Yam takes the place of *báisháo* in relieving spasms. Coldness can congeal in the lower abdomen and uterus. The cold, if left untreated, will lead to qi stagnation, blood stasis, and eventually congestion may arise. Wild Yam is an important herb to rectify the qi and stop spasms, while also resolving congestion and constraint. Wild Yam also opens the network vessels, and its qi moves downward. This is fundamentally important when treating chronic problems of the female reproductive system and will facilitate a more rapid and complete recovery.

Combine with *xiāngfù*, *báisháo*, *chuānxiōng*, and *gāncǎo* for menstrual pain due to liver constraint qi stagnation. This combination is effective as a tincture to relieve acute menstrual pain, and can be given separately for symptomatic relief while a larger formula is used to address both the branch and root of the disorder. If the pain is severe (generally meaning that significant blood stasis is present), add *yánhúsuǒ* and/or Dicentra to strengthen the effect.

Combine with *zhǐshí*, *báisháo*, and *gāncǎo* for abdominal pain due to qi stagnation accompanied by stomach or intestinal heat.

Commentary:

Wild Yam is native to eastern North America from Ontario on south to Texas and Florida, and is also found on Puerto Rico. *D. villosa* is one of about 600 species in the Dioscoreaceae family of plants, which are primarily found in the tropics, but also range into the warm temperate zone. There are many species of this genus used in medicine and for food (around 6–8 species). In some South Pacific areas, they are primary food sources, the accumulation of which is used to create or show wealth within a community.

In Western herbal medicine, Wild Yam is a staple medicinal that was learned by European invaders from the native peoples. This medicinal quickly became a favorite amongst the doctors of the time and has remained an important medicine to this day. An example of its importance to 19th and 20th Century doctors is exemplified by Felter & Llody (1905), "The rhizome of *Dioscorea villosa* is a favorite therapeutical agaent among Eclectic physicians, who have advantageously used it for more than 60 years." It has been used by herbalists in the United States and beyond for nearly two centuries and has a strong reputation for both reliability and safety.

In gynecology, this medicinal is extremely useful. It can be used in any painful menstruation pattern associated with liver constraint, and combines very well with any of the standard Chinese formulas used for this purpose. I routinely add this herb into decoction formulas. It can also be quite effective for vomiting during early pregnancy, particularly when combined with Ginger and Peppermint. For this, I prefer the tincture: two parts wild yam to one part fresh ginger, with three (3) drops of peppermint essential oil added for every 2 ounces of tincture. This can be taken in 5–10 drop dosages every 15 minutes until the vomiting stops. For severe menstrual cramps, I will often combine Wild Yam (3 parts) with Motherwort (3 parts), Peony (fresh California Peony is preferred) (2 parts), Dicentra (1 part), and Licorice (1 part), and give the tincture to the patient who can then carry the bottle with her and use as needed. This is palliative and is only used during the first two, perhaps three, months of treatment until the larger formula can effect a more lasting change on the menstruation, at which point the tincture is no longer needed.

The above instructions are a call for the use of tinctures. Here is where the Western herbal medicine practice of using tinctures surpasses the use of "clunky" decoctions used in standard Chinese medicine. While I generally give decoctions to all my patients, in a case of severe menstrual pain, a decoction may not offer a significant relief of symptoms in the first month. While it is uncommon for this to be true in later months, it is possible. The administration of a tincture allows women to have something on hand that offers speedy relief in an acute situation.

It is important to note that although this herb is related to the Chinese *shānyào* and the popular Mexican species *D. composite* (Mexican Wild Yam), this plant is quite different in action and usage. This is not surprising, given the size of the Dioscorea genus, which includes over 600 species. Thus, *shānyào*, Wild Yam, and *D. composite* have no therapeutic relationship and cannot be used in place of each other. The medicinal actions of these three herbs are actually quite different, particularly the difference between *shānyào* and the Wild Yam of this monograph.

I could find almost no modern therapeutic–related research on Wild Yam. While there is some research concerning the plant's saponins and other chemical constituents, this research is of little use in the clinic. There have been a few minor studies done on this plant for menopausal symptoms. One study done in Australia on the external application of Wild Yam cream found that although there seem to be no side effects, there also seems to be little benefit.[1] There also seems to be scant ethnobotanical literature available.

Translation of Available Source Material:

There are more than 20 species of *Dioscorea* used in Chinese medicine and a significant number of them, although less well–known in the West, have some similarities with the American species described in the monograph above. I have translated some information about several of these species as a point of reference, and tried to note those that, along with similar uses, also have similar ecological requirements and morphology.

D. zingiberensis C.H. Wright *huǒtóugēn* (火頭跟), which shares very similar morphology and ecological requirements to *D. villosa*, is found in Hebei, Hubei, Hunan, Sichuan, Shanxi, and Gansu provinces between 100–1500 meters elevation. It is considered bitter, slightly sweet, cool, and with slight toxicity. It clears the lung and stops coughing, disinhibits dampness and frees strangury, and resolves toxin and disperses swelling. It is used to treat coughing due to lung heat, damp–heat strangury pain, wind–damp lumbar pain, swollen welling–abscess and malign sores, external injuries and sprains, and stings and bites from insects. It is used in decoction at 6–15g or is made as a tincture.

D. glabra Roxb. *hóngshānyào* (紅山藥) also has a similar morphology and range to *D. villosa*, but its range pushes more south, to Guangdong, Guangxi, Hainan, Guizhou, and Yunnan provinces. It resolves toxin and stops dysentery, and quickens the blood and stops bleeding. It is used to treat dysentery, wind–damp impediment pain, lower back taxation detriment, irregular menstruation, flooding and leaking, and external injury with bleeding. It is used in a decoction 9–30g, or as a powder (draft), or as a tincture. Externally, it is ground to a powder and applied topically.

D. esquirolii Prain et Burkill *bǔxuèshǔ* (補血薯) has a very different morphology, although it has similar ecological requirements and is in the same southern range latitudinally to *D. villosa* in Guangxi, Guizhou, and Yunnan, from 600–1430 meters elevation. This species is one in the group with divided leaves and grows from a root tuber rather than a rhizome, the latter being like *D. opposita* (山藥). It is acrid, slightly sweet, and cool. It cools the blood and stops bleeding, and disperses swelling and stops pain. It is used for postpartum abdominal pain, painful menstruation, pulmonary tuberculosis with coughing of blood, and knocks and falls. It is used in 6–15g dosages in decoction or externally applied as a powder. It is often used alone for the above indications.

D. nipponica Makino (穿山龍 *chuānshānlóng*) has similar morphology, ecological requirements, and latitude, growing throughout much of eastern China, but extending farther north than *D. villosa*, all the way into Russia. The rhizome of this plant is an important source of plant steroids for the drug industry. It is bitter and neutral, and enters the liver and lung channels. It dispels wind and expels dampness, quickens the blood, and stops cough. It is used to treat wind-damp impediment pain, numbness and tingling of the limbs, wind-damp-heat, chest impediment heart pain, abdominal pain, chronic bronchitis, knocks and falls, taxation sprains, malaria, swollen welling-abscess, and frostbite. It is decocted either dry (6–9g) or fresh (30–45g), or made into a tincture. Externally, it is used fresh, and is pounded and applied, or the dried herb made into a paste. This species appears to be very similar in usage to *D. villosa*.

D. cirrhosa Lour. (薯莨 *shǔliáng*) has a different morphology and similar ecological requirements, but grows both within and south of *D. villosa*'s latitudinal range, growing throughout southern China as well as in Taiwan, Vietnam, and Thailand. The root is very high in tannin and is used in the fabric industry for dying, which explains part of its function to stop bleeding. It is bitter and cool, with a small amount of toxicity. It quickens the blood and stops bleeding, rectifies qi and stops pain, and clears heat and resolves toxin. It is used for spitting blood, expectorating blood, vomiting blood, nosebleed, blood in the urine, blood in the stool, flooding and spotting, irregular menstruation, painful menstruation, menstrual block, postpartum abdominal pain, stomach duct and abdominal pain and distention, heat-toxin bloody dysentery, watery diarrhea, joint pain, swelling and pain associated with knocks and falls (with or without bleeding), sores and boils, and herpes zoster. It is used as a decoction 3–9g, or squeezed into a juice, or pounded. Externally, it is ground to a powder or pounded for application. This species has many similarities to *D. villosa* ,but its tannin content makes it a very strong medicinal for stopping bleeding.

1. Komesaroff, P. A., et al., (2001). Effects of wild yam extract on menopausal symptoms, lipids and sex hormones in healthy menopausal women. *Climacreric.* 4: pp 144–150.

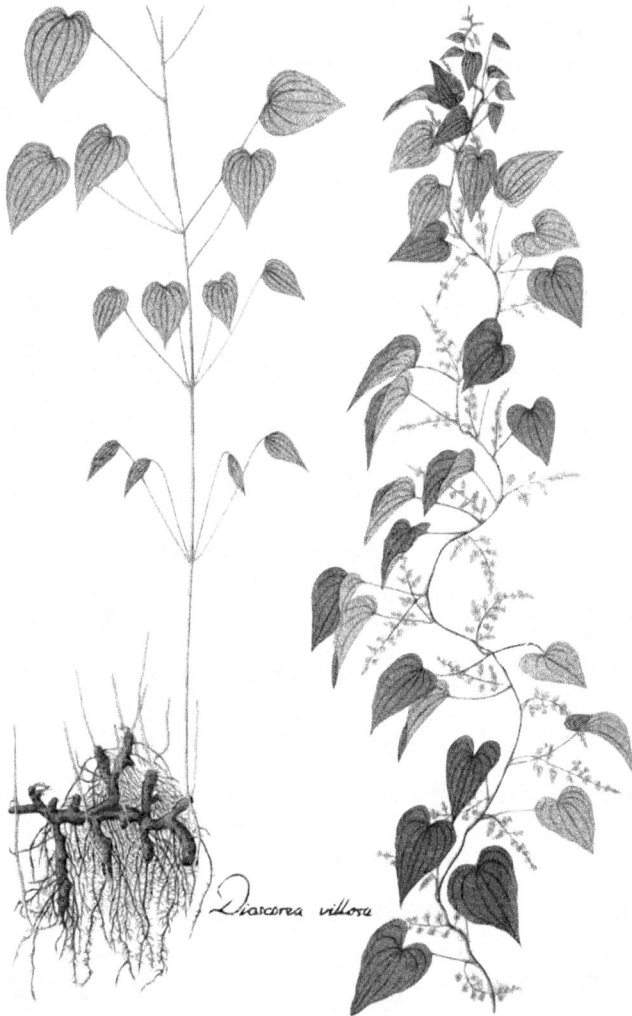

Diascorea villosa

Dill Seed

Anethum graveolens L.
Chinese name: *shíluózǐ* (莳萝子)
Apiaceae
Anethi Graveolens semen
Flavor and Qi: acrid, aromatic, and warm
Channels entered: spleen, stomach, liver
Actions: antibacterial, antifungal, antispasmodic, carminative, warming stomachic

Functions & Indications:

Warms the spleen, disperses food stagnation and cold, and stops pain. Dill seed is used for abdominal pain due to cold, and vomiting (especially due to excessive consumption of raw and cold food). Associated symptoms may include excessive fullness after eating, decreased appetite, and a thick white (possibly greasy) tongue coating. Dill seed warms the spleen and disperses food with its warm acridity and aroma.

Warms the center, disperses cold, and downbears stomach qi. Dill seed is used for counterflow stomach qi with upward belching of sour fluids, vomiting, hiccup, glomus, distention in the stomach duct, and nausea due to cold in the middle burner associated with excessive consumption of raw and cold food. Excessive consumption of raw or cold food can lead to accumulation of cold and dampness in the stomach, which can impair the stomach's normal downward flow of qi. Dill seed is acrid and warm, and can disperse cold in the middle and harmonize the stomach to restore the qi dynamic.

Courses the liver and resolves qi constraint. Dill seed is used for rib–side pain, distention, and abdominal fullness due to liver constraint qi stagnation. Dill seed courses the liver with warm acridity, and opens the abdomen and chest with aroma. This herb has also been used for delayed menstruation due to cold.

Cautions:
Contraindicated for heat/fire patterns. Use caution with yin vacuity.

Dosage and Preparation:

Light decoction or infusion 3–6g; tincture 1–3ml

Major Combinations:

Combine with *Bǎo Hé Wán* for children or adults when there is cold in the stomach.

Combine with Fennel, Mint, and Chamomile for an effectively neutral tea that is generally easy for children to take for a variety of stomach problems ranging from pain to diarrhea to vomiting. Increasing or decreasing any of the herbs appropriately will tip the scale toward warm or cold, as needed. This can also be prepared as a glycerin extract, which is suitable for children and easy for them to take.

Commentary:

This is a commonly used medicinal for children, as it has no toxicity, is not terribly disagreeable in taste, and has a long history of use. Dill is native to the Mediterranean region and has been cultivated since antiquity.[1] Dill is a member of the Apiaceae family (the same plant family as many other warm, acrid herbs used in botanical medicine, such as *chuānxiōng*, *dāngguī*, *huíxiāng*, and many others). This plant family is well known for its spicy/acrid seeds used as spices for cooking such as Coriander, Cumin, Fennel, etc.

Like nearly all other medicinal/culinary plants in this family (and other families) the essential oil of Dill has been found to be effective against a wide range of microbials including bacteria[2] and fungi.[3] Dill seed has been used traditionally throughout Europe and Western and Central Asia as an antispasmodic to relieve colic in young children, which has been substantiated by laboratory findings.[4]

Dill herb and seeds are well known in pickling, and are the primary flavoring of the Dill Pickle. In China, the herb is known as *huíxiāng* (茴香) and is a primary herb used in the famous northern dish *jiǎozi* (what Westerners would call "dumplings" or "pot stickers"). This is a curious fact because *huíxiāng* is what we call Fennel in Chinese medicine, and every dictionary I have referenced states that *huíxiāng* is, in fact, Fennel. However, when going to the market, at least in the North, what you will find is Dill. Neither Dill nor Fennel are native to China. They have very similar morphological features and somewhat similar tastes and odors, thus it is possible that somewhere in history there was a switch that went more or less unnoticed. I have been unable to locate any sources in either Chinese or English discussing this phenomenon.

Gerard (1597) quotes Galen as saying that Dill is "hot in the end of the second degree, and dry in the beginning of the same, or in the end of the first degree." In other words, this medicinal is rather warm and thus, moving, but does not have a strong action to dry. Gerard also states that Dill seed is good for stomach cramps, hiccough, intestinal gas, and engenders mother's milk, as well as increases urination. Although the author has no experience using this medicine for improving mother's milk, given its liver qi moving action, it could help in cases where liver depression qi stagnation is the underlying pathological pattern.

Parkinson (1640) says of Dill seed: "The seed is of more use than the leaves, although they be much used to relish condiments, and is more effectural to digest raw and viscous humors, yet more unpleasant than Fennel, and is used in all medicines that serve to expel wind, and ease torments and pains thereof." Although this is not much different from what Gerard said, Parkinson tells use that Dill seed is used for these types of gastrointestinal disorders.

Culpeper (1653) said, "it stayeth the belly and stomach from casing [vomiting]." It is effectual "to digest raw and vicious humours, and is used in medicines that serve to expel wind, and the pains proceeding therefrom." While this says nothing of the qi of this medicinal, it does say something about the downbearing or rectifying action on the stomach.

Salmon (1710) has much to say about this medicinal. He employs both the herb and the seed, and discusses them separately in his monograph. He says the seed is "hot and dry in the third degree." Of the powder of the seed, he says, "Taken to one dram [~4g] in any fit vehicle, it warms and comforts the stomach and bowels, and powerfully expels wind. Drank mixed with wine, it is good against the hiccough, vomiting, loathing and convulsions of the stomach and other viscera." With regards to the tincture of the seed, he states, "It powerfully warms, comforts, and strengthens the stomach, expels wind, and causes a good appetite and digestion."

It should be noted that when Salmon uses the term "wind", he is not talking about the same "wind" of Chinese medicine; instead, he is talking about gas trapped in the stomach and intestines that the body can release either through belching or flatulence.

Translation of Available Source Material:

Dill seed first appeared in the *Guǎng Zhōu Jì* (4th Century), but has since been lost. The *Hǎi Yào Běn Cǎo* (海藥本草)—written in the early 10th Century by Lǐ Xún (李珣, 907–960) a Persian born in the south of China who lived most of his life in Chengdu[5]—references it, but I am unsure whether Lǐ Xún adds any of his own assessment, or simply transcribes from the *Guǎng Zhōu Jì*. Nevertheless, the *Hǎi Yào Běn Cǎo* states that Dill seed is from Persia, and compares it to Celery seed *mǎqínzǐ* (馬芹子), saying that Celery seed is black and heavy, while Dill seed is brown and light. The text also states that it governs the qi of the diaphragm, disperses food, warms the stomach, and is good for enriching the flavor of food. Lastly, it states that it can be eaten in large amounts without harm, but should not be combined with Asafetida *āwèi* (阿魏) because the Asafetida will overwhelm its flavor. The *Grand Dictionary of Chinese Medicinals* (2009) says it is acrid and warm and enters the spleen, stomach, liver and kidney channels. It warms the spleen and opens the stomach, disperses cold, and stops pain. It is used for abdominal cold and pain, rib-side distention and fullness, vomiting counterflow with low appetite, and cold mounting. As a decoction, it is used in 1–5 gram doses; it is also used as a pill or powder (draught).

1. Bailer, J., T. Aichinger, G. Hackl, K.D. Hueber and M. Dachler, (2001). Essential oil content and composition in commercially available dill cultivars in comparison to caraway. *Industrial Crops and Products*, 14: pp 229–239.
2. Badar, Nazish, Arshad, Muhammad, Farooq, Umer, (2008). Characteristics of *Anethum graveolens* (Umbelliferae) Seed Oil: Extraction, Composition and Antimicrobial Activity. *International Journal of Agriculture & Biology*. 10: pp 329–32.
3. Soundharraja Radhakrishanan Sridhar, et al. (2003). Antifungal Activity of Some Essential Oils. *Journal of Agriculture and Food Chemistry* 51(26), pp 7596–7599.
4. Naseri, M.K. Gharib and Heidari, A. (2007). Antispasmodic Effect of *Anethum graveolens* Fruit Extract on Rat Ileum. *International Journal of Pharmacology*. 3(3), pp 260–264.
5. Chen Ming, (2007). The Transmission of Foreign Medicine via the Silk Roads in Medieval China: A Case Study of *Haiyao Bencao* 海藥本草. *Asian Medicine*. 3: pp. 241–264.

Beth Root (Wake-Robin)

Trillium sp. L.
Melanthiaceae
Trillii radix
Favor and Qi: acrid, slightly sweet, warm
Channels entered: spleen, heart
Actions: astringent, tonic

Functions & Indications:

Quickens the blood and stop bleeding. Beth Root is used for bleeding of various types, but is particularly useful when the bleeding is due to spleen qi unable to contain the blood in the vessels. Beth Root is used for excessive menstrual bleeding, coughing blood, blood in the urine and blood in the stool. Beth Root enters the spleen and heart channels. The spleen rules the blood, and the heart moves it and rules the vessels. When the spleen qi become vacuous it is said that it "can not rule the blood" or the "qi can not contain the blood [in the vessels]"; this will lead to the blood pouring out into the interstices. By entering these two channels, Beth Root's acridity and sweetness can quicken the blood without damaging it. While Beth Root does not directly nourish the blood, when combined with qi and blood nourishing medicinals, it can enhance their action.

Quickens the blood, regulates the menstruation, and stops pain. Beth Root is used for blood stasis due to qi vacuity. Beth Root is used for menstrual pain, irregular menstruation, chest pain, and groin pain. Beth Root enters the blood through both the spleen and heart (see above), giving it a unique role in treating specific types of blood stasis and pain. Beth Root is an important herb for the treatment of qi vacuity blood stasis, but traditionally has very specific uses. Interestingly, Chinese medicine uses two species in nearly the same ways. Beth Root is acrid and warm. Warm acridity can quicken the blood, regulate menstruation, and stop pain.

Cautions:
None noted

Dosage and Preparation:
Fresh plant tincture 2–4ml; decoction 4–10g; drought 3–6g

Major Combinations:

Combine with Bugleweed and Mullien for expectoration of bloody sputum with chest pain. If the phlegm is purulent add *yúxīngcǎo*, Echinacea, and *huángqín*. If the phlegm is copious and clear, add Elecampane and Yerba Santa. If the phlegm is scant and difficult to expectorate, add *báijí*.

For excessive menstrual bleeding due to spleen qi vacuity, this herb can be added to *Gù Běn Zhǐ Bēng Tāng* or *Gǔ Qì Tāng*.

Commentary:

Trillium is in the Liliaceae family with an estimated 43 species in North America and Asia. The genus is biogeographically centered in North America, with 38 of the 43 known species growing there. China has four species (two are endemic), and the genus can be found as far west as India and Japan. Most species of *Trillium* are quite beautiful while in bloom, and some even have rather large flowers. As the name suggests, most of the plant's parts are found in threes, allowing people who live within its range and who spend any amount of time in nature to easily recognize this plant. The "leaves" (only three on a plant) are at the top of a single stem, with the flowering structure emerging above. In reality, these are not true leaves, but rather, bracts subtending the flower, although they act like leaves and have many similar structures to leaves. Beth root is relatively easy to grow and I would encourage gardeners to incorporate it into their garden as it adds beauty, uniqueness, and helps to preserve this important medicinal plant.

This was a very important medicinal in the 19th and early 20th Centuries in North America and, to a certain extent, in Europe. Unfortunately, this led to overharvesting of the plant, particularly in its Eastern North American range. Fortunately (mainly because herbal medicine was not been very popular in North America for much of the 20th Century, and partially because most herbalists were taught not to use it because of its scarcity), this plant has made a reasonable comeback and is now considered "secure" by most sources. However, a new pressure has befallen the plant, in the form of horticulture. The beauty of this plant has led to large-scale wild-harvesting by the nursery market, with no apparent commercial growing taking place. This plant must be monitored in the wild and we must learn to cultivate it in order for it to become a plant we can use long into the future. It is an incredibly valuable plant, having very specific functions that it performs uniquely well, but without proper management it will once again fall into obscurity.

In an article in the *New England Journal of Medicine* in 1820, a Dr. Williams reports that Beth Root is exceedly superior as an astringent but does not tend to cause constipation, even with extreme use, such as in emergencies when large doses are used. He further states that his friend (another doctor) "uses pounds of this medicine in his practice every year, and thinks it is not suppassed by any astringent in the materia medica." He later tells us, "By the common people this root is used in parturition, and it is believed by them to be of great efficacy in expediting the birth of the child."[1]

Cook (1869) states, "Its astringency is not so great as to cause dryness; yet is sufficiently marked (in company with the tonic power) to diminish superfluous discharges [of the mucus membranes], and to prove of the greatest service in bleeding from the lungs, nose, stomach, bowels, kidneys, and bladder, and is equally useful in checking excessive menstruation and lochia."

Felter & Llody (1905) state: "It has been employed successfully in *hemoptysis, hematuria, menorrhagia, uterine hemorrhage, metrorrhagia, leucorrhea, cough, asthma*, and *difficult breathing*, and is said to have been much used by the Indian women to promote parturition." And, "All the varieties have been found efficient, either internally or externally, in *chronic mucous discharges, bronchorrhea, leucorrhea, menorrhagia*, etc." The authors describe eight species, saying that some are more acrid while others are more astringent. They differentiate them therapeutically by noting that the more acrid species are better applied to "...*chronic affections* or the *respiratory organs, phthisis, hectic fever*, etc." while the more astringent species are better used to check excessive flow. Eclectic physicians understood the connection between acridity and the lungs and externally contracted diseases, or at least they alluded to it here without making further connections. Nevertheless, they did make the distinction and this helps us when using this genus. Unfortunately, however, they don't tell us which species are more acrid and which are more astringent.

As noted above, this medicinal was also used by the Native Americans, and later by the European invaders, to prepare a pregnant woman for the birthing process. In Moerman's Ethnobotanical Database, one entry attributed to the Iroquois reads, "Decoction of root taken for 'food for woman in the womb.'" The roots, taken 6–8 weeks prior to the due date, are widely reported to facilitate delivery. I have used this, along with other herbs, in this manner and found that when such a formula is taken, births tend to be shorter and easier with fewer complications. Beth Root is commonly combined with other herbs for this purpose, including Black Cohosh, Blue Cohosh, and Motherwort.

Translation of Available Source Material:

Chinese medicine uses two species of Beth Root interchangeably. There are three species in China and one which is endemic to Taiwan. One species that grows in China but is not mentioned here only grows in the southern mountains of Tibet to 3200 meters. The other two are found under the Chinese name *tóudǐngyīkēzhū* (頭頂一顆珠). *Trillium tschonoshii* Maxim. *yánlíngcǎo* (延齡草) grows between 1600–3200m throughout much of central China from Zhejiang Province to Tibet, and *T. camschatcense* Ker Gawler *jílínyánlíngcǎo* (吉林延齡草) grows in Jilin Province. The former species is considered "vulnerable" in China, according to the *Flora of China*. Both are considered sweet and slightly acrid, warm, with small amounts of toxicity. They are said to tranquilize (鎮靜), stop pain, quicken the blood, and stop bleeding. They are used for high blood pressure, neurasthenia, dizziness and headache, lumbus and leg pain, irregular menstruation, flooding and spotting, bleeding due to external injury, and knocks and falls. They are used in decoction at 6–9g, or as a powder of 3g. They are also applied externally as a powder.

1. Williams, Stephen W., (1820). Botanical History, and Medicinal Properties of the *Trillium Erectum*, &c. *New England Journal of Medicine*. 9(4): pp. 330–332.

Medicinal	Nature	Flavor	Channels	Functions	Indications
European Angelica	warm	acrid, bitter	spleen, stomach, liver	Warms the middle, moves qi and opens the stomach; Resolves liver constraint and stops pain; Warms the lungs & transforms phlegm-cold; Courses the channels, expels wind & dispels cold & damp	abdominal pain with accumulation of cold & damp with associated qi stagnation; pain in the rib-sides & lesser abdomen due to constraint of liver qi; abundant clear or white phlegm wind-cold-damp impediment
Wild Yam	cool	acrid, bitter	liver, lung	Moves qi, resolves constraint, and relieves pain; Diffuses and downbears qi, stops cough and calms panting	menstrual and abdominal spasms and pain; coughing and panting due to non-diffusion and counter-flow of the lung qi
Dill Seed	warm	acrid, aromatic	spleen, stomach, liver	Warms the spleen, disperses food stagnation and cold, and stops pain; Warms the center, disperses cold, and downbears stomach qi; Courses the liver and resolves qi constraint	abdominal pain due to cold, and vomiting; belching of sour fluids, vomiting, hiccup, glomus, distention in the stomach duct, and nausea; rib-side pain, distention, and abdominal
Bethroot	warm	acrid, slightly sweet	spleen, heart	Quickens the blood and stop bleeding; Quickens the blood, regulates the menstruation, and stops pain	menstrual bleeding, coughing blood, blood in the urine and blood in the stool; menstrual pain, irregular menstruation, chest pain, and groin pain

理

血

藥

Rectify Blood Medicinals

The rectifying blood category is a large group of medicinals that are divided into two principle groups; staunch bleeding and quickening the blood. Both divisions have both internal and external application, in the case of external application this is often for acute trauma, and may be used together in formulas to treat bleeding and pain (due to blood stasis).

The staunch bleeding sub-category is further divided into four groups; cool blood and stop bleeding, transform stasis and stop bleeding, stopping bleeding by astriction, and warming the menses to stop bleeding. This materia medica has two medicinals that can be used to staunch bleeding, Bugleweed and Shepherd's Purse. Both of these medicinals are cooling in nature, however the former primarily functions to cool blood and stop bleeding, while the latter is primarily used to transform stasis to stop bleeding.

The quickening the blood sub-category is also further divided into four groups; quickening the blood and moving qi, quickening the blood and regulating the menses, quickening the blood to treat trauma, and breaking blood and dispersing concretions. The medicinals in this sub-category are frequently acrid in flavor and frequently also move qi; even when the later is true, they are frequently combined with qi moving medicinals in formulas. While the symptoms of the staunch bleeding sub-category are obvious, the symptoms requiring the use of the quickening the blood sub-category are not always as obvious. Pain is the most obvious and this sub-category is the most important group of medicinals in the materia medica used in the treatment of pain. However, many chronic illnesses can benefit from the use of medicinals in this category because chronic conditions tend to lead to both qi stagnation and blood stasis.

Calendula

Calendula officinalis L.
Asteraceae
Calendulae Flos
Chinese Name: *jīnzhǎnjú* (金盏菊)
Favor and Qi: acrid, bitter, cool
Channels entered: liver, lung
Actions: anti-inflamatory, vulnerary, antiseptic

Functions & Indications:

Quickens blood, Clears heat, stops pain, and engenders flesh. Calendula is used in external applications for wounds due to knocks and falls. The combination of quickening the blood, clearing heat, and engendering flesh gives Calendula an important place in the materia medica. Wounds and trauma frequently lead to heat, due to accumulation and stagnation of blood and qi. Calendula moves blood with acridity, and although this is not a strong action, it has a definite effect on blood stagnation and will assist other medicinals in relieving pain. Furthermore, with cool bitterness, it clears and drains heat from the local area, assisting the resolution of qi stagnation and blood stasis.

Quickens blood, clears heat, resolves toxicity, and engenders flesh. Calendula is used as an internal application for damaged tissue due to repletion (evil toxin) or yin vacuity heat. This application is essentially the same as for external application. The use of this herb internally uses all the same principles as above, but for treatment of the tissues of the mouth, throat, stomach, and intestines (see combinations below for delineation of usage).

Cautions:
None noted

Dosage and Preparation:
Light decoction 2–6g; fresh plant tincture 1–2ml; externally as a plaster or salve, also as an oil for use in the ear.

Major Combinations:

Combine with Chamomile and Oregon Grape root for heat-toxin in the lower burner. Add Goldenseal and/or *huánglián* for complications associated with dampness.

Combine with Goldenseal, Plantain leaf, and *sānqī* for damp-heat toxin in the intestines with painful, bloody stools. Add Elecampane and *tiānhuáfěn* for watery stools with phlegm. Add *báizhǐ* for more serious pain.

Combine with St. John's Wort, Arnica, *mòyào*, *rǔxiāng*, and Cayenne for external application to knocks and falls. For more severe pain, or pain associated with nerve damage, add Aconite (Chinese or Western). *Hónghuā* may be substituted for Arnica if it is unavailable.

Combine with Garlic and St. John's Wort for middle ear infections. For this, an oil is prepared and applied via a cotton ball placed in the ear.

Commentary:

Calendula is a classic medicinal in the European herbal medicine traditions and is one of the first herbs that many Western herbalists learn to use. It is found in an abundance of external preparations, from skin care to hair care. It is also an important medicinal to help heal tissue that has been damaged by trauma or chronic inflammatory conditions, which includes tissue of the digestive tract. This common "pot herb" is found in many gardens in Europe and America, and I have seen it beginning to be used in plantings in China. It is extremely easy to grow and is self-seeding, so once you plant it, it will remain in your garden as long as you want it there; and when you don't, it is not terribly difficult to remove.

Although Calendula is probably more often used for its external rather than its internal applications, it certainly has a place in the materia medica as an internal medicinal. It has a very positive effect on heat in the stomach and intestines, and is especially useful when that heat is chronic and has led to accumulation of heat toxin and blood stasis. Thus, many of the chronic diseases of the intestines seen clinically today such as IBS, Crohn's Disease, and chronic constipation can benefit from this medicinal. This medicinal does not, however, have any marked effect on dampness and therefore must be combined with the appropriate medicinals to treat these diseases. Think of the big orange Calendula flowers as being a *júhuā* (clear heat), *hónghuā* (quicken blood), and *zǐcǎogēn* (clear heat/resolve toxin and engender flesh) all rolled into one.

Gerard (1597) states: "The flower of Calendula is of temperature hot, almost in the second degree, especially when dry: it is thought to strengthen and comfort the heart." He later says "Conserve made of the flowers and sugar taken in the morning fasting, cureth the tremblings of the heart." Gerard speaks quite clearly regarding Calendula's action on the heart and, by extension, the blood. The heart is the commander of the vessels and blood, thus any medicinal that acts on the heart also acts on the blood. Although he does not mention pain, he does say that it strengthens and comforts the heart, as well as resolving "tremblings" of the heart, which are likely palpitations (see below). On the other hand, Gerard may be referring to Calendula's action to clear heat, which might also cause such symptomology.

Culpeper (1653) writes in similar fashion to Gerard, speaking highly of this medicinal saying:

> "They [Calendula] strengthen the heart exceedingly, and are very expulsive and little less effectual in the small pox and measles than saffron. The juice of the leaves mixed with vinegar, and any hot swelling bathed with it, instantly giveth ease, and assuageth it. The flowers, either green [fresh] or dried, are much used in possets [a drink made of hot milk curdled with ale, wine, or the like, often sweetened and spiced], broths, and drink, as a comforter of the heart and spirits, and to expel any malignant or pestilential quality which might annoy them. A plaister made with the dried flower in powder, hog's-grease, turpentine, and rosin, applied to the breast, strengthens and succours the heart infinitely in fevers, whether pestilential or not."

This describes Calendula's action in clearing heat and resolving toxin, as well as its blood quickening action.

Salmon (1710) states, "The Juice of the Flowers. It is cordial, comforts and strengthens the heart very much, resists poison, and is prevalent against pestilential fevers. [The] dose from half an ounce to an ounce in a glass of generous wine." This is similar to what Gerard and Culpeper said, and is likely to have come from those sources.

Later, Salmon seems to draw directly from Gerard when he states "The Conserve of the Flowers. Taken in the morning fasting, it cures the palpitation or trembling of the heart; and is given as a prophylactic or preservative in time of plague or pestilence. The Distilled Water of the Leaves and Flowers. Dropped into red and rheumatic eyes, it cools the inflammation, stops the rheum, and eases the pain." (Note: The latter statement, e.g. use in the eyes, is also in Gerard's herbal, but he credits another author.)

Homsher, R.D., (1908) discusses Calendula at length, but sticks to its external application both as an antiseptic and a pain reliever. Regarding the latter, he states:

> *"Calendula as a local anodyne is as positive as opium, if not more effectual. It apparently does not affect the sympathetic like opium. In this respect it resembles aconite, the most powerful local anodyne we have of that class. It also resembles belladonna in relieving pain, local congestion and inflammation, but not so dangerous."*[1]

This is indeed high praise for our simple Calendula, and while I am not ready to agree with this to its fullest extent, there is no doubt that Calendula is an important medicinal for pain relief when applied externally.

Felter (1922) states, "[It] prevents or lessens the formation of pus, and promotes the prompt healing of wounds, with the least possible cicatrization [scarring]." He also advises that it should be taken internally "to reinforce its local action, particularly in old ulcers, varicose veins, capillary engorgement of tissues, and chronic suppurative and catarrhal conditions." Felter also says "While of unquestioned value in all of the local conditions named it has been much overrated, and its real medicinal worth obscured by extravagant praise." What he presents in his book is rational use of this medicinal, but this statement warns those who might be taken in by less scrupulous herbalists. This was a time of the "snake oil" doctors who toured the United States, pushing their wares.

The use of Calendula has garnered some attention in modern medicine. A study published in the *Journal of Clinical Oncology* in 2004 states, "Calendula is statistically significantly superior to trolamine [a common external analgesic] for the primary end point, prevention of skin toxicity of RTOG grade 2 or higher, and for all the secondary end points (including allergy, interruption of treatment, patient satisfaction for relief of pain, and dermatitis), with the exception of ease of application, which was considered by the patients to be more difficult with calendula than with trolamine."[2] Another study on external use of Calendula on leg ulcers showed a 41.71% improvement (compared to 14.52% on controls) over three weeks of application.[3]

Translation of Available Source Material:

This medicinal is considered bitter and cold. It clears heat and resolves toxin, and regulates menstruation. It is used to treat inner ear inflammation and irregular menstruation. The *Yunnan Materia Medica* also states that it quickens the blood. It is taken in 5–15 g doses as a decoction and the leaf is used externally to treat ear inflammation.

1. Homsher, R.D (1908). Calendula. *Ellingwood's Therapeutist.* 2(11): pp 8.
2. Pommier, P. (2004). Phase III Randomized Trial of *Calendula Officinalis* Compared With Trolamine for the Prevention of Acute Dermatitis Irradiation of Breast Cancer. *J Clin Oncol* 22(8): pp 1447–1453.
3. Duran, V. et. al., (2005). Results of the clinical examination of an ointment with marigold (*Calendula officinalis*) extract in the treatment of venous leg ulcers. *Int J Tissue React.* 27(3): pp 101–6.

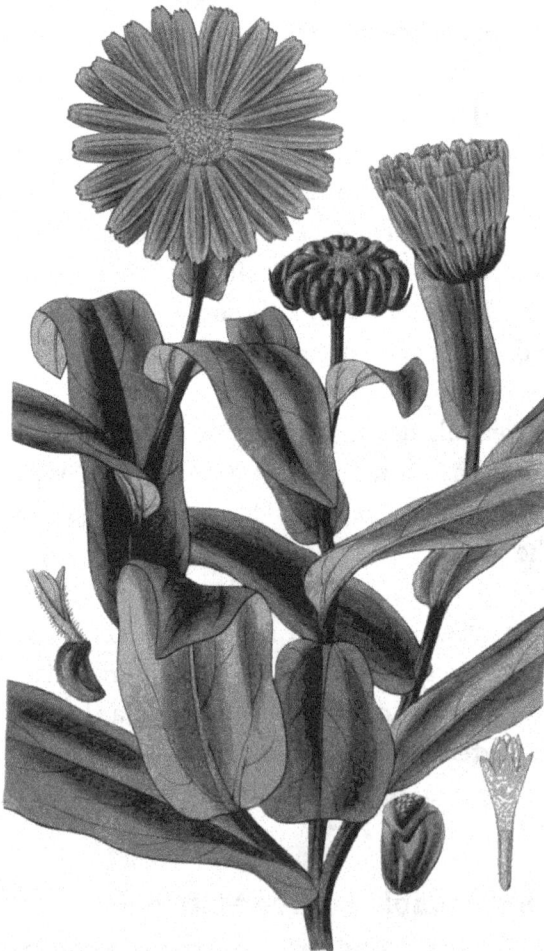

Horse Chestnut

Æsculus hippocastanum L., *A. californica* (Spach) Nutt., *A. chinensis* Bunge, etc.
Hippocastanaceae
Aesculi fructus
Chinese Name: *suōluózǐ* (娑罗子)
Favor and Qi: acrid, bitter, warm
Channels entered: heart, liver, stomach
Actions: anti-oedematous, anti-inflammatory, venotonic

Functions & Indications:

Rectifies qi, quickens the blood, and resolves constraint. Horse Chestnut
is used for qi stagnation and blood stasis causing congestion and pain in
the lower burner, specifically the anus, groin, and legs, with symptoms
such as varicose veins or hemorrhoids. While these hallmark symptoms
in the lower burner are often present when using this medicinal, it also
has a marked qi-moving action when there is fullness and distention
pain in the abdomen and chest. This medicinal can therefore be used to
treat glomus, primarily of a repletion type. (See further explanation of
glomus in the commentary.) To alleviate pain, Horse Chestnut uses
warm acridity to move the qi and quicken the blood, while its bitterness
drains congestion.

Cautions:

Horse Chestnut is slightly toxic and must be used (internally) within the
appropriate dosage range. Common problems associated with overdose are
a burning feeling in the stomach and diarrhea.

Dosage and Preparation:

Dried fruit tincture 0.5-2 ml; decoction 2-6g; externally as a lotion, cream,
or liniment.

Major Combinations:

Combine with Red Root, *huáiniúxī*, and *dānshēn* and use internally for qi
stagnation and blood stasis with painful hemorrhoids. Add Oregon
Grape root and *huángbái* for pronounced heat.

External application of the combination of Horse Chestnut, Collinsonia,
and Calendula is an excellent three-herb *duìyào* for external treatment

of hemorrhoids. To this three–herb combination can be added any number of herbs, depending on the situation: with pronounced heat, add Goldenseal; with pronounced heat and dampness, add Goldenseal and *kǔshēn*; for heat–toxin, add Goldenseal and Echinacea.

Commentary:

Horse Chestnut is a member of the *Æsculus* genus (this common name is often applied to several species within the genus) in the Sapindaceae (Soapberry) family, but was long placed in the Hippocastanaceae family. Sapindaceae is a family of 150 genera and about 1500 species found worldwide, of which the famous lychee berry is a member (*Litchi chinensis*). *Æsculus* is a small genus with 12 species, all but one of which are found in North America and Asia. The one not found on those two continents is the primary medicinal of this monograph, A. *hippocastanum*. This species is native to Southeast Europe but has been planted throughout Europe, North America, and parts of Asia.

Horse Chestnut has a long tradition of use in Europe and has been well–studied. The California species seem to act about the same as the European species. The European species can be found growing throughout much of North America and, thus, is easy to obtain locally, and is the species carried by herb companies.

Horse Chestnut is used both internally as a tincture and externally as an infused oil or other preparation for externally manifesting symptoms such as hemorrhoids and varicose veins. The most frequently used application is as a cream or salve, where the horse chestnut is infused into the product. This is a very effective treatment as a simple (single agent), but combines well with a number of herbs to create very nice products to help relieve the pain of hemorrhoids as well as resolve both hemorrhoids and varicosities.

Parkinson (1640) quotes a Greek author saying, "in the meal of Chestnuts be made into a Electuary with honey, it is very profitable for those are troubled with a cough or with spitting of blood." This shows an action on the blood, but the mechanism is to stop bleeding rather than, specifically, quickening the blood (but stopping bleeding can also be accomplished at times by quickening the blood).

Felter & Llody (1909) state:

> "*Specific medication has taught us that it is a remedy, not for active conditions, but for congestion and engorgement. It is indicated in general by capillary engorgement—a condition of*

stasis—with vascular fullness and sense of soreness, throbbing, and malaise all over the body. An uneasy, full, aching pain in the hepatic region is also an indication. Rectal disorders, such as rectal irritation and hemorrhoids, with marked congestion and a sense of constriction, as if closing spasmodically upon some foreign body, with itching, heat, pain, aching, or simple uneasiness, are fields in which hippocastanum exerts a specific influence. The pile-tumors are purple, large, do not bleed as a rule, but there is a sense of fullness, or spasm of the parts, and a free diarrhea may be present. Not only does it relieve such rectal complaints, but cures disorders hinging upon them, such as rectal neuralgia, proctitis, etc., and the reflexes induced by them, proceeding from the rectal involvement. Among these reflex manifestations may be mentioned dyspnea, asthmatic seizures, dizziness, headache, backache, and disturbed gastric functions amounting to veritable forms of dyspepsia. These conditions pass away when hippocastanum overcomes the rectal difficulties."

This passage supports the monograph above and shows a wider breadth of use for this medicinal. The Chinese species is used in similar ways (see *Translation of Available Source Material* below).

The plethora of modern research can be summed up in a quote from a paper authored by Edward Ernst, who is likely the most vocal anti–allopathic medicine lobbyist in the published literature, "These data imply that HCSE [Horse Chestnut Standardized Extract] is superior to placebo and as effective as reference medications in alleviating the objective signs and subjective symptoms of CVI [chronic venous insufficiency]. Thus, HCSE represents a treatment option for CVI that is worth considering."[1] Coming from Mr. Ernst, this is high praise indeed. Aescin, a constituent present in all or many species of *Aesculus*, has been well studied for its anti–oedematous, anti–inflammatory, and venotonic properties.[2]

Translation of Available Source Material:

There are two species (and one variation) of Horse Chestnut used in Chinese medicine. The *Chinese Dictionary of Medicinals* (2005) lists them all under the same heading as does the *Grand Dictionary of Chinese Medicinals*. The main heading name is *suōluózǐ* (娑羅子), under which fall *Æsculus chinensis* Bge. *qīyèshù* (七葉樹), *Æsculus chinensis* Bge. var. *chekiangensis* (Hu et Fang) Fang *zhèjiāngqīyèshù* (浙江七葉樹), and *Æsculus wilsonii* Rehd.

tiānshīlì（天師栗）. Both sources agree about the flavor, nature and channels entered; sweet, warm, and enters the liver and stomach channels. However, they give slightly different functions and indications. The *Chinese Herbal Pharmacopea* (2003) states that it rectifies qi and loosens the center, and harmonizes the stomach and stops pain. It is used to treat chest and abdominal distention and fullness, and stomach duct pain. The dosage is given at 3–9g. The *Grand Dictionary of Chinese Medicinals* (2009) says that it courses the liver and rectifies qi, loosens the center and stops pain. It is also used to treat the chest and rib-side, breast distention and pain, painful menstruation, and stomach duct pain; dosage 5-10g in decoction, or can be ground and made into a tincture. The *Běn Cǎo Gāng Mù* (1590) says it is sweet, warm, without toxicity. It loosens the center, rectifies qi, and kills worms, and is used to treat stomach pain due to cold, abdominal fullness and distention, gan accumulation and worm pain, malaria, and dysentery.

Case Study

Male, 39 years old
Primary complaint: Varicose veins (spider veins) on lower legs
Other symptoms: Stress (owner of small business), anxiety (vexation), low energy, low appetite, insomnia with occasional night sweats (when very stressed and tired), irregular bowel movements with occasional diarrhea. Otherwise in good health with good eating habits and reasonable exercise, with a history of athletics.
Tongue: pale with a red tip, thin white coat
Pulse: weak, thin, slightly rapid
Diagnosis: spleen and heart qi vacuity, heart yin/blood vacuity with heart yin vacuity heat; also liver constraint qi stagnation and blood stasis.
Treatment strategy: boost qi, nourish blood and yin, calm spirit, harmonize liver and spleen, move blood.

Herbs:

Guī Pí Tāng with modifications	
báizhú	10g
dāngguī	6g
fúlíng	10g
zhìhuángqí	15g

yuǎnzhì	6g
lóngyǎnròu	6g
chǎosuānzǎorén	12g
rénshēn	3g
mùxiāng	10g
gāncǎo	6g
xiāngfù	6g
dānshēn	10g

External:

Cream of Horse Chestnut, Calendula, *hónghuā*, and Cayenne. Made in-house.

Explanation of formula:

Although the patient's primary complaint was varicose veins, he also had other issues that needed to be addressed. Varicose veins are not well-defined in the source literature, but seem to be related to damp-heat, blood stasis, and/or spleen failing to control the blood due to qi vacuity. The primary internal formula (modified *Guī Pí Tāng*) is a classic formula from the Ming Dynasty (*Zhèng Tǐ Lèi Yào*) for spleen qi/heart blood dual vacuity, and is also indicated for spleen failing to control the blood. The formula was administered as a decoction, with the two additions. *Xiāngfù* was added to assist *mùxiāng* to move qi and resolve liver constraint. The liver is thereby more able to order qi, which helps to resolve blood stasis. *Dānshēn* was added to assist *dāngguī* in both nourishing and quickening the blood. Although *chuāngxiōng* is more frequently used as a *duìyào* pairing for liver constraint qi stagnation with blood stasis, *dānshēn* was chosen because of its cooling nature and its ability to treat vexation. The external cream was advised, but the patient refused.

Return visit #1:

Patient returned two weeks later and reported a roughly 25% improvement in his secondary symptoms. He was feeling less anxious and had a bit more energy. His sleep showed only slight improvement. There was no improvement in his varicose veins, which I advised would likely be the case in such a short time and without the external application. The patient had, in the meantime, researched the external cream and now agreed to try it. Pulse and tongue showed little change. The formula was modified slightly by increasing the dosage of *zhìhuángqí* to 30g, *chǎosuānzǎorén* to 15g, and the *yuǎnzhì* to 10g. The patient was told to apply the external cream TID (morning and evening) by massaging it into the affected area.

Return visit #2:

Patient returned two weeks later and reported another 25% improvement, especially in his sleep and energy level. He also reported that the varicose veins had improved (shrunk). Upon visual examination, it was not apparent that they had, but I encouraged him to continue using the cream. The internal formula was not altered.

Return visit #3:

Patient returned three weeks later, but had only taken the internal formula for the first two weeks due to business travel. His symptoms had improved another 20% and he was feeling better than he had since starting the business (about 6 years earlier). He had continued to use the external cream because he was seeing improvement. In fact, he was quite excited to show me his legs. There was noticeable improvement in the varicose veins. He attributed this entirely to the external application of the cream. He said that he would take the internal formula for another two weeks (unless he had a setback) because he was getting tired of preparing and drinking the decoction. He was given more cream and told to call in three to four weeks.

The patient called back in about six weeks and reported feeling "much better" and that his varicose veins had improved by some 60–70%. He was asked to come in when he had time so I could inspect his legs. He came in several weeks later because he had finished the cream. There was an estimated 45–55% improvement, but nevertheless quite significant. He was advised to continue, and also to return to the internal formula. He refused the internal formula, but came back several weeks later for more cream, at which time there was another 5–10% improvement. The patient never returned. We met about one year later at a social function and he told me the varicose veins had improved slightly more, and had not regressed.

Although the external cream included several herbs, Horse Chestnut made up 50% of the formula. The other medicinals in the formula were Calendula, *hónghuā*, and Cayenne. These three primarily support Horse Chestnut in quickening blood. Cayenne also functions as a carrier to assist the medicinals to penetrate transdermally. This formula has been used on many patients with similar results.

1. Pittler, M. & Ernst, E. (1998). *Arch Dermatology*. 134(11): pp 1356–1360.
2. Sirtori, Cesare R. (2001). Aescin: Pharmacology, Pharmacokinetics, and Therapeutic Profile. *Pharmacological Research*. 44(3).

Bleeding Heart

Dicentra formosa (Haw.) Walp.
Papaveraceae
Dicentrae Formosae radix
Favor and Qi: acrid, bitter, warm, slightly poisonous
Channels entered: heart, liver
Actions: sedative, anodyne

Functions & Indications:

Quickens the blood, frees the channels, and relieves pain. Dicentra is used for symptoms of blood stasis due to knocks and falls, painful menstruation, hemorrhoids, abdominal pain, headache, etc. Dicentra is a very good blood quickening, pain relieving medicinal. Warmth can move and activate the blood (and qi) of the channels. Acridity is moving and disperses stasis. Bitter is draining, and enters the heart, which is the ruler of blood and the vessels. The combination of acridity and bitterness with its warm nature allows Dicentra to enter the vessels, quicken the blood, and free the channels to relieve pain.

Frees the channels and relaxes the sinews. Dicentra is used for symptoms associated with unregulated flow of qi in the channels causing pain, tugging and slacking, and spasms. Dicentra is acrid and warm, and is able to penetrate the channels and free the flow of qi and blood. This medicinal is also bitter, which can relax and drain. It warms and activates the qi and quickens the blood to help relax the sinews. The combination of its nature and flavors help to resolve pain and settle tugging and slacking, while also relieving spasms.

Cautions:

This is a relatively strong medicine, therefore, recommended dosage should not be exceeded without careful monitoring of the patient. It is contraindicated in pregnancy, nursing, very weak patients, and should be used with caution in serious cases of blood vacuity. Do not use if the patient is currently using narcotic pain medication. Overdose is likely to cause tachycardia, depression of respiration, drowsiness, and, possibly, nausea due to isoquinoline alkaloids.

Dosage and Preparation:

Fresh plant tincture 0.5–3ml, dry plant tincture 1–4ml, decoction (best if mixed–fried with alcohol) 2–6g

Major Combinations:

This medicinal may be used as a simple for pain control in acute traumatic injury. For this indication, use fresh plant tincture and start with 1ml every 5 minutes for 15 minutes, assessing the status of the pain before each subsequent dose.

Combine with *chuānxiōng* and *xiāngfù* for painful menstruation due to liver constraint and blood stasis. Omit *chuānxiōng*, and add *yùjīn* and Motherwort (or *yìmǔcǎo*) for stasis and constraint leading to fire, with symptoms of blood in the urine, bloody nose, tongue sores, etc. Add *guālóupí* and *zhǐshí* for fullness or stifling sensation in the chest.

Combine with *chuānxiōng*, *hónghuā*, and *báishào* for tugging and slacking, sore aching limbs from injury or excessive use (such as exercise), or pain due to external trauma. Add *dāngguī* for chronic problems with concurrent blood vacuity.

Combine with *sānqī* (1:4) for toothache or for post–dental surgery pain. In the case of toothache, this is a very effective short–term treatment for times when a person is unable to get to a dentist.

Commentary:

Dicentra is a small genus in the Papaveraceae (Poppy) family, comprised of only 18 species in North America and Asia, six of which are found in California. *D. formosa* is the only species with which I am familiar as a medicine, although I have heard reports of herbalists using other species. Many species within this family are well known and used including the opium poppy and the Chinese medicinal *yánhúsuǒ*.

Many gardeners are familiar with the species listed below, *D. spectabilis* (see *Translation of Available Source Material* below) (Note: This genus has apparently been renamed *Lamprocapnos*, but this has not become universal in the literature yet, so, it may be worth looking for both names in botanical guides if one is not listed.).

This species has a wide range and is quite common. It grows in all the mountainous areas (below 2200 meters) of California, from Santa Barbara to the Southern Sierra Nevada, and into British Columbia, Canada. It prefers damp shaded areas, but it also grows in drier areas in the summer which may have been wet earlier in the season, and/or are seeps.

The roots and rhizomes are harvested in the early spring or autumn, and generally tinctured fresh. This medicinal is very similar in action to the related *yánhúsuǒ*.

This plant has surprisingly little ethnobotanical information available regarding its uses, and almost no modern research has been done on it. Without these data, we must rely on botanical relationships and our experience.

Translation of Available Source Material:

There is one species of Dicentra listed in the *Grand Dictionary of Chinese Medicinals* (2009), *Dicentra spectabilis* (L.) Lem *hébāomǔdāngēn* (荷包牡丹根). This plant has a renamed genus, and is now known as *Lamprocapnos spectabilis* (Linnaeus).1 (The name change is not noted in the *Jepson Manual of Higher Plants of California* (2012), which covers the area where 6 of the 16 worldwide species grow.) This species grows in the Northeast part of China, as well as North Korea and extreme Southeast Russia, and has a long history of cultivation. In fact, it is the species (or a cultivar version) with which most gardeners are familiar. There is surprisingly little about the Chinese species in the Chinese literature. The *Grand Dictionary of Chinese Medicinals* says it harmonizes the blood, expels wind, and [is used for] anesthesia. It expels wind, moves blood, and relieves pain. It is also used to treat wounds with pain and toxicity, and stomach pain. The *Lǐng Nán Cǎi Yào Lù* (2009) says that it dissipates blood, disperses sore toxin, expels wind, and harmonizes the blood. Note: *Lǐng Nán*, as in the title of the book, is a collective term for Guang Dong and Guang Xi Provinces (southern-most China), which is a bit curious considering the plant is from the Northeastern part of the country. The herb can be used internally after being mix-fried with alcohol, or administered as a tincture.

1. Fukuhara, (1997). *Plant Syst. Evol.* 206: pp 415.

Bugleweed

Lycopus virginicus L., *L. europaeus* L., and others
Lameaceae
Lycopi herba
Other names: Water Horehound or Gypsywort (*L. europaeus*)
Chinese name: *L. lucidus zélán* (澤蘭)
Favor and Qi: bitter, cool
Channels entered: heart, lung, liver
Actions: anti–inflammatory, anti–hypertensive, sedative

Functions & Indications:

Clears the lungs and stops bleeding. Bulgleweed is used for symptoms of coughing of blood due to heat, mostly associated with phlegm and/or toxicity. Although this herb is mostly employed for chronic coughs with bleeding, it can also be used for acute cough with bleeding. Bugleweed is bitter, which allows it to move the qi of the lung downward, improving the diffusion and depurative downbearing action of the lung, in order to clear the lung; with cool bitterness, Bugleweed clears heat to stop bleeding due to heat.

Clears the heart and resolves vexation. Bulgleweed is used for heart vacuity with or without heat signs associated with yin vacuity (this could also include effulgent yin vacuity fire), and with or without vacuity of blood or qi, leading to vexation, palpitations, shortness of breath, fear of heat, weakness, and a rapid pulse. Bugleweed enters the heart channel and resolves vexation with cool bitterness.

Quickens the blood and relieves pain. Bulgleweed is used for pain of numerous conditions where static blood is the cause, such as painful menstruation, chest bi, and external injury. The heart governs blood and the vessels. Bugleweed enters the heart channel and quickens the blood to help relieve pain due to blood stasis. This medicinal is not as strong in this action as its cousin *zélán*, but is especially useful when these symptoms are combined with vexation due to yin vacuity.

Cautions:

There are none noted in the literature.

Dosage and Preparation:

Fresh plant tincture 2–4ml; infusion or light decoction 3–10g

Major Combinations:

Combine with Mullein and *báimáogěn* for yin vacuity cough with blood in the sputum; for more severe yin vacuity, *tiānhuāfěn* can be added; for more severe coughing, add *xìngrén* or Wild Cherry bark.

Combine with Lemon Balm, Motherwort, and *shēngdìhuáng* for heart vexation with palpitations due to heart yin vacuity; add *huánglián* for symptoms associated with effulgent yin vacuity fire.

Combine with Motherwort and *zhǐshí* for painful menstruation with concurrent vexation, fullness of the chest, and irritability. Add *chuānxiōng* or *dānggui* for more severe menstrual pain due to blood stasis. Add *xiāngfù* for more severe menstrual pain due to qi stagnation. Add *yùjīn* for heat patterns with severe menstrual pain.

Commentary:

Bugleweed is an unscented member of the mint family. The genus, *Lycopus*, has 10–14 species (depending on the source), with four species found in China and ten in North America, including *L. europaeus* (a non-native species from Europe). The genus can be found on all continents except Africa and Antarctica, with its center of distribution in North America. It should be noted that the uses of the single Chinese species (*L. lucidus*) are very similar to, sometimes the same as, both the herbs in this monograph. Many authors state that *L. virginicus* and *L. europaeus* can be used interchangeably, but the author only has experience with *L. virginicus* and the Chinese species *L. lucidus* (*zélán*). Most species have rhizomes, so cultivation from the wild is quite easy, making this a very sustainable resource.

Culpeper (1653) says of *L. europeans*, "The decoction of the leaves and flowers made in wine, and taken, dissolveth the congealed blood in those that are bruised inwardly by a fall, or otherwise, and is very effectual for any inward wounds, thrusts or stabs in the body or bowels; and is an especial help in all wound-drinks, and for those that are liver-grown (as they call it.)" Here, Culpeper discusses this plant's use in the treatment of blood stasis, which is similar to our Chinese medicinal understanding, at least in these particular injuries. At the end, he says "and especial help...for those that are liver-grown," which means an enlarged liver. This seems to indicate a direct action on the liver and the blood. Culpeper also says "It is wonderful in curing all manner of ulcers and sores, whether new and fresh, or old and inveterate; ...gangrenes and fistulas..." It is difficult to say whether he used it both internally and externally, or only externally. He likely saw this as a plant that would quicken the blood, and thus bring fresh blood supply to the area and assist healing since this was a common understanding at the time.

Interestingly, Salmon (1710) states, "As to the qualities of [*L. europeans*], authors have said nothing, but this I have found by experience, that it is an excellent vulnerary, whether inwardly taken in juice, essence, decoction, wine, or tincture, or outwardly applied in oil, balsam, ointment, cerate, or cataplasm, etc."

William Cook (1869) states (of *L. virginicus*), "It is indeed distinctly soothing, but acts upon the nervous peripheries and not upon the brain. Over-sensitiveness and irritability are relieved by it; but no stupor or sedation is induced. It relaxes the capillaries at the same time that it soothes arterial excitement; and thus slowly diverts the circulation outwardly, and relieves a too frequent and hard pulse, and lessens labored efforts of the heart." He seems to be describing a medicinal that clears heat, particularly when the heart is involved, but also is soothing and relaxing without narcotic effects. This puts this medicinal in a similar category as plants such as Lemon Balm and Motherwort (see Garran, 2008). They are all in the mint family, but only Lemon Balm is aromatic, and they all have similar cooling, calming, and (to some extent) nourishing qualities, although Motherwort is likely the only one of the three with overt nourishing properties (nourishes blood). All three act on the heart and have a long history of use for problems associated with heat entering the heart (channel) and causing various symptomology such as vexation, irritability, insomnia, etc. Not surprisingly, these three are also commonly used in *duìyào* combinations.

In Chinese medicine *yìmǔcǎo* (Chinese Motherwort) and *zélán* (Chinese Bulgleweed) are also commonly combined. *Commonly Used Paired Medicinals* (2007) states, "*yìmǔcǎo* regulates the menstruation and quickens the blood, disinhibits water and disperses swelling; *zélán* quickens blood and dispels stasis, disinhibits water and disperses swelling. This two medicinals used together, [treat] the blood and water, while concurrently regulating, together they create a strong blood quickening and water disinhibiting effect."

In his *Discussion of Chinese Medicinals* (2009) Yán Zhèng-huá adds that although *zélán* can be used for both hot and cold conditions, adding *yìmǔcǎo* when there is blood heat and stasis will lead to very good results in the clinic.

Although I could find no reference in the Chinese literature regarding the use of *zélán* for any sort of heart, chest, or vexation conditions, one source does support a similar use for nosebleed and coughing of blood (*Rì Huà Zǐ* circa 935). Most sources list *zélán* as slightly warming, while I list Bugleweed as cooling, which could potentially account for the difference in use, since vexation and the other conditions noted in the monograph are all generally associated with heat.

Ellingwood (1915) offers the following "*Specific Symptomatology*" for *L. virginica*: "In diseases of the heart, either functional or organic, marked by irritability and irregularity of the organ, dyspnea, feeling of oppression in the cardiac region, its administration is followed by gratifying results." Referring to inflammatory processes in the chest, he ads "...it not only effectually reduced the excessive heat, but in so doing, it did not depress in the least the vital forces of the patient." This is very important in showing the medicinal's definite action without being overly moving, cooling, or otherwise causing disturbance of the qi dynamic (a common issue when using medicinals that treat these types of patterns).

This genus shows promising results in the treatment of hyperthyroidism, as does one of the herbs it is commonly paired with, Lemon Balm. Yarnell and Abascal (2006) note the thyroid suppressing properties of several species within this genus, stating "These effects include the ability to inhibit binding of the stimulating antibodies of Graves' disease to the thyroid cells; blocking thyroid–stimulating hormone (TSH) production; decreasing peripheral T4 deiodinization; and possibly inhibiting iodine metabolism."[1] Hyperthyroidism affects approximately 1.3% of the population of the United States, but that number goes up 4–5 times in women over the age of 60.[2] Other studies show that the different ethnic groups are affected equally, although those of African decent seem to have a slightly lower incidence of this disease.

Translation of Available Source Material:

There is only one species, with one variation, listed from the *Lycopus* genus in Chinese medicine, *Lycopus lucidus* Turcz., and *L. lucidus* Turcz. var. *hirtus* Regel. This is the herb that is known as *zélán* (澤蘭), an important herb in the Chinese materia medica. It was first discussed in the *Shén Nóng Běn Cǎo*, where it is said to treat a variety of ailments including swelling and pain, spontaneous bleeding, and sores with pus.

1. Yarnell, E & Abascal, K., (2006). Botanical Medicine for Thyroid Regulation. *Alternative and Complementary Therapies.* 12(4): pp 107–112.

2. Hollowell, J.G., et al. (2002). Serum TSH, T(4), and thyroid antibodies in the United States population (1988 to 1994): National Health and Nutrition Examinations Survey (NHANES III). *Journal of Clinical Endocrinology and Metabolism.* 87(2): pp 489–499.

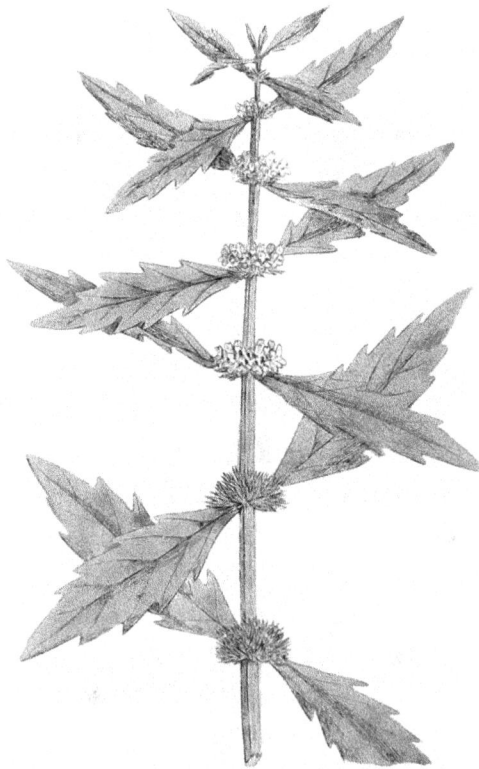

Blue Cohosh

Caulophyllum thalictroides (L.) Michx.
Berberidaceae
Caulophylli thalictroides rhizoma et radix
Chinese name: 類葉牡丹 or 紅毛七 (*C. robustum*)
Favor and Qi: acrid, bitter, warm
Channels entered: liver, spleen
Actions: emmenagogue, antispasmodic, antimicrobial

Functions & Indications:

Quickens the blood and resolves qi stagnation. Blue Cohosh is used for the treatment of menstrual disorders where there is blood stasis and qi stagnation. Blue cohosh is a very important herb for serious menstrual disorders such as profuse bleeding, menstrual block, or dysmenorrhea with serious qi stagnation leading to full/congested feeling in the lower abdomen. However, it is also frequently used for less serious conditions. Blue Cohosh's warm acridity both quickens the blood and moves qi to resolve stagnation.

Warms the channels, expels wind, transforms dampness, and scatters cold. Blue Cohosh is used for wind–cold–damp impediment, especially of the lower limbs. Blue Cohosh enters the channels and *luò* (經絡 *jīngluò*) and expels wind, dampness, and cold. It has an affinity for the lower part of the body and is efficient at relieving pain. This is a lesser known use of this medicinal. Blue Cohosh is acrid, bitter, and warm. With bitter acridity, it courses wind and transforms dampness, while penetrating the channels and *luò* with warm acridity to scatter cold.

Blue cohosh is known to facilitate labor when taken approximately 6 weeks prior to the due date. The action is also known to prevent premature delivery by its "tonifying" action on the reproductive organs. For this, is it often combined with Black Cohosh, Trillium, Mitchella, and sometimes other herbs such as Black Haw. Ellingwood (1915) states, "It has caused many cases [of pregnancy] to overrun their time a few days, and yet easy labors and excellent recoveries have followed." It is also used during labor when contractions are insufficient. For this, it is given every ten minutes at 10–20 drops of tincture until labor normalizes, at which time it can be discontinued."

Cautions:

Blue Cohosh has a long history of safe and effective use as a medicinal plant, but in recent years there have been several case reports suggesting that the use of Blue Cohosh is linked to serious problems when used during pregnancy. However, at this time, these reports cannot be substantiated, and without any concrete information, and in consideration of its long history of use, there seems to be no reason to be overly cautious with this medicinal.

Dosage and Preparation:

Infusion 3–6g; tincture 1–3ml; 3–6g decoction

Major Combinations:

Combine with *sānqī* and Cotton Root bark for excessive menstrual bleeding associated with qi stagnation and blood stasis.

Combine with Black Cohosh, Cramp Bark, and *hónghuā* for painful menstruation due to blood stasis. For painful menstruation associated with liver constraint qi stagnation, add to *Chái Hú Shū Gān Sǎn*. This is especially good when there is a sense of fullness and congestion in the lower abdomen, and pain and congestion in the legs associated with the menses.

Combine with Black Haw and Trillium for threatened miscarriage.

Combine with *huáiniúxī* and *Angelica brewerii* for lower back and leg pain due to cold in the channels.

Combine with *xùduàn* and *dùzhòng* for lower back and leg pain associated with kidney yang vacuity cold.

Commentary:

This Berberidaceae family plant is native to nearly all of eastern North America, excluding Texas, Louisiana, Mississippi, and Florida. The genus, *Caulophyllum*, has only two species; *C. thalictroides* (discussed here) and a Chinese species, *C. robustum* (see below for more information). In fact, some sources suggest that *C. robustum* is merely a subspecies of *C. thalictroides*. This plant is relatively slow growing and requires part to full shaded moist forests in order to thrive. Although the flowers are rather inconspicuous, the leaves have a blue-green hue and the fruit-like seeds slowly turn blue as they mature, making this an attractive ornamental in the late summer and autumn. This plant spreads by rhizomes, but grows slowly and won't flower for 3–4 years if planted from seed. Although transplanting may be possible, sources suggest that this plant does not like to be moved, so it may be best to use the slow growing seedlings.

According to Felter & Llody (1898), this is one of the oldest medicinal plants used by Europeans which is native to North America. It was first mentioned in the botanical literature in 1743, and the medical literature in 1813. The Native Americans, probably the Algonquins, introduced this plant to the foreigners.

This is a warming herb which also courses the channels, evidenced by numerous quotations such as the following, "In delayed menstruation in young girls, as where the woman has taken cold or menstruation stops from other cause than pregnancy, tuberculosis, or anemia, [Blue Cohosh] will restore it promptly."[1]

Blue Cohosh has a long reputation for use in the later stages of pregnancy, in combination with other herbs, as a preparation for giving birth. This was likely learned from Native Americans, and is probably why it used to be called "Squaw Root". The following is an example of a very popular formula used in the late 19th and early 20th Centuries, and is still used in today (because of the ecological status of Helonias root, a lily that is either threatened or endangered in all of its range, this medicinal is often substituted or left out of the formula).

Compound Syrup of Mitchella:
Partridgeberry (*Mitchella repens*) 4pts
Helonias (*Helonias bullata*) 1pt
Cramp Bark (*Viburnum opulus*) 1pt
Blue Cohosh (*Caulophyllum thalictroides*) 1pt

There is a specific preparation technique listed in Felter & Llody (1898), which is basically a combination of a percolation tincture (25% brandy) and an infusion, with the addition of sugar, and flavored with sassafras essence. This formula is recommended for "all cases where the functions of the internal reproductive organs are deranged, as in *amenorrhoea, dysmenorrhoea, menorrhagia, leucorrhoea,* and to overcome the *tendency to habitual abortion.*" For the latter complaint, it is advised to take 2–4oz. three times a day; during pregnancy it is used only 1 or 2 times per day.

Translation of Available Source Material:

Caulophyllum robustum Maxim. hóngmáoqī (紅毛七) is a yellow-flowered plant with blue-black berries and is found in the forested mountains throughout Central and Western China, even into the high elevations of parts of Tibet. The root and rhizome are used and it is prepared as a decoction (3–15g), as a tincture, or ground to a powder. The *Grand Dictionary of Chinese Medicinals* (2009) says that it is bitter, acrid, and warm. Functions are to quicken the blood and regulate the channels, expel wind, and move qi and stop pain. It is used for unregulated menstruation, channel pain, postpartum blood stasis with abdominal pain, pain and swelling of the stomach duct and abdomen, knocks and falls, and painful wind–dampness impediment.

Folk Medicine of Guizhou (1965) says it is slightly cold, bitter, acrid, and astringent, and is used to treat stomach-qi pain and external hemorrhoids. This opposite classification of temperature (qi) is quite interesting, but certainly not surprising. It is possible that this is a different species or that when found in a different region/ecosystem, its qi is different. However, as noted in the introductory material in the beginning of the book, this difference of opinion regarding qi and nature is not uncommon in the Chinese literature.

A Compilation of Commonly Used Folk Medicines (1959) states that it is used to treat blunt trauma, eliminate wind-dampness, disperse accumulations and swellings, treat sinew and bone pain, and free the channels and quicken the network vessels.

The *Shaanxi Chinese Herbal Medicine* states that its functions are to quicken the blood and disperse stasis, expel wind and stop pain, lower blood pressure, stop bleeding, and as a remedy for aconite poisoning. It is used to treat unregulated menses, pain in the lower abdomen associated with the menses, postpartum blood stasis with pain, arthritis, "work" related injuries [I assume this means something like injuries due to over-work or injuries common in farm work], tonsillitis, and high blood pressure.

Selected Herbs From Shanxi, Gan Su, Ning Xia, and Qing Hai (1971) has three combinations, each of which uses alcohol, but each in a slightly different way. The first is a simple tincture in which the medicinal is used as a "simple" or single remedy. It says to make a tincture with the herb (10g powder:300ml alcohol and steeping for 7 days) and taking this twice a day at 10ml dosage for joint inflammation and knocks and falls.

The second is also a simple formula using only this medicinal, where 3 grams of herb is ground to a power and dissolved in alcohol, and taken for stomach pain.

The third is a formula for the treatment of irregular menstruation and consists of *hóngmáoqī*, *báisháo*, *chuānxiōng*, and *fúlíng*, 10g each, cooked in yellow wine and water.

Unfortunately neither the second nor third combinations tell us how much alcohol to use, or in the case of the last formula, the ratio of water to wine. However, it is somewhat safe to assume that since the amount of alcohol was given for the first one, this can be used in the following situations as well, particularly the second one.

1. Arthur Weir Smith, Ed. *The Medicinal Plants of North America.* Berwyn, IL. D.H. Rosenberg, MD pp 40, 1914.

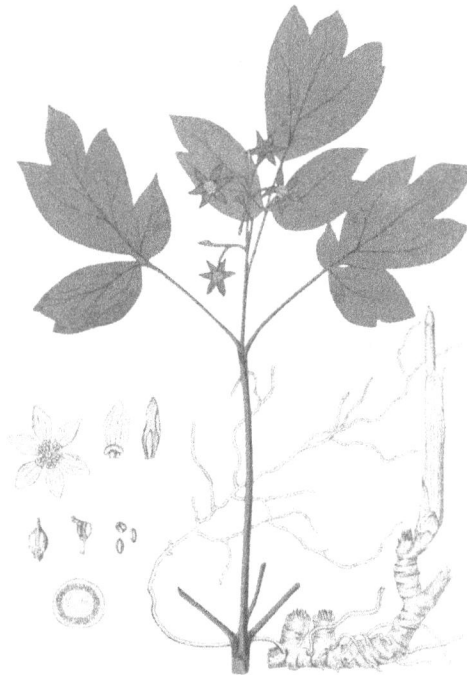

CAULOPHYLLUM THALICTROIDES. Michx.

Shepherd's Purse

Capsella bursa-pastoris (L.) Medik.

Brassicaceae

Capsellae Bursae-pastori herba

Other names: *jìcài* (薺菜)

Favor and Qi: sweet, bland, cool[1]

Channels entered: liver, spleen, urinary bladder[2]

Actions: hemostatic, anti–inflammatory, antihypertensive, antihistaminic, anti–hepatotoxic, anti–herpetic, anti–diabetic

Functions & Indications:

Cools the liver and stops bleeding. Shepherd's Purse is used for patterns of liver heat or liver fire causing frenetic movement of blood, with symptoms such as spitting blood, spontaneous external bleeding (including nosebleed), expectoration of blood, blood in the urine, flooding and leaking,[3] excessive postpartum bleeding, and blood in the stool. Shepherd's Purse enters the liver channel and is cooling. It effectively cools the liver to stop bleeding from liver heat or liver fire. Excessive postpartum bleeding and blood in the stool is more likely associated with spleen vacuity rather than liver heat, although the two patterns could easily be concurrent. Western herbal medicine has a long tradition of using this medicinal to stop these two types of bleeding, and experience shows that liver heat does not need to be present as a pattern diagnosis in order to utilize this medicinal. The medicinal enters the spleen channel, is sweet, and thus can stop bleeding via this energetic mechanism.

Calms the liver and brightens the eyes. Shepherd's Purse is used for liver fire surging upward, causing symptoms of red painful eyes, bleeding in the fundus of the eye, and high blood pressure.[4] Shepherd's Pulse is cool and enters the liver channel. This liver opens to the eyes and connects to the *dū* channel at the vertex of the head. By cooling the liver, Shepherd's Purse downbears heat from the head and *dū* channel, and can therefore lower blood pressure.

Clears heat and disinhibits dampness. Shepherd's Purse is used for damp–heat conditions with symptoms including dysentery, kidney inflammation with water swelling, and chyluria.[5] Shepherd's Purse is cool and bland. Blandness can disinhibit water and help to drain dampness. Cool blandness can be used to eliminate heat and dampness, especially in the lower burner.

Cautions:
There are no known cautions for this herb.

Dosage and Preparation:
Decoction: dried herb 15–30g; fresh herb 60–120g; fresh plant tincture 2–4ml (in serious bleeding this should be repeated every 15 minutes until the bleeding slows to at least half). The fresh plant tincture should be made each year. Although the Chinese materia medica lists the dry material as useful, most Western herbalists view it as very weak or inert.

Major Combinations:
Combine with *sānqī* and cotton root bark for flooding and leaking. Add Cramp Bark for concurrent cramping pain.

Combine with *huāngqín* for nosebleeds due to upward flaring of liver fire. This combination is also useful for expectoration of blood in the sputum. If, in the latter situation, there is thick, yellow or greenish sputum, add *yúxìngcǎo* and Echinacea

Combine with Golden Rod for reddish urination with short voidings of dark yellow urine. Add Marshmallow for painful, burning urination.

Combine with Mullein and *tiānhuāfěn* for coughing of blood with thick, difficult to expectorate sputum.

Commentary:
Shepherd's Purse is one of only four members of the *Capsella* genus; a name that comes from the Latin (meaning case or box) owing to the shape of its seed capsule that resemble a medieval purse. The genus is part of a the large and diverse Brassicaceae or Mustard family (338 genera and 3780 species), a family that is well-known for the many vegatables humans enjoy, including but not limited to broccoli, colards, kale, radish, bok choi, rape seed (Canola oil), and many others. Shepherd's Purse is native to Europe and SW Asia but is one of the most common weeds on Earth.

Shepherd's Purse is used in Chinese medicine, although it is not a primary herb. It is also consumed regularly as a spring vegetable known as *jìcài* (薺菜), which is the most common name for this medicinal, although there are a number of others. This member of the Mustard family is a common weed throughout most of the Northern Hemisphere, preferring trampled grounds such as pathways, but also popping up in newly tilled or disturbed areas. It is very easy to identify, owing to the heart shape of its seed pod, combined with an obvious rosette and relatively simple, though slightly branched, flowering stem. It is should picked before the flowering stem emerges (just the rosette) when using as a food. It gets tough and more bitter once the flowering stem arises, but can be harvested anytime for use as a medicine.

There is research showing the seed can be used to kill mosquitoes, which seems like an interesting application until one realizes the small size of the seed and the process for harvesting that seed. However, owing to the simplicity of cultivating this plant, a mechanized harvesting and willowing of the seeds could potentially offer an excellent way to deal with those pesky critters. I have been unable to find the original reference for this function, but it is noted many times throughout the literature. Apparently, the seeds are placed in water, and a mucilaginous substance from the seeds attaches itself to the mosquito larvae and suffocates them before they can emerge from the water. Considering the apparent safety of this method, it seems that there should be further study into the applications of Shepherd's Purse for mosquito control.

Gerard (1597) says of the temperature of Sheperd's Purse, "They are of temperature cold and dry, and very much binding." He credits three German writers with is assignment, but says that two other authors (one French and the other Spanish) say they are hot and dry (See commentary on this below under the entry for Salmon.). Gerard states that this medicinal stops bleeding in any part of the body by application of either the decoction or the juice. And, also says it is good for healing "green and bleeding wounds" and any "inflammations newly begun." Gerard very likely used this herb frequently. It is exceptionally common and has excellent therapeutic advantage for stopping bleeding.

Culpeper (1653) said this medical is "of a cold, dry, and binding nature..." and, "It helps all fluxes of blood, either caused by inward or outward wounds; as also flux of the belly, and bloody flux, spitting and pissing of blood, stops the terms in women..." There is nothing surprising here, as what Culpeper wrote is consistent with nearly every other authors' comments regarding this medicinal. However, other than mentioning that it makes a good ointment "for all wounds, especially wounds in the head," he does not mention the method of preparation. He often explicitly states that he is using fresh herb in other monographs, which means that he was either not using it in this way, didn't feel it was of particular importance, assumed it was obvious, or simply neglected to mention it.

Salmon (1710) notes some disagreement with regard to the nature of this medicinal and tries to rectify it. "Dodoneus, Matthiolus, and Ruellius say that Shepard's Purse is cold and dry, but Lobel and Pena hold them [Shepard's Purse] to be hot and dry, judging so from the taste of the seed, it having a little heat upon the tongue. Doubtless though the seed may be hot and dry in the first degree, yet the plant itself is temperate in respect to heat or cold, and dry in the second degree."

Shepard's Purse is a Cruciferaceae (Mustard) family plant, and like so many other plants within that family, the seed pods and seeds are spicy to the taste. This is interesting in so far as to gain a further understanding of how classical Western herbalists viewed and determined the nature of medicinal plants. Noteworthy is that Gerard, and then Salmon follows suit, calls this medicinal cold and dry, and although they don't say so specifically, it appears to be due to the fact that this medicinal stops bleeding, which by virtue of the medical theory of the time would require a cooling medicinal. It is also interesting to note that Salmon (and Gerard above) obviously had access to quite a few sources and was comparing them when he wrote his book.

Translation of Available Source Material:

Chinese medicine uses the exact same species as used in the West. [Rather than include translation here, I have translated sources and included them in the monograph above, and provided literature citations. If there is no citation, it comes from my experience with the herb.]

1. *The Grand Dictionary of Chinese Medicinals* (2009)
2. ibid
3. ibid
4. ibid
5. ibid

Mullein Flower

Verbascum thapsus L. and others
Scrophulariaceae
Verbasci flos
Chinese name: *máoruǐhuā* (毛蕊花)
Favor and Qi: acrid, bitter, warm
Channels entered: liver, heart, lung
Actions: diuretic, expectorant

Functions & Indications:

Moves qi and resolves blood stasis. Mullein flower is used for pain due to qi stagnation and blood stasis, such as earache, hemorrhoids, and knocks and falls. For this function, the flower is used both internally and, externally as an oil or liniment. Mullein flower is acrid warm. The combination of acrid flavor and warm qi can quicken the blood and move qi to effectively relieve pain. This medicinal is not narcotic, it is quite useful and similar in action to herbs such as *hónghuā*, and can be used as a substitute or as a *duìyào* for an effective pain-relieving combination.

Cautions:

None noted. Always use caution when using this, or any medicine, if putting it into the ear canal. The oil of this flower is one of the most common products to apply in a child's ear when they have an earache. Be sure the oil is neither too hot nor too cold; just above body temperature is the best.

Dosage and Preparation:

Infusion or light decoction 2–6g; fresh plant tincture 1–3ml; oil infusion as needed.

Major Combinations:

When infused in oil and used to treat ear infections, it is most commonly combined with garlic.

Combine with *hónghuā* and St. John's Wort for pain due to traumatic injuries; Add *sānqī* and Yarrow for bruising and bleeding. This combination can be used both internally and externally. Although

Mullein flower, *hónghuā*, and Yarrow can be used to produce an oil for external use, *sānqī* does not extract well in oil, so an alcoholic liniment should be prepared.

Combine with Horse Chestnut and St. John's Wort as an oil or salve for hemorrhoids. Add Yarrow and Plantain for bleeding.

Commentary:

Mullein flower is best known in North America as an ingredient in oil for external application to treat earaches in children. However, I have found this medicinal quite serviceable both internally and externally for the treatment of various types of pain. Externally, it is an excellent ingredient in liniments for knocks and falls, and internally for pain due to qi stagnation and blood stasis. For information on botany see the entry under Mullein leaf on page 131.

Culpeper (1653) stated, "And the oil made by the often infusion of the flowers, is of very good effect for the piles." I take "often infusion" to mean that the oil was infused several times with new flowers. This would naturally make the oil stronger medicinally than simply infusing it once. What we don't know is how much of the flowers he was infusing into the oil, i.e. the ratio of flowers to oil. In modern day herbal pharmacy, the general rule of thumb is to put as many flowers into the oil as the oil will cover. Heat is sometimes used today, which makes a stronger product, but Culpeper makes no mention of using heat, not even the sun (which is used by many folk herbalists).

Cook (1896) mentions a preparation whereby the flowers are allowed to sit in the sun in a jar, and oil exudes from them, after which this oil is collected and used in preparations. I have never made this preparation, but it seems like an interesting way to extract the oil—rather simple, but apparently effective.

I have also found the alcohol extraction of the flowers to be quite serviceable in combination with *hónghuā* and St. John's Wort in liniments where there is broken skin from external trauma. Although the alcohol is a bit painful at first, it is a good first aid when there is chance of infection and your ability to clean the wound is hampered by current conditions; think backpacking, or other outdoor sporting events where clean, hot water may not be readily available. I also like to add Yarrow to this combination!

Some ethnobotanical research has shown that this species as well as a number of other Verbascum species flowers are used for other lung complaints such as shortness of breath, pain the chest, cough, and panting (asthma).[1] While I have yet to use this medicinal for these indications, there is a substantial amount of ethnobotanical data suggesting that these uses warrant further investigation and are most likely to show results in the clinic.

Translation of Available Source Material:

See translation material in the Mullein leaf monograph.

1. Jaric S. et al. (2007). *Journal of Ethnopharmacology* 111: pp 160–175.

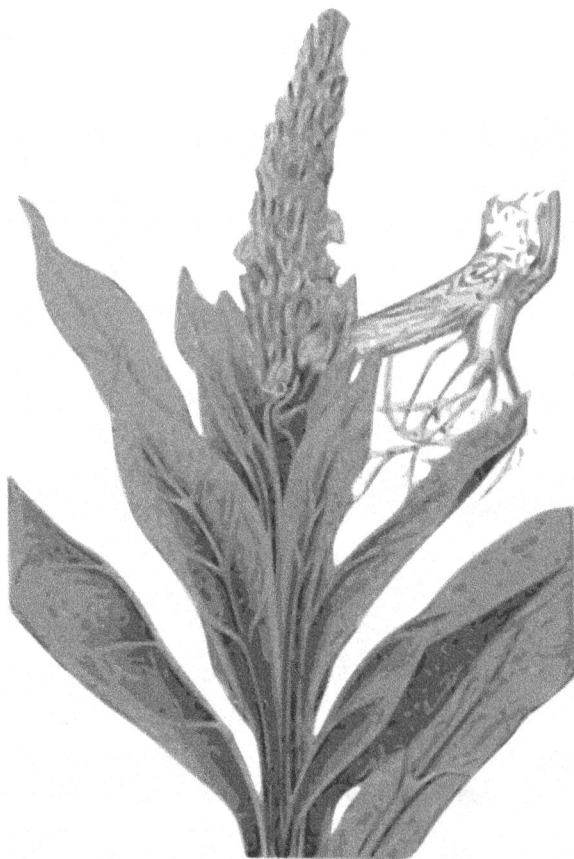

VERBASCUM THAPSUS . Linn.

Medicinal	Nature	Flavor	Channels	Functions	Indications
Calendula	cool	acrid, bitter	liver, lung	Clears heat, quickens blood, stops pain, and engenders flesh; Clears heat, quickens blood, resolves toxicity, and engenders flesh	external application for wounds due to knocks and falls; damaged tissue of the mouth, throat, stomach, and intestines, with or without bleeding
Horse Chestnut	warm	acrid, bitter	heart, liver, stomach	Rectifies qi, quickens the blood, and resolves constraint;	varicose veins or hemorrhoids, glomus
Bleeding Heart	warm	Acrid, bitter, slightly poisonous	heart, liver	Quickens the blood, frees the channels, and relieves pain; Frees the channels and relaxes the sinews	Pain from knocks and falls, painful menstruation, hemorrhoids, abdominal pain, headache, etc.; pain, tugging and slacking, and spasms
Bugleweed	cool	bitter	heart, lung, liver	Clears the lungs and stops bleeding; Clears the heart and resolves vexation; Quickens the blood and relieves pain	coughing of blood due to heat; vexation, palpitations, and a rapid weak pulse; static blood causing pain such as menstruation, chest bi, and external injury

Medicinal	Nature	Flavor	Channels	Functions	Indications
Blue Cohosh	warm	acrid, bitter	liver, spleen	Quickens the blood and resolves qi stagnation; warms the channels, expels wind, transforms dampness, and scatters cold	menstrual disorders where there is blood stasis and qi stagnation; wind-cold-damp impediment, especially of the lower limbs; facilitate labor
Shepard's Purse	cool	Sweet, bland	liver, spleen, urinary bladder	Cools the liver and stops bleeding; Calms the liver and brightens the eyes; Clears heat and disinhibits dampness	nosebleed, expectorating blood, blood in the urine, flooding & leaking, postpartum bleeding, & blood in the stool; red painful eyes, bleeding in the fundus of the eye, & high blood pressure; dysentery, kidney inflammation
Mullein Flower	warm	acrid, bitter,	heart, liver, lung	static blood is the cause of pain such as menstruation, chest bi, and external injury	pain due to qi stagnation and blood stasis, such as earache, hemorrhoids, & knocks & falls

補

虛

藥

Supplement Vacuity Medicinals

The supplementing vacuity category is an extremely important category of medicinals that is one of most intriguing groups of medicinals in Chinese medicine. This category is used to supplement and boost right qi, support vacuity and weakness, and treat vacuity of qi, blood, yin and yang. The category is divided into four sub-categories; supplement qi, supplement blood, supplement yin, and supplement yang.

Sweet flavor can supplement, therefore many of the medicinals in this category are sweet. Many, especially in the supplement blood and supplement yin sub-categories, can also be cloying in nature and care must be used when employing them; moving qi, strengthening the spleen, and/or dispersing food medicinals are almost always included in formulas with these medicinals.

These medicinals are generally taken over long periods of time either as decoctions, pills, or other preparations. Many people consider this category of medicinals to be important for most people as they age to be taken in small doses on a daily basis; this is the basis for many medicinal wines frequently consumed in China.

Care should be used when a person has an acute pathogen so that it is not get detained in the body. Likewise, care should be used when treating chronic illness that the illness is not being supplemented or boosted (making the illness worse). However, it is a misconception to think that these medicinals should never be used in acute illnesses. If a patient is ill and also has a significant vacuity it may be necessary to supplement in order for them to overcome and completely resolve the illness.

The medicinals in this materia medica are both well-known and, perhaps, somewhat obscure to many herbalists. However, I believe they represent significant therapeutic action and although some, like Licorice Fern and Pine Lousewort may not be easily procured, it is my hope that this information will further develop medicinals in the West within this extremely important category.

Gotu Kola

Centella asiatica L.
Asteraceae
Centellae herba
Chinese name: *jīxuěcǎo* (積雪草)
Favor and Qi: sweet, slightly bitter, cool
Channels entered: kidney
Actions: vulnerary, antiinflammatory, tonic

Functions & Indications:

Boosts essence, improves memory, and sharpens the wit. Gotu Kola is used for kidney vacuity with dulled wit, poor memory, slow reflexes, etc. Gotu Kola has a long history of use (especially in India's native medicine, Ayurveda) as a rejuvenate tonic for all types of disorders associated with kidney depletion in Chinese medicine. Gotu Kola is sweet, slightly bitter, and cool; its nourishing sweetness combined with mild bitterness offers the most common combination of flavors found in supplementing herbs.

Clears heat, cools the blood, and engenders fluids and flesh. Gotu Kola is used for patterns of damage to fluid, humor, or flesh caused either by heat or traumatic injury. Gotu Kola is particularly effective in treating tissue damage from various etiologies, and its cool nature further assists by clearing heat. Damage to fluids or flesh is generally caused by either heat damage or traumatic injury. In the case of external injury, heat often arises because the external trauma causes qi and blood stagnation, which usually engenders heat. Furthermore, if the flesh is cut, the inside of the body is opened up for easy invasion of external toxin. Gotu Kola can be used in either acute or chronic stages of these injuries, and can be used either internally or externally, although I find internal application to be more beneficial. Injury due to heat is generally internal, often causes bleeding, and affects systems such as the lung, stomach, and intestines. Gotu Kola is an excellent application in these patterns. Gotu Kola is sweet, slightly bitter, and cool. Coolness and bitterness can clear heat, while sweetness can nourish and engender fluids and flesh. The combination of these flavors and nature make Gotu Kola an excellent herb for treating both acute and chronic damage to both fluid and flesh.

Cautions:

Use this herb cautiously for those with vacuity cold, especially spleen/stomach cold.

Dosage and Preparation:

Decoction 10–15g, fresh plant tincture 2–4ml, up to 60ml fresh juice. Both tradition and modern science seem to agree that water extracts (i.e., decoctions) or fresh juice are the best for its kidney nourishing functions, and water extracts are preferred (both internally and externally) for use in healing wounds. In one study looking at the treatment of nerve damage, alcoholic extracts were shown to be the only extract effective for the regeneration of nerves.[1]

Major Combinations:

Combine with *shēnghuángqí*, *sānqī*, and *dānshēn* for slow-healing sores or deep wounds, including those from surgery or traumatic injury. Add *shānzhīzǐ* for local heat and swelling. Exclude the *shēnghuángqí* and add *dāngguī* for external application.

Combine with Comfrey, Plantain, Calendula, Goldenrod, Chaparral, *mòyào*, *zǐcǎogēn*, *dāngguī*, and St. John's Wort as an all-purpose external application for skin abrasions and minor cuts. This is a formula that combines some of the best botanical medicines from North America, Europe, the Middle East, and China to form a very effective application that can be prepared as a wash, paste, or salve.

Combine with St. John's Wort for nerve damage. This combination can be used both externally and internally, as a tincture.

Combine with Plantain and Calendula for abdominal or upper abdominal pain due to ulceration of the GI tract.

Combine with Golden Rod and *huángbǎi* for scant, burning urination associated with kidney yin vacuity. Remove *huángbǎi* and add Oregon Grape Root and *huángqín* for repletion patterns.

Combine with *báirénshēn* and *gǒuqǐzi* for kidney exhaustion with essence depletion associated with poor memory, impaired learning ability, dullness of thinking, etc.

Combine the fresh juice with a wide variety of fruits and vegetables for a refreshing and nourishing drink. This can be an especially valuable supplement for those in need of extra nutrition such as athletes, those recovering from major surgery or illness, chronically ill patients such as those suffering from cancer and receiving chemotherapy, or the elderly. It should be noted that this is a fresh juice and can damage the spleen of patients with spleen vacuity or dampness. To avoid this Ginger or other warming herbs can be added to the juice to help the spleen and stomach receive and transform this nutrition into usable food for the body.

Commentary:

Gotu Kola is a member of the genus *Centella* in the Apiaceae family, which is a small genus of less than 20 species mostly found in South Africa. The genus is not a common morphological representation of the family which usually has very obvious umbrella shaped inflorescense and include plants like *dāngguī*, Parsley, and carrot. *Centella asiatica* is a creeping low-growing plant that sends out stolons that generate roots at nodes, these nodes create a rosette of stems with the characteristic roundish leaf that helps to explain another common name for the plant, Asian Pennywort. It is a native of Asia from India east through SE Asia, but is now found as a week throughout the South Pacific islands, parts of Southeastern United States, tropical and subtropical areas of Central and South America, and some areas of Africa.

This plant is widely used around the world and in systems within its native range such as Ayurveda,[1] Thailand,[2] and Indonesia[3] as well as, more recently, in Western herbal medicine. Its place in Chinese medicine is quite fringe, which is curious. It is found commonly in all the southern provinces of China, and can be assumed to have been in most of that area since the time of antiquity. The *Shén Nóng Běn Cǎo Jīng* (circa 200CE) states that it is bitter, acrid, and cold, and treats great heat, sores, flat and welling abscesses, acute redness and swelling of the skin, and bodily heat. It is discussed in *Newly Revised Materia Medica* (659), and again in other important materia medicas, including modern textbooks used in China. The *Běn Cǎo Gāng Mù* (1590) has a more complete explanation of this medicinal, and even includes it in two formulas, one for "Lower Abdominal Pain in Women" the other for "Blood Disease in Men." However, these formulas are not named, nor are the ingredients given.

To my knowledge, there are no prominent modern formulas that utilize this medicinal, and I have not seen it prescribed in a Chinese clinic or hospital.

It is a very common weed throughout the tropics and some sub-tropical area. In fact, while I lived in Hawai'i, I noticed that many people were constantly trying to rid their lawns of this plant; meanwhile, I was cultivating it in my little garden as a groundcover below the basil and other plants.

The body of modern research is relatively large with studies focusing on its wound healing, cognitive, and nerve regenerative actions. The list of studies on its wound healing properties is long, but the following from a review paper sums it up very well:

> "In numerous pharmacodynamics studies involing animal experiments and in vivo experiments with human fibroblasts, the clinical, mechanical, cellular and bio-chemical effects of Centella asiatica have been investigated. The topical application of Centella extracts has shown to be associated with accelerated wound healing in abnormal conditions of the skin associated with a reduction in granuloma weight, and an increase in the force needed to produce rupture (rupture strength) of the wound. In addition, further studies have revealed a dose-dependent increase in the synthesis of collagen, intracellular fibronectin content, an increase in mitotic activity of the germ layer, and an enlargement of the kerato hyaline granules in the scar tissue."[4]

The above is relatively convincing and comprehensive in scope showing Gotu Kola should have a place in the treatment of wounds. In a study done in 2012, aqueous extracts were shown to improve scratch wounds to corneal tissue,[5] suggesting a low cost and effective way for people approach eye injuries. There has been work done showing Gotu Kola can increase the growth of nerve tissue. In a paper published in 2005, the authors summarize their findings by saying, "In summary, our findings clearly demonstrate the therapeutic efficacy of oral administration of the ethanolic extracts of *Centella asiaitica* for accelerating nerve regeneration in the peripheral nervous system *in vivo*."[6] In a study done with the aqueous extracts (prepared as a solid or powered extract similar to those used in Chinese medicine, but with no binder added) was shown to have significant positive outcomes in rats with Alzheimer's disease. The authors conclude the paper with the following statement, "In conclusion, the present study demommstrates that *C. asiatica* significantly prevented cognitive impairment and attenuated the oxidative stress induced by brain glucose metabolism impairment in i.c.v. STZ–treated rats by its neuroprotective property. However, the possibility of an effect of *C. asiatica* on neurotransmitters in improving cognitive deficits cannot be ruled out."[7] Finally, in a study done in India with an extract using undisclosed solvents showed, "The repetitive administration of *Centella asiatica* further to 2 showed the significant increase in % accuracy of both numeric working memory and wor recognition. In addition, *Centella asiatica* also showed significan increase in reaction time of both numeric working memory and spatial memory." And, "It is very striking that *Centella asiatica* improves not only the cognititive performance but also the mood. The high dose of *Centella asiatica* could increase calmness and alertness after 1 and 2 months of treatment. In addition, the significant increase in calmness was also observed after *Centella asiatica* treatment at medium and high doses for 2 months."[8] Medium and high doses were 500mg and 750mg respectively, once a day.

These data show that there appears to be a difference in the method of extraction of this medicinal, aqueous or ethanol. However, most herbalists, if possible prepare Gotu Kola as a fresh plant extract, and I certainly recommend this. This may be worth investigating since the opinion of many prominent herbalists and botanical pharmacists (in most cases), is that production of fresh plants offers not only a more potent representation of the plant, but also tends to yield both water and alcohol soluble constituents. Also, the ethnobotanical literature suggests the traditionally healer prefer the fresh plant over the dried, and often administer this medicinal as a juice. Further investigation is warrented.

Translation of Available Source Material:

This medicinal first appeared in the *Shén Nóng Běn Cǎo Jīng*, and has held a place in many other materia medicas through history. As noted above in the commentary, I find it quite curious that it is not part of regular practice in today's Chinese medicine. Here, I will present some information from the *Grand Dictionary of Chinese Medicinals* (2009) and, although much of what you will find here is also found in the above monograph, you will notice that I have some slightly different ideas about the mechanism of action, or how it functions according to Chinese medical theory. It is considered bitter, acrid, and cold, and is said to enter the lung, spleen, kidney, and urinary bladder channels. It is ascribed the functions of clearing heat and disinhibiting dampness, quickening the blood and staunching bleeding, and resolving toxin and dispersing swelling. It is used to treat heat effusion, cough, throat swelling and pain, intestinal inflammation, dysentery, damp–heat jaundice, water swelling, strangury patterns, blood in the urine, spontaneous external bleeding or nosebleed, painful menstruation, flooding and spotting, clove toxin, scrophula, swollen and toxic boils and sores, herpes zoster, swelling and pain due to knocks and falls, bleeding due to external injury, and snake and insect bites.

Although there is no doubt that this medicinal can be used for the above conditions and symptoms, I believe this is too narrow a view, and Chinese medicine practitioners should learn to use this medicinal and include it in other ways.

Case Study

Male, 33 years old

Primary complaint: poorly healing wound from auto accident and subsequent surgery; pain.

Other symptoms: Patient is over–all good health, slightly over–weight, gets regular exercise, eats fatty diet, no other health complaints. Patient suffered a serious auto accident in which his left leg was badly injured; flesh, nerve, and bone injury were incurred in the lower thigh and knee area. The patient lost a significant amount of blood and there is numbness on the lateral and posterior aspect of the lower leg and lateral aspect and sole of foot. Motor skills were difficult to assess because of the injury, but there appears to be loss of motor function of two lateral toes.

Tongue: dry, cracked, pale

Pulse: thin, only slightly weak

Diagnosis: acute blood vacuity; wound is open, hot (inflamed), and damp with small amounts of pus, patient is taking antibiotics. Wound is healing very slowly; doctors are concerned but only treating with antibiotics and regular debridement.

Treatment strategy: nourish blood, generate flesh, quicken blood, treat numbness.

Herbs:

Dāngguí Bù Xuè Tāng with modifications

huángqí, dāngghuī, jīxuěcǎo, dānshēn

Formula given as a powered extract (granules). Primary formula 50%, Gotu Kola (*jīxuěcǎo*) 40%, *dānshēn* 10%. Dosage 6g TID

External:

Plaster of Gotu Kola (powdered extract), Gotu Kola (fresh plant tincture), St. John's Wort (fresh plant tincture), Calendula (powdered). Made in-house.

Explanation of formula:

Dāngguí Bù Xuè Tāng is the most important formula in Chinese medicine for blood vacuity due to acute loss of blood. Gotu Cola (also a Chinese medicinal available as a powered extract) is well-known for its ability to engender flesh and heal wounds, as well as mend nerves. *Dānshēn* cools the blood and supports *dāngguī* to nourish the blood. It is also known to improve microcirculation, thus helping to heal wounds. This combination also works to quicken the blood and relieve pain without damaging right qi. The external formula was made by taking the powdered extract of Gotu Kola and adding ground Calendula, then moistening it with the two tinctures. This was allowed to dry so that the alcohol would evaporate, then moistened with saline when applied. While Gotu Cola is well-known for wound healing, research shows that alcohol extracts are better for healing nerves. Calendula is a primary medicinal for wound healing, quicken blood, and stops pain. St. John's Wort is also an excellent wound healing medicinal, clears heat, stops pain, and helps to heal nerve damage. Because of concerns from the doctors, the external application was not applied the first week.

Return visit #1:

After one week the patient showed significant improvement. Pain was much reduced as was redness and swelling. There was also significant improvement in granulation of the wound. This impressed the doctor enough to request to know what I was doing. The patient gave approval for us to communicate, and after a 20 minute conversation with him, I convinced him to allow the patient to apply the external preparation.

Return visit #2:

One week later there was marked improvement in the wound. No change in treatment.

Return visit #3:

Continued improvement and the patient suggested that he was feeling some sense of tingling in his lower leg and foot where there had only been numbness before. Patient's tongue was no longer dry and cracked and was close to normal color. I advised the patient to continue with the internal formula until he ran out (about 10 days) and call me if he needed anything.

Patient called in two weeks and said he had stopped both the internal and external treatment. He was still having tingling in his lower leg and foot, but now that he could move his lower leg more easily, there was impaired function in his two most lateral toes and ankle. The wound was about 70% healed. I advised him to continue with the external treatment and added a fresh plant tincture of Gotu Kola 70% and St. John's Wort 30% as an internal therapy.

Patient called two weeks later, wound now 90% healed, there was improvement in the sensation of the back of the leg and foot, mostly tingling and sensitivity to hot and cold. I advised the patient to use Castor oil packs in the area surrounding, but not in, the wound. I also advised him that when the wound was completely healed to continue both the tincture and the Castor oil packs, but at that time he could apply the Castor oil packs to the area of the healed wound.

Patient called 3 weeks later, the wound was completely healed over. He had marked improvement in both sensations and motor skills of the lower leg. I advised him to continue treatment for one month and contact me. He called back in two weeks to tell me, other than muscle atrophy and weakness, he felt about 85% improvement in all other symptoms related to nerve damage. He wanted to ask if he needed to continue the Castor oil packs because they were messy. I advised him to do them for one more week, but to continue the herbs for another month, regardless of how he felt. He agreed.

The last time I saw this patient, about one year later, he had full motor control and sensory abilities in his lower leg. Scaring appeared minimized considering the original wound, and he was back to good health.

1. Dash, Vaidya Bhagwan & Kashyap, Vaidya Lalithesh. *Materia Medica of Ayurveda: Based on Ayurveda Saukhyam of Todarānanda.* New Delhi, India: Concept Publishing Company, 1980.

2. Brinkhaus, B., et al., (2000). Chemical, Pharmacological and clinical profile of the East Asian medical plant *Centella asiatica. Phyomedicine.* 7(5): pp 427–448.

3. ibid

4. ibid

5. Idrus, Ruszymah Bt Hj, et al., (2012). Aqueous extract of *Centella asiatica* promotes corneal epithelium wound healing in vitro. *Journal of Ethnopharmacology.* 140(3): pp 333–338.

6. Soumyanath, A. et al. (2005). *Centella asiatica* accelerates nerve regeneration upon oral administration and contains multiple active fractions increasing neurite elongation in–vitro. *Journal of Pharmacy and Pharmacology.* 57(9): pp 1221–1229.

7. Kumar, Veerendra MH & Gupta, YK, (2003). Effects of *Centella asiatica* on cognition and oxidative stress in an intracerebroventricular streptozotocin model of Alzheimer's disease in rats. *Clinical and Experimental Pharmacology and Physiology.* 30: pp 336–342.

8. Wattanathorn, Jintanaporn, et al., (2008). Positive modulation of cognitive and mood in the health elderly volunteer following the administration of *Centella asiatica. Journal of Ethnopharmacology.* 116(4): pp 325–332.

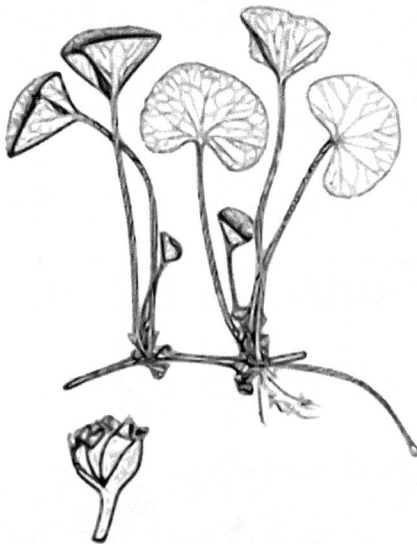

Stinging Nettle Seed

Urtica dioica L.
Urticaceae
Urticae Dioicae semen
Favor and Qi: sweet, slightly bitter, neutral
Channels entered: kidney, liver
Actions: nutritive tonic

Functions & Indications:

Supplements qi, benefits the kidney, and engenders essence. Stinging Nettle seed is used for kidney qi vacuity and depleted essence leading to lethargy, fatigue, loss of appetite, weight loss, muddled thinking, low sex drive, etc. Stinging Nettle seed is sweet and slightly bitter. This is a common combination of flavors for medicinals that supplement such as *rénshēn*. Sweetness nourishes, while the slight bitterness gently drains in order to prevent stagnation from the supplementing action.

Cautions:

None noted

Dosage and Preparation:

Tincture 2–4ml; decoction or draft 3–10g

Major Combinations:

Combine with *rénshēn* and *shúdìhuáng* for kidney qi vacuity and essence depletion with fatigue, loss of appetite, and weight loss. Add *huángqí* and *báizhú* for severe loss of appetite and lethargy. Add *yínyánghuò* for marked loss of sex drive, especially combined with muscle weakness and pain.

Commentary:

Stinging Nettle is a common plant found throughout North America and Europe and, typically, it has been the leaf which is used in medicine (see Garran 2008). Stinging Nettle is one of 45 species in the genus *Urtica*, which is in the Urticaceae family (Stinging Nettle). The family is found throughout much of the world with its biogeographical center in Asia. China has some 14 species with three endemic, while North America only has four species. *U. dioica* is found in North America, Europe, North Africa, Central Asia, and into China. The plant has been widely used as food, medicine, cordage, fodder, and is considered to be a primary plant in bio–dynamic and ecological agriculture practices.

Stinging Nettle seed is not widely used, compared to the leaf, or even the root, the latter of which has gained repute as a medicinal for prostate problems (BPH) over the last decade or so. However, the seed of this plant has been shown to reduce serum creatinine levels, thus improving renal glomerular function in patients with kidney disease.[1] When treating kidney failure, this is clinically significant and should be considered by practitioners as an important medicinal.

Dioscorides (2000, *trans.*) states, "A decoction of the seed (taken as a drink with *passum* [raisin wine]) is an aphrodisiac and opens the womb. Mixed in with honey it helps asthma, pleurisy and pneumonia, and fetches up stuff out of the chest. It is mixed with antiseptic preparations." This is likely the source for both Culpeper and Salmon's information on this medicinal (see below). The first sentence is likely the source of Salmon's comment (discussed below) regarding Stinging Nettle seed's apparent action on the kidney, as understood by Chinese medicine. However, Dioscorides merely states that it functions as an "aphrodisiac," not necessarily that it can be used for physiologically depressed sexual desire or function. Since Dioscorides does not explain in detail, we have no way to ascertain his precise meaning. However, because Dioscorides specifically says "incites sexual union" and "encourages lust" in other plant monographs, one may loosely assume that he ascribes the improvement of decreased sexual function to Stinging Nettle seed, "aphrodisiac," rather than simply heightened libido for anyone, "incites sexual union" and "encourages lust".

Gerard (1597) says, "The seed of [Stinging] Nettle stirs up lust." And is used in combination with other medicinals [he does not say which ones] to "draw out of the chest raw humors." The former statement is likely the origin of Salmon's statements below and likely is derived from Dioscorides. Gerard continues his discussion on Stinging Nettle seed's use for lung complaints with: "It is good for them that cannot breathe unless they hold their necks upright, and for those that have the pleurisy, and for such as be sick of the inflammation of the lungs..." What is interesting about this statement is that he is very specific in the condition necessary for the patient to breathe, which suggest evidence of a kidney qi vacuity. If the patient must sit up straight in order to breathe, this suggests that the kidney qi is too weak to draw the breath in and down.

Parkinson (1640) only mentions the seed briefly in his monograph saying that they can be pounded and snuffed up the nose to staunch bleeding. While he discusses very similar symptomology to Gerard in his monograph, he suggest the leaves or roots to be used rather than the seed.

Culpeper (1653) mentions the use of the seed several times, primarily in combination with the leaves (for a monograph of the leaves, see Garran 2008). However, he makes an interesting statement about the seeds as separate medicine, "The seed drank, is a remedy against the stinging of venomous creatures, the biting of mad dogs, the poisonous qualities of hemlock, henbane, nightshade, mandrake, or such like herbs that stupefy or dull the senses (Gerard also mentions quicksilver, aka mercury); as also the lethargy, especially to use it outwardly, to rub the forehead or temples in the lethargy,...with a little salt." Although I would not recommend this as an antidote for poisons, it is good information that, in an emergency, might be beneficial. This action may also speak to its action on the kidney, as noted above, to improve the renal glomular functions if there was damage caused by the toxins in these plants mentioned. Even though he seems to be particularly fond of using this medicinal externally (combined with salt) for lethargy, he also says to use it internally, which supports the usage described in the monograph above, as a medicinal to treat vacuity detriment. Culpeper also states, "...the seed, provoks urine and expells the gravel and stones in the reins or bladder..." Although I would suggest that this action applies more to the leaves, this reference shows that the seeds have an affinity for the kidney.

Salmon (1710) echoes much of what Culpeper wrote, however, he states, "...the seed is the strongest [compared to the leaf], or more effectual." Also, the seed "provokes lust." However, Salmon seems to favor its internal use, for lethargy, "being taken with a little salt" and recommends that the powerful seed be taken in 4-6g dosages in a glass of "generous wine."

There is not much difference between the monographs of latter three authors, and one might wonder how much of what Salmon and Culpeper wrote was merely taken from Gerard (or perhaps some other author), and how much was from their own clinical experience. However, what we have from Salmon is a dosage for the seeds, as well as another method of administration, which is very much in line with some modern usages. Furthermore, the phrase, "provokes lust" can be reasonably assumed to refer to "sex drive," which originates in the kidney according to Chinese medicine (essentially a function of kidney qi). Thus, one might also reason that Stinging Nettle seed supplements the kidney qi and/or engenders essence.

A final note is the use of salt when preparing this medicinal. The use of salt in Chinese medicine *páozhì* (preparation of medicinals) is used to prepare medicinals that are being guided to the kidney. The *Dictionary of the Study of Chinese Medicinals Preparation* (2004) states:

> "Salt processing enters the kidney: salt's flavor is salty, it's nature is cold. Salty [flavor] goes to the kidney, therefore after medicinals undergo salt processing they are more likely to enter the kidney, and they are more efficacious for treating symptoms of the kidney channel."

All the authors above mention specifically that Stinging Nettle seed is used for various kidney ailments, both Culpeper and Salmon mention the use of salt in its preparation (albeit external, although Salmon leaves the question open to whether or not this should be only external or also internal) for the use of Stinging Nettle seed for lethargy. While this may be a bit of a stretch, it does show a possible connection to these authors' understanding of this medicinal in a Chinese context.

1. Treasure, J. (2003). *Journal of the American Herbalist Guild*, 4(2): pp 22–25.

Licorice Fern

Polypodium glycyrrhiza D.C. Eaton
Polypodiaceae
Polypodii Glycyrrhizae rhizoma
Favor and Qi: sweet, slightly bitter, slightly cool
Channels entered: lungs, kidney
Actions: antitussive, nutritive tonic

Functions & Indications:

Nourishes yin and supplements lung qi. Licorice Fern is used for chronic cough with weakness, dry cough, and panting. Licorice Fern is also used for shortness of breath and sweating upon exertion. Licorice Fern is sweet and slightly bitter. Sweet can nourish while bitter can drain. The combination of sweet and slightly bitter is a important combination for supplementing medicinals.

Opens the chest and assists the lung with its dupurative downbearing action. Licorice Fern is used for symptoms of oppressive sensation in the chest, cough, panting and wheezing, and shortness of breath. As noted above this medicinal has the classic supplementing combination of sweet and slightly bitter. This combination of flavors allows supplementing while gently draining so that stagnation is less likely. When using this medicinal to open the chest, an alcohol extract is used because the alcohol better extracts the bitter flavor and adds a qi moving function from the warm acrid nature of alcohol. Thus, the primary flavors acting in this preparation are bitter, which can drain, and acrid, which can move, but also sweet that helps to improve the function of the lung. The warm acridity of the alcohol extract opens the chest while the more strongly bitter extraction of the alcohol assists with the dupurative downbearing action of the lung.

Cautions:

None noted

Dosage and Preparation:

Decoction 2–6g (up to 10g); dry plant tincture 1–4ml

Major Combinations:

Combine with *wŭwèizĭ* for symptoms of chronic cough due to lung yin and qi vacuity. Add *màiméndōng* or Marshmallow for dry cough.

Combine with *zhĭshí* and *jiégĕng* for an oppressive sensation in the chest with cough and a short, string–like pulse.

Combine with *guālóu* and Yerba Santa for chest oppression combined with abundant white sputum and a pale tongue with a thick greasy coating.

Commentary:

This monograph examines *Polypodium glycyrrhiza* and although a related species, *P. vulgare*, can be used as a substitute. The latter medicinal is not nearly as good as a qi supplementing medicinal, although it is a good yin supplementing medicinal and functions better as a heat clearing medicinal. While both herbs clear heat (especially yin vacuity heat), *P. glycyrrhiza* acts more like a supplementing medicinal than *P. vulgare*. Both seems to have a similar action to open the chest, but *P. glycyrrhiza* is the species that I have the most experience with and is the species I harvest myself. I have worked to some extent with *P. vulgare*, but since it does not seem to have the same supplementing action as P. glycyrrhiza I have chosen to avoid it.

Polypodium is a genus of about 160 species. A number of these species are used in medicine in Europe, Asia, and the Americas. The prefix "poly" means "many" and "podium" means "feet," thus we have "many feet." *P. glycyrrhiza* is a species that is only found in the Western mountain areas of North America and, perhaps, the northern part of Russia. It prefers the old-growth forests and will grow epiphytically on trees, or as a lithophyte on rocks, on dead logs, and even on the ground. Its preferred habitat is forests dominated by big-leaf maple (*Acer macrophyllum*). This species' preference for old-growth forest calls into question its sustainable harvest and use because of the rapidly shrinking old-growth forests and the imperative to preserve them. That said, it is a common species within its range and will, if given enough time, colonize second-growth forests. While the author is not aware of any cultivation of this medicinal, he believes that, given the right habitat, Licorice Fern could be cultivated.

The Native Peoples within its range have a long history using this plant both as a medicine as well as a food. Ethnobotanical research reports its use for cough, sore throat, and colds as well as a number of other ailments.[1,2,3,4]

Within the main body of the monograph there are two functions which are quite different. The first is a supplementing function, while the second is a moving function. This is a clear example of how a water extraction and an alcohol extraction can give two different medicines. As the botanical Latin name (*P. glycyrrhiza*) implies, this plant has a very sweet root. In fact there has been some research into the chemistry of the sweet components of this plant.[5,6] This chemistry is water soluble (and slightly alcohol soluble) and therefore water extractions, i.e. decoctions, better represent this fraction of the medicine. Other aspects of the medicinal, such as it's bitter qualities can be better extracted with alcohol and water. So, although a hydro–alcoholic extract will be less sweet, and therefore less nourishing, it will be more bitter and, as noted in the monograph above, also carry with it the warm acrid nature of the alcohol. Therefore, when using this medicine for the different functions indicated in the monogrpah, it is important to apply these different methods of preparation.

Additionally, although I have not tried this, I suspect that the alcohol mix–fried version of this medicinal, then prepared as a decoction, might yield similar medicine to that of the tincture. This method of preparation is used for many medicinals in Chinese medicine. They are first prepared by mix–frying them with alcohol prior to decotion, i.e. *dānggūi* is first mix–fried in alcohol to improve its blood quickening properties. The use of alcohol can be used to our advantage, whether using the Chinese traditional *páozhì* technique, or the Western traditional tincture technique. An example of how using the tincture technique might benefit clinical outcome is the Chinese medicinal *xiāngfù*, which when extracted with alcohol offers the practitioner a stronger qi moving medicinal than the water extraction. It is important to note that many supplementing medicinals do not extract well as tinctures, e.g. *huángqí*, which although is useful as an alcoholic extraction is far less effective than a water extraction (decoction). This is primarily due to the chemical constituents (polysaccharides) of these medicinals only being soluble in water, or only poorly soluble in alcohol.

Translation of Available Source Material:

There are two species of *Polypodium* used in Chinese medicine, as the same medicinal, *P. vulgare duōzújué* (多足蕨) and *P. virginianum dōngběiduōzújué* (东北多足蕨). However, some botanical literature suggests these two are actually the same species. (See more information on *P. vulgare* in the *Commentary* section above.) The *Grand Dictionary of Chinese Medicinals* (2009) lists it as sweet, bitter, and cool. It has the function of resolving toxin and abating heat (fever), expelling wind and disinhibiting dampness, and stopping cough and pain. It is used to treat children's fever, panting and cough, urinary tract infection, wind–dampness joint pain, and toothache. Externally, it is used to treat Stinging Nettle rash, swelling and toxin of sores and boils, and injuries due to knocks and falls. Internally, it is prepared as a decoction in 10–30 gram dosages. Externally, it is boiled first, then pounded to a paste and applied.

1. Compton, B.D. (1993). *Upper North Wakasha and Souther Tsimshian Ethnobotany*. Ph.D. Dissertation, University of Columbia.

2. Turner, N.J. (1973). The Ethnobotany of the Bella Coola Indians of British Columbia. *Syesis* 6: pp 193–220.

3. Turner, N.J., Thompson, L.E., Thompson, M.T., and York, A.Z. *Thompson Ethnobotany: Knowledge and Uses of Plants by the Thompson Indians*. British Columbia Provincial Museum Memoir No. 25. British Columbia Provincial Museum, Victoria, British Columbia, pp 321.

4. Gunther, E., *Ethnobotany of Western Washington*. University of Washington Press, Seattle. pp 71. 1973.

5. Kim, Jinwoong, Pezzuto, John, M., Soejarto, D. Doel, Lang, Frank A., Kinghorn, A. Douglas. (1988). Polypodoside A, An Intensely Sweet constituent of the Rhizomes of *Polypodium glycyrrhiza*. *Journal of Natural Products*. 51(6): pp 1166–1172.

6. Kim, Jinwoong & Kinghorn, A. Douglas. (1989) Further Steroidal and Flavonoid Constituents of the Sweet Plant, *Polypodium glycyrrhiza*. *Phyochemistry*, 28(4): pp 1225–1228.

Red Baneberry

Actaea rubra (Aiton) Willd.

Ranunculaceae

Acteae rubrae rhizoma et radix

Favor and Qi: sweet, slightly bitter, slightly acrid, warm

Channels entered: liver, spleen

Actions: antispasmodic, antiinflammatory

Functions & Indications:

Nourishes the liver, enriches blood, and relaxes the sinews. Red Baneberry treats a variety of symptoms associated with liver blood vacuity, such as scant menstruation (especially with associated painful menstruation), tugging and slacking, sinew hypertonicity, and pain. Red Baneberry is sweet, slightly bitter, and slightly acrid. Sweetness nourishes, while the combination of slightly bitter and acrid, along with its warm nature, allows it to nourish without causing stagnation. Bitter and acrid flavors are the two flavors with the most significant action to move qi and blood in the body and warm nature inherently moves. The liver stores the blood and governs the sinews. When liver blood is vacuous menstruation can become scant and the liver is unable to properly nourish the sinews. This leads to symptoms such as tugging and slacking (spasms) and pain. Red Baneberry nourishes the liver blood while also moving the blood. This not only helps to relieve the pain or discomfort associated with these symptoms, it also facilitates the nourishment of the blood in the sinews.

Quickens the blood and resolves stasis. Red Baneberry treats blood stasis due to, or in combination with, blood vacuity. This medicinal is particularly important for lower burner stasis associated with menstrual disorders or other conditions associated with the liver channel. Although this medicinal is sweet and nourishing, as noted above, it is also warm, slightly bitter, and acrid, which give it an active nourishing property (somewhat similar to *dānggui*) that is not likely to cause stagnation. This combination of flavors and nature make this medicinal very valuable when treating stasis caused by blood vacuity. For this function the medicinal should be alcohol mix–fried.

Cautions:

The berries are said to be poisonous, although birds eat them freely and are the main means of seed distribution for the plant. Although some older texts report that the root is toxic, I could find no modern literature supporting any toxicity of the root.

Dosage and Preparation:

Fresh plant tincture 2–4ml; decoction 3–10g

Major Combinations:

Combine with *dāngguī* and *shēnghuángqí* for scant menstruation due to blood vacuity.

Combine with Wild Yam and Motherwort for painful menstruation with blood stasis due to blood vacuity. Add *chuāngxiōng* to strengthen the blood moving effect.

Combine with *dùzhòng*, *xùduàn*, and *huáiniúxī* for pain and stiffness (especially with spasms) of the lower back and legs due to liver and kidney vacuity.

Commentary:

Red Baneberry is part of the *Actaea* genus within the Ranuculaceae family (Crowfoot). Ranuculaceae is a mid-size family with 60 genera and about 1700 species. The family is well represented in medicine (Chinese and otherwise) with a few very prominate species including species from the gerera *Aconite* (*fùzǐ*), *Clematis* (*wēilíngxiān*), *Acteae* (*shēngmá*), *Anemone* (*báitóuwēng*), and others. Ranunculaceae is found around the world and some species are common and weedy. The family also has many ornamental species and cultivars owing to their sometimes showy flowers. See below for more on the genus *Actaea*.

Red Baneberry in an important medicinal that is currently under-utilized. It is found throughout North America with the exception of the southeastern portion of the United States, and is often abundant. This plant prefers thickly wooded areas, but is sometimes found in the open or along the edges of forests. It survives logging activity, and I have often found it in the remains of a clear-cut. Since it is generally found in sloped areas, I prefer to dig roots from the bottom 1/3 of the slope (not all the roots), since gravity will easily allow for the seeds from the plants above to repopulate the harvested area. This medicinal is currently not widely available in commerce but has gained some popularity amongst a growing number of Western herbalists.

This plant was formerly considered poisonous by many people, as evidenced by literature from the 19th and 20th Century. However, the Cheyenne Nation have long known this to be an important medicine. In fact, the plant is said to hold the power of their cultural hero and prophet, Sweet Medicine or Sweet Root Standing. To the Cheyenne, Red Baneberry is known as Sweet Medicine. Hart (1980) writes, "Sweet Medicine reputedly lived 445 years with the Cheyenne. Upon his death, he transformed his sacred powers into this plant. To this day, Cheyennes keep this root in the Sacred Arrow, Sacred Hat, and Sun Dance bundles, thus benefiting from Sweet Medicine's sacred powers." Cheyenne women used it, and perhaps still do, to increase milk flow. Cheyennes also believed that when Red Baneberry was taken by children, they would mature with good mentality, and be strong and patient.[1] This interesting ethnobotanical link to the culture of the Cheyenne people, and points to not only the plant's safety, but also to Red Baneberry's nourishing and supplementing properties. Although I have never used this medicinal to supplement blood for women with poor milk production, Fù Shān states in his classic gynecology text, *Fù Qīng-zhǔ Nǚ Kē* (mid–17th Century), "Without first having blood, milk can not be engendered, without also having qi, milk can not be engendered." This is yet another link to this medicinal being a blood nourishing medicinal. The connection between Cheyenne traditional usage and Chinese medical theory offers us another way to draw conclusions on how to classify Western medicinals in Chinese medicine.

In the past, there was a distinction between the genus of this plant and that of Black Cohosh (*A. racemosa*) and *shēngmá*, the latter two being classified as Cimicifuga. However, these two genera have now been reunited (*Cimicifuga* was a division that was created in the early 20th Century). The *Cimicifuga* and the *Souliea* genera have been eliminated and merged into *Actaea*. This is not that important for the clinician, but what it tells us is that plants formerly known as *Cimicifuga* and those that have always been in the *Acteae* genus are more closely related than we had previously thought. With this merging of genera, we now have one genus that consists of about 24 species, and we can use these species' botanical relationship as a tool to learn how to use new species by examining what we already know about plants like Black Cohosh (see Garran 2008) and *shēngmá*. Also noteworthy is that the *Grand Dictionary of Chinese Medicinals* (2009) lists three species of Cimicifuga* as *shēngmá: C. heracleifolia, C. dahurica,* and *C. foetida.* Another species, *C. acerina,* is known as *xiǎoshēngmá* (小升麻) (Sieb. Et Zucc.). Lastly, a plant known as *yěshēngmá* (野升麻) is listed as *C. simplex* Wormsk. All these species are used in more or less the same way, although, each has some of its own unique characteristics.

Translation of Available Source Material:

Actaea asiatica Hara *lǜdòushēngmá* (綠豆升麻) first appeared in the *Wàn Xiàn Zhōng Běn Cǎo* (1977) although it's use can be assumed to predate that reference. It has a very wide range, between 350–3100 meters throughout much of China from Inner Mongolia to Yunnan in the south, and to Tibet in the west. The *Grand Dictionary of Chinese Medicinals* (2009) says it is acrid and slightly bitter, and neutral. It dissipates wind–heat, outthrusts papules, and resolves toxin. It is used to treat wind–heat headache, wind–papules, measles not outthrusting, whooping cough, and dog bite. The *Gān Sù Zhōng Yào Shǒu Cè* (1959) calls this herb *lèiyèshēngmá* (類葉升麻) and says it is acrid, bitter, and slightly warm. It dispels wind–dampness, effuses the exterior, and outthrusts papules. It treats wind–damp pain, measles not outthrusting, and skin wind–papules, etc. This text also gives a formula for using this herb for skin wind–papules: *lèiyèshēngmá* 10g, *jīngjiè* 6g, *fángfēng, niúbàngzǐ, huángqín, báizhí* each 10g.

It would appear from this formula, and from other uses given in various texts, that this medicinal is used similarly to *shēngmá.* This is not surprising since the two plants are very similar in genetics and appearance. See more about this genus in the commentary above.

Souliea vaginata (Maxim.) Franch., known as *huángsānqī* (黃三七), has also been brought into the *Actaea* genus along with *Cimicifuga.* It first appeared in the *Shǎnxī Zhōng Cǎo Yào* (1971). In that book, it is considered bitter and cool. It drains fire and dries dampness, clears the heart and eliminates vexation, is antibacterial and disperses inflammation, and fortifies the stomach. It is used for throat inflammation, conjunctivitis, stomatitis, steaming bone tidal heat, being easily flustered and heart palpitations, vexation and disquietude, bacterial dysentery, intestinal inflammation, and toxic swollen welling–abscess.

*It is common for non–scientific publications to continue to list old genera names long after the change has been made in the botanical (taxonomy) literature.

1. Hart, J.A. (1980). The Ethnobotany of the Northern Cheyenne Indians of Montana. *Journal of Ethnopharmacology* 4: pp 1–55.

Blueberry

Vaccinium sp. L.
Ericaceae
Vaccini fructus
Favor and Qi: sweet, neutral
Channels entered: kidney, liver
Actions: nourishing

Functions & Indications:

Nourishes the liver, enriches blood, and benefits essence. Blueberry is very good for the treatment of liver blood vacuity with symptoms of poor night vision, lack of vision acuity, and dry eyes. This medicinal may also be used in cases of spleen qi vacuity leading to liver blood vacuity, with symptoms of varicose veins, bruising easily, and other similar symptoms. Blueberry is sweet and neutral and, unlike many similar medicinals, does not tend to be cloying, thus it is generally very well tolerated.

Cautions:

None noted

Dosage and Preparation:

Decoction 6–30g

Major Combinations:

This medicinal may be added to any formula used to treat liver blood vacuity, especially when treating eye diseases.

Commentary:

Blueberries are in the large (about 500 species) and diverse genus *Vaccinium*, which is part of the large family (120 genera with some 4100 species) known as Ericaceae or Health family. The family is represented around the world (except Antarctica and is not well represented in the tropics) and tends to prefer poor acid soil where it depends on micorrhizal associations to thrive. Most, if not all the fruits produced by the species of this genus are edible, and some are highly prized and commercially important. Blueberry is one of these, but this name actually represents several species. Another species, commonly known as Bilberry (*V. myrtillus*) is a famous species in Europe known for its exceptional nutritional value. Not to be forgotten is the Cranberry, *V. macrocarpum*, which, Blueberry and Cranberry, both a food and medicinal plant (see Garran 2008). Rododendrons and Azaleas, famous for their ornamental value are also part of this family.

Most people think of Blueberries as a tasty berry that they add to pancakes or smoothies. The idea to use it as a medicinal came quite naturally to me while thinking about what Western herbs fit into the supplementing category of Chinese medicine. The Bilberry (noted above) is a close European relative and is also very nourishing. Bilberry has become quite well-known for its positive influence on the vessels and thus in a general way the cardiovascular system. There is ample evidence that this (and other) species benefit the vessels through mitigating the oxidative stress from LDL.[1,2] Kay and Holub (2002) state in the conclusion of their study:

> *"In conclusion, we have demonstrated that supplementation with a freeze-dried wild blueberry powder increased serum antioxidant status following the consumption of a high-fat meal. Increasing the serum antioxidant status has been suggested as a possible method of reducing the risk of many chronic degenerative disorders. In vitro analysis of the blueberry shows it to have hightly active antioxidant characteristics. The present study provides physiological evidence for the enhancement of postprandial serum antioxidant status in human volunteers consuming a blueberry-supplemented meal."*

Blueberries and related *Vaccinium* species have also show to be benefitial in type-2 diabetes by their action on the pancreatic β-cells.[3,4] Martineau, et al., (2006) conclude:

> *"V. angustifolium extracts were found to exert positive effects on pancreatic β-cells. The β TC-tet cellular system used here is well suited to distinguish effects on insulin secretion from effects on proliferation. In growth-arrested pancreatic β cells, leaf and stem extracts exerted a subtle anti-diabetic effect on GSIS [glucose-stimulated insulin secretion] consisting of bothan increase in maximal secretion as well as a leftward shift in the glucose-insulin secretion dose-response curve, without a significant effect on basal secretion. These are highly desirable properties in an anti-diabetic medications...Perhaps more*

246 Part II Materia Medica

> *important than the effects of the leaf and stem extracts on GSIS is the considerable effect of the fruit extract on proliferation of replicating β cell decompensation in advanced T2DM [type-2 diabetes]."*

While none of the research cited above specifically directly supports my claim that Blueberries nourish the liver blood or kidney essence, it might be supposed that, in the first case, deterioration of the vascular system is directly related to both the liver blood and kidney essence. And, it also might be supposed the type-2 diabetes is related to these systems. In fact, most modern TCM books that use an integrated model site liver and kidney vacuity as primary diagnosis for type-2 diabetes. Of course this is only conjecture and we must use our clinical experience to best judge how this medicine truly works within the framework of Chinese medicine.

Unfortunately, purchasing dried Blueberries without added sugar or oil is next to impossible. My solution to this problem is to purchase fresh berries and dry them myself in order to use in the clinic. This also makes for a very tasty snack while in the pharmacy putting formulas together! They can be a relatively expensive addition to a formula, but a major benefit. And, beyond the medicinal action, the flavor of Blueberries is almost universally tolerated if not appreciated, which can be very benefitial when dispensing raw herbs for decoction.

I have noted in other monographs about supplementing medicinals that it may be difficult to ascertain their exact function and Blueberry is no different. I have used Blueberry for many years as a dried medicinal, and frequently add it to formulas when indicated, but the formulas are generally complexes of other supplementing medicinals that make it difficult to evaluate the efficacy of Blueberry by itself. However, I feel strongly that my ideas are pretty close to clinical reality. Blueberry has a long history of use as a food and is closely related to the European Bilberry, which is very well researched and shown to have positive effects on a number of systems that can be directly or indirectly related to liver blood and kidney essence.

1. Laplaud, PM, et al., (1997). Antioxidant action of *Vaccinium myrtillus* extract on human low density lipoproteins in vitro: initial observations. *Fundamental & Clinical Pharmacology*. 11(1): pp 35–40.
2. Kay, Colin D. & Holub, Bruce J., (2002). The effect of wild blueberry (*Vaccinium angustifolium*) consumption on postprandial serum antioxidant

status in human subjects. *British Journal of Nutrition*. 88: pp 389–397.

3. Martineau, Louis C., et al., (2006). Anti–diabetic properties of the Canadian lowbush blueberry *Vaccinium angustifolium* Ait. *Phytomedicine*. 13(7): pp 612–623.

4. Grace, Mary H., et al., (2009). Hypoglycemic activity of a novel Anthocyanin–rich formulation from Lowbush Blueberry, *Vaccinium angustifolium* Aiton. *Phytomedicine*. 16(5): pp 406–415.

Pine Lousewort

Pedicularis semibarbata A. Gray
Scrophulariaceae
Pediculari semibarbatae planta
Favor and Qi: sweet, slightly bitter, cool
Channels entered: stomach, lung, kidney
Actions: antiinflammatory, sedative, calmative, muscle relaxant, demulcent

Functions & Indications:

Enriches yin, moistens dryness, and clears vacuity heat. Pine Lousewort is used for lung and stomach yin vacuity with thirst, dry cough, dry mouth, and a dry red tongue with little or no coat. Pine Lousewort is sweet, slightly bitter, and cool. Sweetness can nourish and engender yin, while bitterness can drain. Pine Lousewort enriches yin with sweetness and drains vacuity heat with cool bitterness.

Enriches kidney yin, benefits the heart and liver. Pine Lousewort is used for kidney yin vacuity, particularly when it affects the heart and liver, with symptoms such as dizziness, low back pain, afternoon heat effusion, bleeding gums, headache, irregular menstruation, insomnia, heart palpitations, and vexation. The pulse is fine and rapid, and the tongue is red with little coat. Although the primary action is to enrich kidney yin, this pattern is always seen in combination with other organ systems' pathology, and when present is a contributing factor to vacuity of the heart and liver. This medicinal is sweet and slightly bitter. Sweet is nourishing and supplementing, while bitter is draining. This herb is only slightly bitter, which acts to gently drain, thereby avoiding stagnation that can be caused by supplementing medicinals. Its sweet flavor is thick, thus settles deep into the yin to nourish.

Cautions:

None noted in the literature, however caution should be used with those with spleen qi/yang vacuity with dampness.

Dosage and Preparation:

Decoction 3–10g; fresh plant tincture 2–4ml

Major Combinations:

Combine with *tàizǐshēn* and Licorice Fern for dry, weak cough due to lung qi and yin vacuity.

Combine with *báirénshēn* or *xīyángshēn* and *shúdìhuáng* for kidney yin vacuity with weakness, night sweats, aching lower back, and thirst.

Commentary:

This species of *Pedicularis* is not discussed by any of the authors in the Western United States who use this genus, most notably Michael Moore, who championed this genus as a medicinal in the late 20th and early 21st Centuries. This is most likely because it is a low growing plant with only a basal rosette of leaves, with a few leaves on the flowering stem, and lacks the aerial portions that most herbalists like to use (the flowering tops are the portion used on most other species). With only a rosette of foliage, and flowers that rarely grow more than four (4) centimeters above the ground (even on a large plant), one might think it uninteresting, or at least not worth the time and effort to gather, unless of course you considered harvesting the roots along with the rest of the plant!

Many years ago, when I was going to the Sierra Nevada and the Coast Range of Northern California on a regular basis, this seemed like the only Pedicularis I could ever find (I was trying to find Elephant's Head (*P. groenlandica*). On one of these trips, I mistakenly pulled up an entire plant while attempting to pinch off a leaf. The area was unusually sandy and the root was pretty long and robust. When I arrived at camp that night, I decided to take this plant and simmer it into a tea. The sensation I had was a palpable relaxation, and a rather soothing feeling in the mouth and stomach. The next day I decided to harvest some whole plants, including the roots. I made a quart of tincture with some fresh whole plant; the rest I dried (about 3 pounds) and used in decoctions. At first, I just used it on myself to see what more I might notice. While camping, I had made a tea with the leaves, then the whole plant, and experienced a whole body relaxation, similar to how other species are described and used, but hadn't made a strong decoction with a dose similar to what we use in Chinese medicine. So I started with 3, then 6, then 9 grams, and eventually cooked as much as 20 grams of the whole dried plant and drank it over the course of an hour or so. This experiment was spread out over several weeks, and I noticed that I felt "looser," "moister," and generally more relaxed, but never spaced out or feeling a sense of any narcotic effects. Since I experienced no symptoms of toxicity, and I knew many species to be medicinal, I started using it in the clinic, adding it to formulas for yin vacuity of the kidney, liver, lung, or stomach diagnostic patterns.

It is impossible for me to say to what degree this medicinal helped any of those patients because I always combined it in a formula with other herbs. However, I have used it as a leading herb a few times, and I believe it is worth further investigation.

It is important to be mindful of where this plant is harvested, and the quantities being removed from any one area. This species is primarily found in the dry pine forests of California, with only a few ajoining counties of Nevada and Oregon reporting its presence. In my experience, it is most frequently associated with various species of the Ericaceae (Heath) family. Although the plant's range is large, it also is a relatively sensitive ecosystem due to lack of rainfall. This plant generally is quite common, and once you tune into it, you may find yourself seeing it often when you are within its habitat.

I suspect that there are other species within the genus that might be able to used in this way, but have done no further experimentation. For more information on the *Pedicularis* genus, please refer to page 273-5 in the commentary under *Pedicularis*.

Translation of Available Source Material:

The *Grand Dictionary of Chinese Medicinals* (2009) lists three species (*P. davidii*, *P. decora*, and *P. dunniana*) as interchangeable under the heading *tàibáishēn* (太白蔘). The root is the part used of these species; it is gathered from August to October. It is listed as sweet, slightly bitter, warm, and slightly toxic, with functions of nourish yin and supplement kidney and boost qi and strengthen the spleen. It is indicated for spleen/kidney dual vacuity, steaming bone tidal heat [effusion], joint pain, and no thought of eating. It is used in decoction at 9–15g, but may also be used in 30–60g dosages.

The *Gui Zhou Collection of Herbal Folk Remedies* (1965) uses the root of *P. henryi* Maxim. to supplement vacuity and weakness, for treat symptoms of liver vacuity, night sweating, and sores that haven't healed for a long time. It also lists the whole plant of *P. rex* Clarke as a medicinal to supplement vacuity and boost detriment, and clear heat and resolve toxin. It is used to treat kidney vacuity with dizziness, smallpox, and Stinging Nettle rash.

Medicinal	Nature	Flavor	Channels	Functions	Indications
Gota Cola	cool	sweet, slightly sour	kidney	Boosts essence, improves memory, and sharpens wit; Clears heat, cools the blood, and engenders fluids and fresh	dulled wit, poor memory, slow reflexes, etc.; damage to liquid, humor, or flesh caused either by heat or traumatic injury
Stinging Nettle Seed	neutral	sweet, slightly bitter	liver, kidney	Supplements qi and benefits the kidneys	lethargy, fatigue, loss of appetite, weight loss, muddled thinking, low sex drive, etc.
Licorice Fern	cool	sweet, slightly bitter	lung, kidney	Nourishes yin and supplements lung qi; Opens the chest	chronic cough with weakness, dry cough, and panting; oppressive sensation in the chest, cough, panting and wheezing, and shortness of breath
Red Baneberry	warm	sweet, slightly bitter, slightly acrid	liver, spleen	Nourishes the liver, enriches blood, and relaxes the sinews; Quickens the blood and resolves stasis	scant menstruation, tugging and slacking, sinew hypertonicity and pain; painful menstruation, scrotal pain, etc.

Medicinal	Nature	Flavor	Channels	Functions	Indications
Blueberry	neutral	sweet	liver, spleen	Nourishes the liver and enriches blood	poor night vision, lack of vision acuity, and dry eyes;
Lousewort	cool	sweet, slightly bitter	stomach, lung, liver, kidney	Enriches yin and moistens dryness; Enriches liver and kidney yin	thirst, dry cough, dry mouth, dry tongue with little or no coat; dizziness, low back pain, afternoon heat effusion, bleeding gums, headache, irregular menstruation, insomnia, heart palpitations, and vexation

安

神

藥

Calm Spirit Medicinals

The calm spirit category of medicinals is used to calm and settle the spirit–mind, i.e. the conscious mind. These medicinals are used for patterns where the spirit–mind is neither calm nor settled with disquietude causing the person a range of symptoms that range from simple anxiety to psychological diseases, which can arise from either vacuity or repletion.

In the Chinese materia medica this category is divided into two sub–categories. The first is what I call the bones and stones or the heavy settling the spirit–mind medicinals, none of which are found in this materia medica. The second, the nourish heart and calm spirit medicinals, is what is found in this materia medica. However, at least two medicinals in this materia medica, Hops and Pasque Flower lean much more heavily toward calming the spirit–mind rather than being particularly nourishing.

Common symptoms associated with a disquieted spirit–mind are heart palpitations and fearful throbbing, excessive dreaming, forgetfulness, heart vexation with sleeplessness, etc. and are associated with most modern psychological disease diagnoses.

Medicinals in this category tend to be sweet and neither too warm or too cold, however as noted above, two medicinals in this materia medica are slightly outside of the standard when it comes to Chinese medicinals in this category, and their placement here is, to some extent, arbitrary (which by the way is true for most medicinals in most categories). Many of the classic Chinese medicinals in this category nourish the heart, boost the liver, and calm the spirit. While this is certainly true for Lemon Balm and Pedicularis, Hops and Pasque Flower are not so much nourishing as they are calming. This is also true of at least one medicinal in the first materia medica, Kava, which although is not particularly nourishing, most definitely has a calming action. These types of medicinals seem to be absent from the Chinese materia medica and one has to wonder if this is not because such an action might have been considered toxic by Chinese herbalists and therefore these types of medicinals were never developed.

Hops

Humulus lupulus L.

Canabanaceae

Hummuli lupuli strobile

Chinese name: *píjiǔhuā* 啤酒花

Favor and Qi: bitter, aromatic, warm

Channels entered: heart, spleen, stomach

Actions: digestive tonic, hypnotic, diuretic

Functions & Indications:

Quiets the spirit. Hops is used for a wide range of patterns with symptoms such as irritability, irascibility, sleeplessness, and vexation. Hops has a decided action on quieting the spirit and can be applied in most patterns where the above symptomology exists. It is particularly useful when there are stomach problems associated with the pattern (see below). It is also important to note that although Hops is warm, it can be used in heat conditions when formulated appropriately. In fact, Hops can be extremely useful in these conditions because they tend to be more serious, i.e. liver constraint transforming into fire, and rapid reduction in symptoms such as irritability and sleeplessness will have a marked effect on the patient's health. Although Hops is warm, its strong bitter flavor downbears qi, and the aroma both transforms turbidity and opens the orifices of the heart, thus calming the spirit.

Harmonizes the stomach and liver, and disperses food. Hops is used for symptoms of sour belching, stomach qi ascending counterflow, sour taste in the mouth, nausea, and vomiting. Hops is a bitter aromatic, whose bitterness downbears stomach qi and aroma transforms stagnant food.

Stops pain. Hops is used for a wide variety of pain conditions, both internally and externally. That being said, I have very little experience using this herb to alleviate pain.

Cautions:

Hops is strongly aromatic and bitter, and should be used with caution in yin vacuity, especially stomach yin vacuity.

Dosage and Preparation:
Tincture 1–4ml; decoction 2–6g

Major Combinations:

Add to *Wēn Dǎn Tāng*, particularly when there is pronounced irritability, nervousness, or sleeplessness. Although Hops is warm, it is a strong bitter and helps to downbear turbid yin, allowing for the clear yang to rise.

Combine with Chamomile and Bǎo Hé Wán for children with abdominal pain or sleeplessness associated with food stagnation. Add Catnip for agitation with weeping and crying.

Combine with Skullcap, *yuǎnzhì*, and Calamus for manic behavior patterns associated with phlegm–turbidity. Add Goldenseal and *huángqín* for phlegm–heat–turbidity patterns.

Combine with Skullcap and California Poppy for anxiety, irritability, and difficulty sleeping due to constraint of liver qi. This combination can be used to try these symptoms and others that arise when patients are trying to quit smoking, drugs, or alcohol; for these cases add Wild Oat to the combination.

Add to *Liù Jū Zǐ Tāng* for spleen/stomach vacuity sleeplessness with lack of appetite, copious phlegm, and fatigue, with inability to fall asleep. Add to *Bǔ Zhōng Yì Qì Tāng* for the same pattern without the copious phlegm.

Add to *Dà Chái Hú Tāng* for spleen/stomach (large intestine) disharmony with anxiety, irritability, fullness in the chest, constipation and other symptoms related to this pattern. Use Hops when the anxiety and irritability are particularly pronounced, and especially if the person's sleep is difficult or disturbed.

Commentary:

Hops is native to Europe and West Asia, growing as a perennial vine which inhabits thickets on forest margins in the wild, but is extensively cultivated. Hops is one of the most consumed herbs in the world, next to tea and coffee, because of its use in the production of most beer. Hops is a warm, acrid, and bitter herb but most people find them pleasant to consume, so they are easily incorporated into formulas or even given as a simple. Hops make a good addition to a decoction as well as a good tincture.

Gerard (1597) says that Hops is hot and dry in the second degree and is good for old sores and scabe, and further states:

> *"The decoction of Hops drunk, opens the stoppings of the liver, the spleen, the kidnys, and purges the blood from all corrupt humours, causing the same to comeforth with the urine. The juice of Hops opens the belly, and drives forth yellow choleric humours, and purges the blood for all filthiness. The manifold virtures in Hops do manifestly argue the holsomness of beer above ale; for the Hops rather make it a physical drink to keep the body in health, than an ordinary drink for the quenching of our thirst."*

Gerard is equating the "hotness" of Hops and its bitterness with a purging action, ridding the body of all manner of "corrupt humours." Like Chinese medicine, Gerard viewed heating medicinals, in general, to be stimulating and moving. That Hops "opens the belly" and eliminates "yellow choleric humours" is a direct association with Hops action on the stomach and liver and supports my statements above with regards to harmonizing the liver and stomach.

Culpeper (1653) says of Hops, "This, in physical operations, is to open obstructions of the liver and spleen, to cleanse the blood, to loosen the belly, to cleanse the reins from gravel, and provoke urine." This statement seems to support the second function I have applied to this medicinal. While the phrase, "cleanse the blood," is quite nebulous, I think it speaks to Hops' bitter nature, which helps to move the liver qi. Since the liver stores the blood, when the liver qi becomes constrained this may have been viewed as "unclean blood" by physicians such as Culpeper.

He also says, "A syrup made of the juice and sugar, cureth the yellow jaundice, easeth the head-ache that comes of heat, and tempers the heat of the liver and stomach, and is profitably given in long and hot agues that rise in choler and blood." Here we have a clear sense that Culpeper was discussing heat patterns, even from the Chinese point of view, which leads us to consider why we would use a medicinal that is warm in such patterns. This is when it is important to remember that we always work with formulas. Warm herbs are moving, as a general rule, and Culpeper seems to be discussing a condition where heat has caused qi to either become stagnant or to move in a counter-flow direction. Thus, he understood that using a medicinal such as Hops would provide relief from such a pattern.

Translation of Available Source Material:

There are three species of hops in China. One is the European species, *Humulus lupulus*, one endemic, *H. yunnanensis*, and *H. scandens*, lùcǎo (葎草), which is native but also grows in Korea, Japan, and Eastern Russia. The *Grand Dictionary of Chinese Medicinals* (2009) says *H. scandens*, lùcǎo (葎草) is sweet, bitter, and cold; and enters the lung and kidney channels. It clears heat and resolves toxins, and disinhibits urine and frees strangury. It is used to treat lung heat with cough, lung welling–abscess, vacuity heat with vexation thirst, hot strangury, water swelling, inhibited urination, damp–heat diarrhea, heat toxin hemorrhoids, and itchy skin. I have used this plant as a tincture. It has a similar aroma and flavor to Hops, but is much weaker. Its action is also much weaker compared to Hops. It is a very common weedy plant in Northeast China and can be found commonly in vacant lots and fields in and around Beijing. I, unfortunately, didn't realize how weedy it was when I allowed it to grow in my garden one year and the next year had to contend with its nasty vines, which have small, but very sharp, saw–type "teeth" and easily tear through the skin of the arms and legs while working in the garden. Management has been painful and slow!

While there is a significant amount of research on Hops in the literature, nearly all of the work done in the last 30 years has been on the phytoestrogens in hops, which have no bearing on this monograph. There has been a small amount of research on the antibacterial activity of Hops.[1,2] Most of the sedative effects have been studied either using combinations of herbs or by injection of extracts or fractions of the medicinal, which although may be somewhat interesting, do not offer much support for the oral administration of Hops. However, one study using ethanol extracts by oral administration did show analgesic and increased sleeping times.[3] The authors conclude, "The traditional use of hop preparations in nervousness, anxiety and sleep disorders was clearly confirmed by our own findings in three test models." And finally, one study on the effects of Hops on the gastric secretions showed that there was a dose dependant increase in gastric secretions without a parallel increase in stomach acid.[4]

1. Simpson, W.J., Smith, A.R., (1992). Factors affecting antibacterial activity of hop compounds and their derivatives. *Journal of Applied Bacteriology.* 72: pp 27–334.

2. Oshugi, M., et. al. (1997). Antibacterial activity of traditional medicines and an active constituent lupulone from Humulus lupulus against *Helicobacter pylori. Journal Traditional Medicine.* 14(2): pp 186–191.

3. Schiller, H., Forster, A., Vonhoff, C., Hegger, M., Biller, A., Winterhoff, H., (2006). Sedating effects of *Humulus lupulus* L. extracts. *Phytomedicine.* 13(8): pp 535–541.

4. Kurasawa, Takashi, et al., (2005). Effect of *Humulus lupulus* on Gastric Secretion in a Rat Pylorus–Ligated Model. *Biol. Pharm. Bulletin.* 28(2): pp 353–357.

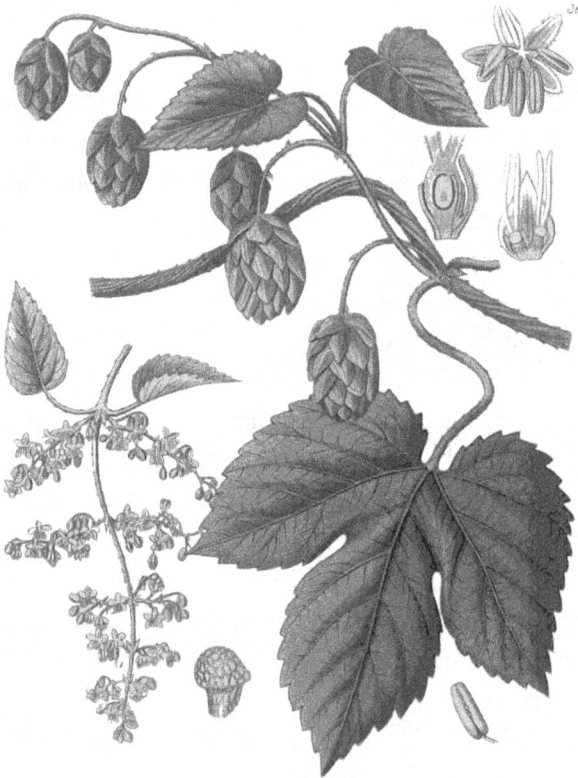

Humulus Lupulus L.

Lemon Balm

Melissa officinalis L.

Laminaceae

Melissae folium

Favor and Qi: acrid, bitter, slightly sweet, cool

Channels entered: stomach, liver, heart

Actions: anxiolytic, antiinflammatory, diaphoretic

Functions & Indications:

Eliminates vexation. Lemon Balm is used for heat vexation in the chest due to effulgence of liver fire with other symptoms including red eyes, lip and mouth sores, and headaches. Lemon Balm is bitter and cool. Bitter coolness can clear heat and eliminate vexation. This function of Lemon Balm is ancient and is reflected in the commentary by Culpeper in which he says that Avicenne, the great 11th Century Persian scholar and physician, notes this as well.

Clears heat, dispels wind, and resolves the exterior. Lemon Balm is used for externally contracted wind–heat that has not been properly resolved, leading to heat vexation. Also for simple wind–heat invasions without the complication of vexation. Lemon Balm is acrid and bitter. Acridity can resolve the exterior and bitterness can clear heat. Lemon Balm very effectively resolves the exterior without being overly releasing, causing excessive sweating. At the same time, Lemon Balm is bitter and cool, thus helping to drain the lung. These two qualities are what *Wēn Bìng* therapeutics require when treating all *wèi* aspect illnesses, i.e., to resolve the exterior and drain the lung. This function also applies to *shàoyáng* presentations of *Shāng Hán Lùn* therapeutics and can be added to *Xiǎo Chái Hú Tāng* in cases where heart vexation is prominent, and to assist in venting the pathogen.

Opens the stomach, facilitates the flow of qi in the middle, and stops pain. Lemon Balm is used for children (or adults) with a variety of digestive issues generally caused by intemperate eating with symptoms such as stomach pain, bloating, headache, lack of appetite, and inability to sleep. Lemon Balm is acrid and bitter. Acrid can move and open, bitter can drain and move qi downward, with acridity and bitterness Lemon Balm opens the stomach, moves the qi, and relieves pain.

Importantly, Lemon Balm is cool, and coolness clears heat. In children, who are naturally yang in nature, these conditions are almost always associated with heat. This is a very commonly used herb for children, both because it is relatively gentle in small doses and because its flavor is quite agreeable even to the sensitive palettes of children.

Cautions:
None noted

Dosage and Preparation:
Infusion or light decoction 1–3g (up to 10g); 1–4ml fresh plant tincture; 2–6ml glycerin extract

Major Combinations:
Combine with *Xiǎo Chái Hú Tāng* for patients with a *shàoyáng* pattern with pronounced heart vexation.

Combine with *Yín Qiào Sǎn* for wind–heat invasion combined with heart vexation.

Combine with *Sāng Jú Yǐn* for wind–heat fettering the lungs, combined with cough and irritability.

Combine with Catnip for digestive pain in children who are agitated and perhaps having difficulty sleeping.

Combine with *méiguīhuā* for liver constraint with vexation, irritability, and difficulty sleeping.

Combine with St. John's Wort and Cedar for internal and external application for herpes simplex with lip or genital sores. The three combine very nicely to make an oil or tincture that can be used both internally and externally. The combination of these herbs comes from the Western herb tradition and is based on the antiviral effects of these three herbs.[1,2,3] All three herbs can resolve toxin; Lemon Balm and St. John's Wort are cool, clear heat medicinals, while Cedar is a warm herb that is used to treat many different pathogens that Chinese medicine views as "toxin." St. John's Wort is well-known for healing wounds and generating flesh, and the cedar provides movement of blood locally to facilitate healing. Lemon Balm acts as a cool herb that assists St. John's Wort to clear heat, and works together with Cedar to facilitate movement with its acridity. They all work together to resolve toxin.

Commentary:

Lemon Balm is well known as a pleasant tasting tea for everyday use. As a tea it gently cools the body and calms the spirit without being overly cooling or damaging to the spleen. Lemon Balm is a European plant from the Mint family that has found its way to North America and is now naturalized in many places along creeks and other wet areas. It is easily cultivated in most temperate zone environments. It can be a little weedy, but can be reasonably managed in gardens.

Lemon Balm is generally a mild herb but doesn't always need a heavy dosage to have a positive effect. Quality of this herb is very important, be sure that the herb is fragrant and not musty; otherwise the tincture works nicely and preserves the action better. The tea is both wonderfully pleasant and effective, which makes it a good herb to just have around. I recently made a red wine vinegar with this herb and it was quite pleasant, the whole family liked it. I use it on salads and other vegetables for a nice herbal twist to a meal.

Parkinson (1640) writes extensively about Lemon Balm and says much of what Culpeper echoes 13 years later. However, he attributes much of this information to the Greek physicians, quoting Serapio (Greek—1st Century CE) as saying:

> *"It is the property of Baulme [Lemon Balm], to cause the mind and heart to become merry, to revive the fainting heart falling into swoonings, to strengthen the weakness of the spirits and heart, and to comfort them, especially such who are overtaken in their sleep, there with taking away all motion of the pulse, to drive away all troublesome cares and thoughts out of the mind, whether those passions rise from melancholy or black cholar, or burnt phlegm...Avicen confirmeth in his book of medicines."*

This passage shows an interesting connection in the minds of 17th Century writers between the heart/spirit and dreams. While we can not necessarily draw a direct line between these ideas and theories in Chinese medicine that discuss this connection, this does show a similar line of thinking. What makes this so important is that when classifying a medicinal from outside of China, these connections help us to understand the medicinal from the perspective of the Chinese medical paradigm.

Culpeper (1653) writes, verbatim, what Parkinson wrote in the quote above, but adds: "It is very good to help digestion, and open obstructions of the brain, and hath so much purging quality in it, (saith Avicen) as to expel those melancholy vapours from the spirits and blood which are in the heart and arteries, although it cannot do so in other parts of the body." From this we can see that Culpeper relied on two older authors to draw his conclusions about this medicinal. Culpeper also mentions several other authors in his monograph. An interesting note is that we can see a possible connection between the small intestine and heart of Chinese medicine with the reference to the digestion and "obstructions of the brain" as well as "expel those melancholy vapours from the spirits and blood." The small intestine governs transformation, and when the small intestine is not functioning well, the clear and turbid are not properly separated. This can lead to turbidity rising and obstructing the heart spirit leading to symptoms similar to when Culpeper discusses above.

Salmon (1710) states, "It is approved against fainting and swooning, fits, poisons, sickness at the heart, and hypochondriack melancholy." Throughout the classic herbal literature there are mentions of "melancholy," "swoonings," "heart," and finally the most specific "sickness *at* [emphasis added] the heart," and "hypochondriack melancholy." Melancholy is generally described as what we now define as "depression" in the emotional sense of the word. In his classic *The Anatomy of Melancholy* (1621), Robert Burton describes the symptoms of "windy Hypochoncriacal Melancholy" as, "The symptoms alone vexeth many. Some again are black, pale, ruddy, sometimes their shoulders, and shoulder blades ache, there is a leaping all over their bodies, sudden trembling, a palpitation of the heart, and that cardiac passio, grief in the mouth of the stomach, which maketh the patient think his heart itself acheth, and sometimes suffocation, *difficultas anhelitus*, short breath, hard wind, strong pulse, swooning." Earlier in his work he describes the causes as primarily centered around the liver (being over-heated or obstructed) and the stomach and/or spleen (generally being cold). Although it is impossible to draw a straight line between this description and the Chinese medicine term "vexation" (see below) I am suggesting that there is a significant enough correlation to use the term vexation in the above monograph in reference to how to understand the clinical application of this medicinal.

Vexation is a common symptom seen in the Western clinic. Vexation is generally a term that is coupled with other terms such as heat, heart, thirst, anguish, and the locational "heat vexation in the chest." Vexation is a subjective feeling or "onrest or irritability" and although it can occur in vacuity, repletion, hot, or cold conditions, it is most often associated with heat of one kind or another.[4] The etymology of the character sheds some light on this. The character is made up of two parts, *huò* (火), which is fire, and *xiè* (頁), which means head. The *Explanation of [Simple] Graphs and [Complex] Characters (Shuō Wén Jiě Zì* 說文解字 published ~100AD) says, "煩, 熱頭痛也 " "Vexation, [leads to] hot headache." showing a clear connection between heat (and pain) with vexation.

In one study done using a commercially prepared product (30% ethanol; 70% water), the product, which is made exclusively with Lemon Balm (extraction method not disclosed), showed moderate anti-anxiety effects when taken for an undisclosed period of time.[5] This study was done on rats. Although it is difficult to extrapolate from this study, based on the known traditional information, this study does confirm (to some extent) and validate that traditional knowledge.

Translation of Available Source Material:

A related species, *Melissa axillaris, bíxuècǎo* (鼻血草), is classified in the *Grand Dictionary of Chinese Medicinals* as bitter, astringent, and neutral. Functions are; cool the blood and stop bleeding, and clear heat and resolve toxin. Indications are; spitting blood, nose bleed, flooding and spotting, vaginal discharge, leprosy, itchy skin, scabies, snake bite, and bad breath.

1. A. Allahverdiyev, et. al. (2004). Antiviral activity of the volatile oils of *Melissa officinalis* L. against *Herpes simplex* virus type-2. *Phytomedicine* 11(7–8): pp 657–661.
2. Axarlis, S., et. al. (1998), Antiviral *In vitro* activity of *Hypericum perforatum* L. extract on the human cytomegalovirus (HCMV). *Phytother. Res.*, 12: 507–511.
3. Beuscher N, Kopanski L. Reinigung. (1986) und biologische Charakterisierung von antiviralen Substanzen aus *Thuja occidentalis. Planta Med.* 52: pp 555–6 (*article in German*).
4. Wiseman, Nigel, and Feng Ye. *A Practical Dictionary of Chinese Medicine.* Brookline, MA: Paradigm Publications, 1998. pp 654–655.
5. Ibarra, Alvin, et al., (2010). Effects of chronic administration of *Melissa officinalis* L. extract on anxiety-like reactivity and on circadian and exploratory activities in mice. *Phytomedicine.* 17(3): pp 397–403.

Pasque Flower

Anemone occidentalis S. Watson, *A. patens* L., others
Ranunculaceae
Anemoni herba seu radix
Favor and Qi: acrid, bitter, aromatic, warm
Channels entered: heart, liver
Actions: sedative, antispasmodic

Functions & Indications:

Opens the heart orifice and calms the spirit. Pasque Flower is used for a variety of mental/emotional conditions where phlegm, turbidity, or heat has combined to confound the heart orifice and cause disturbances in the heart/spirit. This medicinal has a piercing nature and can give nearly immediate (though perhaps temporary) resolution to a variety of complaints, including vexation, emotional depression, inability to think clearly, anxiety, as well as mania and withdrawal (including drug induced). Anemone is very warm, acrid, and aromatic; with warm aroma, it opens the orifices of the heart, and with acridity, it moves stagnation caused by congestion due to phlegm–turbidity; with bitterness, it can drain downward to remove turbidity.

Rectifies the qi and regulates the menses. Pasque Flower is used for stopped or painful menstruation caused by liver constraint qi stagnation with symptoms of stopped or painful menstruation, headache, vexation, irritability, irascibility, fullness in the chest and rib–sides, and a string–like pulse. Anemone moves liver qi and resolves constraint with warm acridity, thus allowing the qi to flow smoothly and the body to return to normal functioning.

Cautions:
This medicinal should not be used for thin, vacuous patients. There have been reports of these types of patients temporarily losing consciousness when using the herb, although there seemed to be no lasting negative effects.

Dosage and Preparation:
Fresh plant tincture 3–30 drops

Major Combinations:

Combine with California Poppy for liver constraint with symptoms of anxiety, panic attacks, and vexation.

Combine with *shíchāngpú* and *yuǎnzhì* for mania and other serious mental–emotional disorders associated with clouded spirit, phlegm obstructing the orifices of the heart, or other syndromes where there is accumulation of phlegm, turbidity, or dampness causing any of the above symptoms.

Combine with Skullcap for anxiety and vexation associated with drug or alcohol withdrawal. Using this combination in a ratio of 1:4 (Pasque Flower:Skullcap) can be a very effective method of relieving symptoms, but other herbs are often needed and any withdrawal from drugs or alcohol should be monitored by an expert and often need hospitalization or placement in a special clinic.

Commentary:

There are two genera, *Pulsatilla* and *Anemone*, that have plants called "Pasque Flower," which is somewhat of a problematic situation. However, as Ren et al. (2010) explain, the plant often labeled as *Pulsatilla chinensis,báitóuwēng* is actually *Anemone chinensis*.[1] This is an important distinction when comparing these plants for medicinal use across cultures and systems of medicine. Futhermore, the Flora of North America notes that the genus *Pulsatilla* and *Hepatica* should both likely be classed as Anemone. *Anemone* has approximately 150 species in the genus, mostly in northern temperate and arctic regions of the world. The genus is part of the Ranuculaceae or Crowfoot family, which has been further discussed in the *Commentary* section of Red Baneberry on page 241.

Pasque Flower has a long history of use in both Western and Chinese herbal medicine, although the method of preparation differs significantly between the two systems of medicine. Chinese medicine uses a decoction of the entire plant of *Anemone chinensis*, while modern Western herbalists use a tincture (*Anemone pulsatilla* being the most commonly used species), and most prefer the fresh plant tincture, considering it far superior to the product prepared from the dried material. While the entire plant can and is used, the above ground portions, harvested in full bloom, or even once gone to seed, are most commonly used. The root is considered stronger, but the plant is strong medicine to start with, so for ecological reasons there is no need to dig the entire plant when the herbaceous part will suffice.

I was trained in California and lived much of my adult life in either California or Oregon, before moving to Hawai'i and then China. The species of Anemone most frequently used by West Coast herbalists is *Anemone occidentalis*, a locally abundant species and the one with which I have the most experience. *A. patens* and *A. chinensis* also work similar to this species.

Gerard (1597) lists 10 species that he calls "Wind Flower," another common name for Pasque Flower. However, based on the drawings and descriptions, not all these are true *Anemone* species, rather they seem to be either other related Ranunculaceae family plants, or poppies. He says that, "All the kinds of *Anemones* are sharp, biting the tongue, and of a binding quality." There is no doubt that these plants exhibit this quality, and in fact one must be very careful when harvesting or processing fresh *Anemone* because it can cause significant eye and sinus irritation. Gerard says that the leave (juiced) and snuffed up the nose "purge the head mightly," which Salmon repeats with further elucidation (see below). I would not recommend this. He also says that, "The juice mundifies [purges and purifies] and clenses maligne, virulent, and corrosive ulcers." This application is one that the author has no experience with, but can imagine that the fresh juice would act in this way and might have very appropriate applications in these cases, although modern herbalists rarely are called on to address such an issue.

Culpeper (1653) states, "The leaves provoke the terms mightily, being boiled, and the decoction drank." The phrase, "the terms" refers to menstruation. This medicinal has a long history of use in delayed and irregular menstruation, and Culpeper emphasizes that it is a very strong medicinal in this function. In contrast, I would not suggest such a strong action, but it certainly has use in menstrual disorders.

Salmon (1710) says this medicinal is hot and dry in the third degree and is specific for "apoplexies, epilepsies, lethargies, madness, [and] vertigo proceeding from a cold and moist humor or distemper of the head and brain." Later, he describes the use of the juice (the juice is probably the closest to our modern fresh plant tincture) by saying:

> *"The juice being snuffed up the nose morning and evening, but chiefly at bed time, it mightily purges the head and brain, and brings away abundance of cold, moist, phlegmatic humors, and thereby frees the patient of apoplexies, epilepsies, lethargies, and most other cold distempers of the head, brain, and nerves, caused*

by those humors lodged in the head, in the cavities of the brain, or between the meninges thereof, viz. between the "pia" and "dura mater."

To my knowledge, this is the most complete and clear description we have from an early author of using this medicinal in the way that modern Western herbalists employ it today. Modern Western herbalists, almost exclusively, employ the fresh plant tincture of this medicinal. And, although this preparation method is different it is likely quite similar in action and can have profound therapeutic actions.

In the Felter & Llody (1909), had this to say:

"Pulsatilla is a remedy of wide applicability, but more particularly for those conditions in which the mind is a prominent factor. A gloomy mentality, a state of nerve depression and unrest, a disposition to brood over real or imagined trouble, a tendency to look on the dark side of life, sadness, mild restlessness, and a state of mental unrest generally denominated in broad terms "nervousness," are factors in the condition of the patient requiring Pulsatilla. A Pulsatilla patient weeps easily, and the mind is inclined to wander—to be unsettled. The pulse requiring Pulsatilla is weak, soft, and open, and the tissues have a tendency to dryness (except when the mucous tissues are discharging a thick, bland material), and, about the orbits the parts appear contracted, sunken, and dark in color. The whole countenance and movements of the body depict sadness, moroseness, despondency, and lack of tone. Hysteria of the mild and weeping form may be a symptom. The whole condition is one of nervous depression, the nutrition of the nerve centers are at fault. With such symptoms, Pulsatilla may be confidently prescribed in the conditions and disorders enumerated in this article."

Contemporary herbalist, 7Song, writes (in an article on his website):

"It is important for the herbalist to distinguish between panic disorder and other stress-type syndromes. I have not seen it work well for the fear that accompanies public speaking or interviews. I see it work most proficiently when the panic comes on suddenly, often without obvious provocation and the person has a sense of impending terror. These are often cardinal symptoms of panic attack."[2]

The above quotes are very much in line with my experience with this plant. An example of a clinical encounter follows:

I was called to help a friend one night. She is a single mom with a pre-teen son who has a history of behavioral problems. She was in a panic and asked me to come over right away because her son was acting very strangely. I was at her home within a couple of minutes. When I arrived, her son was mumbling and largely non-communicative. This had occurred suddenly and was, as far as she could tell, the result of the child's repeated behavioral problems at school coming to a head that day. Honestly, Anemone was not my first thought. My first thought was that he needed to be assessed by professional psychiatrists, but this was out of the question. When it occurred to me to try the Anemone, I had to find a way to get the boy to take it. He would not allow anyone to touch him. Finally, after over 10 minutes, I instructed my friend on how to administer the tincture while I would physically restrain her son. The tincture was nearly two years old, and was made with *Anemone chinensis* in a 40% vodka solution (that's all I had at the time), so I was not confident in the strength of the tincture. I instructed her to administer about 10-15 drops. Once this was accomplished, I left him on his bed and stood back. After an initial flurry of yelling and violent movements, there was a clear shift in him. Within 1-2 minutes he was significantly calmer, and by that time his uncle, with whom he has an excellent relationship, arrived, and his mother and I were able to step back. Disaster averted!

Translation of Available Source Material:

As noted above, the Chinese species is well known and since there is reliable literature in the English language I see no need to translate more here.

1. Ren, Yi et al., (2010). *Botanical Journal of the Linnean Society*. 62: pp. 77–100.
2.http://7song.com/files/Herbalists%20View-%20Anemone%20for%20 Panic%20 Attacks.pdf (accessed 24 April, 2013).

Pedicularis

Pedicularis densiflora Benth., *P. groenlandica* Retz., and others
Scrophulariaceae
Pedicularis herba et flos
Common Name: Indian Warrior (*P. densiflora*), Elephant's Head (*P. groenlandica*)
Favor and Qi: sweet, bitter, slightly acrid, cool
Channels entered: liver, heart
Actions: anodyne, muscle relaxant, sedative

Functions & Indications:

Calms the spirit, settles and nourishes the heart, and resolves constraint. Pedicularis is used for symptoms of emotional constraint leading to symptoms of vexation, heat vexation, fullness or stuffiness in the chest, anxiety, insomnia, irritability, etc. Emotional constraint can lead to qi stagnation and disharmonious interaction between the organs system, particularly the heart, liver, and kidney. Pedicularis is sweet, bitter, slightly acrid, and cool. Sweet can nourish, bitter can drain, while acridity moves. Pedicularis is cool in nature and has a sweet and bitter flavor, so it can cool the heart when it becomes over-heated from constraint, while nourishing it to both settle the heart and calm the spirit. The acrid flavor can move and Pedicularis gentley moves qi to help resolve constraint.

Relaxes the sinews, quickens the blood, and relieves pain. Pedicularis is used for muscle tension and pain due to a variety of causes ranging from physical strain or trauma to tension due to emotional issues. The root of pain is stagnation of qi and/or stasis of blood. When blood becomes static, this can lead to heat. Bitterness and coolness drain and clear heat, acridity moves and opens. The combination of these flavors with its cool nature allows Pedicularis to relax the sinews, quicken the blood, and relieve pain.

Cautions:

This is a hemiparasitic plant, therefore great care must be taken when harvesting. It is critical to pay close attention to what other plants are growing around it, and avoid any potential interactions with toxic plants.

For example, I used to live near an area with a lot of *P. densiflora* (Indian Warrior), and one large stand near my house was also home to a species of *Senecio*, some of which are known to have toxic compounds. Although I couldn't be sure if there was any relationship between the plants, I avoided harvesting from that area. It is also important to remember that different stands may have quite a lot of variation in quality, so once a particular area is found to be good, I suggest harvesting from that same area for consistent medicine.

Dosage and Preparation:

Fresh tincture 2–6ml; fresh juice 10–60ml; dry herb tea 6–15g; flowering tops (in bud) of Elephant's Head, Little Elephant's Head, and Indian Warrior can be smoked, as can Parrot's Beak leaf.

Major Combinations:

Combine with California Poppy and Skullcap for anxiety and tension due to emotional upset.

Combine with *sānqī* and Arnica for muscle pain and tightness due to external trauma; add *chuānxiōng* and *hónghuā* for more severe pain.

Combine with Red Baneberry or Black Cohosh for muscular pain with spasms. Add Lobelia for severe spasms.

Commentary:

Pedicularis is a genus that is biogeographically centered in the Himalayas.[1] This genus is part of the Scrophulariaceae or Figwort family (it recently was moved to the Orobanchaceae/Broomrape Family, but most sources still list it as Scrophulariaceae), which consists of 500–600 species. The genus is circumboreal, mostly in the Northern Hemisphere, and approximately half (271) are endemic to China. The *Grand Dictionary of Chinese Medicinals* has four separate materia medica monographs totaling seven species (see translation material below). There are at least 36 species in North America, one-third of which have recorded uses. I could find no ethnobotanical information about any European species. In short, considering that Pedicularis is the largest genus in the Scrophulariaceae family (which is likely also true of the Orobanchaceae) and clearly has wide usage throughout Asia and North America, there is relatively little knowledge about its use.

The species listed in this monograph are all, generally, used interchangeably, although many herbalists seem to favor the Elephant's Head (*P. groenlandica*). I prefer the Indian Warrior, but that may be because; 1) my convenient access to stands of this plant, 2) its large size, which makes harvesting much easier, and 3) the habitat it grows in is significantly less ecologically sensitive. Indian Warrior's geographic range is significantly smaller than that of the other major species (*P. groenlandica*). It is found only in California and Southern Oregon. Within its range, however, it is quite common and often creates large carpets of scarlet (from the flowering heads; both the flowers and the bracts are scarlet colored) on the forest floor or shrubby hillside where it colonizes. Although Elephant's Head can be found throughout the Western Mountain States and much of Canada, it prefers boggy areas and wet meadows at high elevation (dependent on latitude), which are far more ecologically sensitive than the drier areas preferred by Indian Warrior. That being said, there is no reason to believe the proper harvesting of Elephant's Head is not ecologically sound. I know of several herbalists who have been harvesting and monitoring stands of Elephant's Head in Oregon for over two decades and they report that there appears to be no decline in those stands in spite of annual harvesting.

There is very little information on this genus in the literature, either ethnobotanical or scientific, as it relates to medicinal use. There are some records of use throughout North America and Asia, but the information is not very detailed. One example is this record from India about *P. longiflora*, "Used against all kinds of kidney and urinary disorders, soothing, and controls urine discharge, inflammation and bleeding in the kidney."[2] This description is actually very detailed compared to others, such as "stomach disorder" for *P. pectinata* (also from India).[3]

In North American this botanical medicine seems to have only recently gained some notoriety, but only amongst herbalist. The source for this all seems to come from one of the fathers of modern American herbal medicine, Michael Moore. There are a few ethnobotanical records, but unfortunately they are both scant and lacking detail. The Cheyenne Nation of Montana used *P. groenlandica*, "For coughs, the patient drank an infusion made by long boiling the pulverized leaves and stems."[4] Naturopathic doctor Eric Yarnell from Seattle uses *P. bracteosa* for chronic pelvic pain and prostatitis.[5] Well-known herbalist Michael Moore writes, "By itself, it is one of our safest and most effective skeletal muscle relaxants."[6]

Some modern research suggests that a few species may have "good" to "very good" antioxidant properties and might be beneficial for liver damage. (I have chosen not to cite studies because they all involve the use of animals.) There are also a number of papers (in Chinese) that discuss the chemical constituents of various species of Pedicularis, which focus mostly on iridoids, phenylpropanoids, and flavonoids, as well as other chemistry, but that is beyond the scope of this book. Most research on this genus seems to be from China, although I was able to find one paper from Iran (in English) that looked at two of the nine species present in that country.[7] In this paper the authors are looking at the chemistry of their native species based on research that has been done in China. They also state that the medicinal properties of the Iranian species are unknown.

Taken as a whole, the genus *Pedicularis* is very large with a few well defined species regarding medicinal actions, yet a few more species with limited information on their usefulness, and a lot of species with little to no information. Given that the species we have information about seem to show significant usefulness, it is the opinion of the author that further investigation should be done on this genus to determine which species might be useful and to further develop what we know about those we already use.

Translation of Available Source Material:

Approximately half of the *Pedicularis* genus is endemic to China, however there are only scant references to any of these plants being used in Chinese medicine. The largest entry is for at least three different species all referred to as *tàibáishēn* (太白蔘). The *Grand Dictionary of Chinese Medicinals* (2009) is the source for nearly all the material I can find in Chinese about this plant. *Grand Dictionary of Chinese Medicinals* lists the following three species: P. davidii, dàwèimǎxiānhāo (大衛馬先蒿), P. deora, měiguānmǎxiānhāo (美觀馬先蒿), and P. dunniana, dèngshìmǎxiānhāo (鄧氏馬先蒿) (for more on these species see Lousewort entry on page 271). There is also brief mention of a fourth species, P. rudis, yěmǎxiānhāo (野馬先蒿). All of these species grow at the intersection of the Qing Hai Plateau and Central China, in or near the provinces of Qing Hai, Shaanxi, Gansu, and Sichuan; some grow beyond this range. They are all high elevation plants, with *P. davidii* growing down to the lowest elevation of 1750m. The *Grand Dictionary of Chinese Medicinals* lists them as sweet, slightly bitter, warm, and slightly toxic (Note: I did not find any other sources that mentioned toxicity. This leads me to believe that the Chinese have found that it can be toxic, but perhaps didn't realize that the genus is hemiparasitic. As noted above, this could lead to toxicity if the plants are growing with other toxic plants by *Pedicularis* up-taking toxic constituents from these plants.) It enriches yin and supplements the kidney, boosts qi, and fortifies the spleen. It is used to treat spleen–kidney dual vacuity, steaming bone tidal heat [effusion], joint pain, and no desire for food or drink. The *Handbook of Frequently Used Chinese Medicinals from Northern China* (1971) only lists *P. davidii*. The root is harvested in the autumn, sliced and dried prior to use. The preparation method is to mix-fry it with wheat bran until the root turns yellow; discard the bran and store for use. This source also gives us the following three clinical nuggets: For body weakness and dizziness, combine this herb with *dǎngshēn* (15g each) and *xìxīn* (3g) as a decoction; for whole body and joint pain with feverishness of the palms and soles, combine 250g with pig's feet and cook as a soup to eat; for vacuity taxation tidal heat, combine with *cháihú*, *qínjiāo*, and *huángbǎi*.

1. Wolfe, Andrea D., et al. (2005). Phylogeny and Biogeography of Orobanchaceae. *Folia Geobotanica* 40(2–3): pp 115–134.

2. Ballabh, Basant, et al. (2008). *Journal of Ethnopharmacology.* 118(5): pp 331–339.

3. Singh, K.N. & Lal Brij. (2008). *Journal of Ethnopharmacology* 115(3): pp 147–159.

4. Hart, Jeffrey, A. (1981). *Journal of Ethnopharmacology.* 4(1): pp 1–55.

5. Yarnell, Eric. Sylvan Institute of Botanical Medicine. *Urology Series.* 2012.

6. Moore, Michael. *Medicinal Plants of the Pacific West.* Red Crane Books. pp 68. 1993.

7. Khodaie, Laleh, et al. (2012). *BioImpacts.* 2(1): pp 47–53.

Medicinal	Nature	Flavor	Channels	Functions	Indications
Hops	warm	bitter, acrid	heart, spleen, stomach	Quiets the spirit; Harmonizes the stomach and liver, and disperses food; Stops pain	irritability, irascibility, sleeplessness, and vexation; sour belching, stomach qi ascending counterflow, sour taste in the mouth, nausea, and vomiting; internally and externally for pain
Lemon Balm	cool	acrid, bitter, slightly sweet	stomach, liver, heart	Clears heat, resolves the exterior, and eliminates vexation; Clears heat and eliminates vexation; Opens the stomach, facilitates the flow of qi in the middle, and stops pain	Externally contracted wind-heat, vexation; vexation, red eyes, lip and mouth sores, and headaches; fullness in the abdomen, burping, acid reflux, pain in the middle
Pasque Flower	warm	acrid, bitter, aromatic	heart, liver	Opens the heart orifice and calms the spirit; Rectifies the qi and regulates the menses	vexation, emotional depression, inability to think clearly, anxiety, mania & withdrawal (drug induced); stopped or painful menstruation, headache, vexation, irritability, irascibility, fullness in the chest & rib-sides, & a string-like pulse
Pedicularis	cool	bitter, slightly acrid	liver, heart	Relaxes the sinews, quickens the blood, and relieves pain;	vexation, heat vexation, fullness or stuffiness in the chest, anxiety, insomnia, irritability, etc.; muscle tension and pain

開竅藥

Open the Orifices Medicinals

The open the orifices category is made up of strongly aromatic, mobile, and penetrating medicinals. These medicinals are used to open the orifices and arouse the spirit. They treat blockage patterns (heat block, damp block, or phlegm block) with clouded spirit. This category is also sometimes called aromatic open the orifices, or open the orifices with aroma, or open the orifices and arouse the spirit.

Spirit–mind clouded and confused has both repletion and vacuity patterns. Repletion patterns are blockage patterns and are caused by heat, cold, dampness, or phlegm. The combination of either heat or cold with dampness or phlegm is almost always present, but predominance of one must be determined for appropriate treatment strategies to be established. This should not be overly difficult as the signs and symptoms associated with these patterns are the same as any other pattern, e.g. heat patterns exhibit a red face, forceful pulse, and a red tongue, etc.

Vacuity patterns here are also known as desertion patterns. Desertion patterns are any disease where there is a critical damage to yin, yang, qi, or blood. This can come from two primary causes, either acute damage such as severe blood loss or an extremely traumatic event, or the gradual collapse of essential qi due to an enduring illness, the former is known as fulminant desertion and the latter is known as vacuity desertion.

Treatment for each of this diverse group of patterns is likewise diverse, however when the spirit–mind is clouded the medicinals in this category are always useful.

Lavender

Lavandula angustifolia Mill.

Lamiaceae

Lavandulae herba cum flos

Chinese Name: *xūnyīcǎo* (薰衣草)

Favor and Qi: acrid, bitter, slightly sweet, warm

Channels entered: heart, liver

Actions: antiinflammatory, anxiolytic

Functions & Indications:

Disperses phlegm, eliminates vexation, and settles the liver. Lavender is used for anxiety, restlessness and sleeplessness due to liver wind rising to the head and bringing with it phlegm, rheum, or turbidity. Although Lavender is warm, it settles the liver by dispersing internal wind and moving qi. Lavender is an effective medicinal for quieting the spirit in small doses, but can have a reviving action on the spirit in larger doses (in part due to its action of dispersing phlegm). It can have a profound action on those with vexing anxiety that lead to restlessness and sleeplessness. Lavender's warm acridity disperses phlegm, phlegm-rheum, or phlegm-drool, to help resolve vexation and disquieted spirit, manifesting in symptoms such as restlessness and sleeplessness.

Moves qi and relieves constraint, gently moves the qi of the liver and resolves liver constraint qi stagnation. Lavender is used for abdominal or menstrual pain, especially when associated with headache and vexation due to liver constraint. Lavender is warm, acrid, and bitter. Warmth moves and activates, while acridity can dissipate and move; bitter can drain and move downward. The symptoms of headache and vexation due to liver constraint are pathologically related to qi stagnation and the liver's inability to properly regulate the flow of qi. Lavender effectively moves the liver qi and relieves constraint to treat these conditions. Although the pattern often includes, or is a function of, heat or fire, and Lavender is warming, its qi is "mild or thin" (薄 *bó*) thus can disperse. This medicinal can be used in combination with cooling medicinals very effectively.

Quickens blood and engenders flesh. Lavender is used for external application to burns and "degraded tissue." For this, the essential oil of this medicinal is generally used. Lavender essential oil is used in a variety of external preparations for the treatment of burns and traumatic skin injuries.

Cautions:

Use the essential oil internally with extreme caution. Immoderate use of the tea can cause abdominal pain.

Dosage and Preparation:

Fresh plant tincture 2–4 ml; essential oil 0.1–0.5 drops; infusion 1–4g. Although this herb can be used as a tea, it is mostly commonly used either as a tincture or an essential oil. Alternatively, the dried flowers are used in such applications as pillows to aid those with stubborn sleeplessness (see commentary below).

Major Combinations:

Add to *Suān Zǎo Rén Tāng* for sleeplessness with vacuity heat vexation.

Combine with *huángqín* and Skullcap for vexation associated with emotional upset, stuffiness in the chest, and headache due to liver constraint.

Combine with *xiāngfù* and *zhǐshí* for vexation associated with menstrual pain or abdominal pain.

Combine with *xiāngfù*, Motherwort, and *yùjīn* for (heat) vexation associated with menstrual pain due to liver constraint and liver heat.

For external application to burns, combine with Calendula, St. John's Wort, and *zǐcǎogēn*.

Commentary:

There are two main species of Lavender used in medicine, and a hybrid known as Lavandin. These species are not exactly the same and the hybrid is a reasonable combination of the two from a medicinal point of view. However, when one wishes to be more penetrating with therapy either *L. spica* or Lavandin should be employed. *L. angustifolia* is significantly less penetrating in action, perhaps due to the former's significantly higher levels of camphor in its chemical profile. That said, *L. spica* is considered a synonym for *L. angustifolia* in the academic literature.

Lavender is one of the most ubiquitous herbs from the Mediterranean region, and the only such aromatic Medierranean herb which is not generally used in food; other such herbs include Rosemary, Thyme, Basil, etc. It is found in numerous products, from skin care to medicinal products, from pillows to help you sleep to potpourri sachets for bringing its pleasant odor into your home. A common folk remedy for difficulty sleeping is to put good quality lavender flowers into a sachet and place it around the pillow area of one's bed; sometimes people simply put the flowers directly into their pillow. The pleasant odor of this flower also has a very calmative effect, and people usually report a more restful sleep. For this application, the essential oil can also be used. The essential oil placed in an infuser (a small glass instrument that will infuse the essential oil into the air of a room) is a common and simple way to use this medicinal's essential oil and is especially useful for children or those unable to take medications by mouth. Many people prefer this method, which allows the addition of other essential oils as needed.

Gerard (1597) writes of the temperature of Lavender:

> *"Lavender is hot and dry, and that in the third degree, and is of a thin substance, consisting of many airy and spiritual parts. Therefore it is good to be given any way against the diseases of the head, and especially those which have their original or beginning not of abundance of humors, but chiefly of a quality only."*

While I believe that Lavender can and does have an action on "abundance of humors," Gerard also recognized that the over-all quality of Lavender is "thin" (see above for more explanation of this concept in Chinese medicine and how it applies to the therapeutics of Lavender), and I agree. I believe that while the light and thin nature of Lavender does, in fact, have a profound effect on the head, its ability to pierce phlegm is a matter of dosage. When using the tincture, or essential oil, Lavender very effectively cuts phlegm and helps to resolve it.

Parkinson (1640) states, "Lavender is especially good for all grief and pains of the head and brain that proceed from a cold cause, such as stroke [or like symptoms], drowsie or sluggish malady, cramps, convulsions, and palsies, as also those that are given to faint often." Although Parkinson does not state that specifically that this herb is warm, he definitely alludes to this by stating these ailments are, "from a cold cause." Gerard (above) and Salmon (1710) actually specifically states that this herb is "hot and dry in the third degree," which suggests that authors of this era considered this plant to be very warming.

Culpeper (1653) has a fairly lengthy monograph on this herb. He leads with (most likely quoting Parkinson without giving him credit), "Lavender is of a special good use for all the griefs and pains of the head and brain that proceed of a cold cause..." Later he says of the distilled water, "...it is not safe to use it where the body is replete with blood and humours, because of the hot and subtil spirits wherewith it is possessed." These statements clearly show that Culpeper considered the medicinal to be warm. This warmth, and (I would add) acridity, are what make it an effective herb for resolving constrained qi. In another part of the monograph, he states "It strengthens the stomach, and freeth the liver and spleen from obstructions, provoketh women's courses, and expelleth the dead child and after-birth." This statement clearly supports my supposition that it moves the qi, while also suggesting that it quickens the blood.

Grieve (1931) reports,

> *"Its use in the swabbing of wounds obtained further proof during the War, and the French Academy of Medicine is giving attention to the oil for this and other antiseptic surgical purposes. The oil is successfully used in the treatment of sores, varicose ulcers, burns and scalds. In France, it is a regular thing for most households to keep a bottle of Essence of Lavender as a domestic remedy against bruises, bites and trivial aches and pains, both external and internal."*

Many of these uses continue today, although it is no longer used as an antiseptic for surgical purposes, it is used externally for a variety of sores, ulcers, and burns. The latter I consider to be a very important use, and strongly advocate the inclusion of this essential oil in products for the external application to burns.

Lavender has undergone a significant amount of modern research. Most of this has been done showing Lavender's affects on the neurological system. Studies showing both safety and positive result abound. In one review paper it states, "The evidence for oral [administration of] Lavender is promising [for anxiety/stress]..."[1] Two-hundred twenty-one (221) patients diagnosed with "anxiety disorder" in a randomized controlled study were given 80mg/day oral Lavender oil for 10 weeks. The authors of the study conclude, "Lavandula oil preparation had a significant beneficial influence on quality and duration of sleep and improved general mental and physical health without causing any unwanted sedative or other drug specific effects."[2] A study done on wound healing, treatment of episiotomy, the Lavender group show significant improvement over standard treatment in pain, swelling, and redness.[3] Unfortunately healing time was not measured.

1. Perry, R., Terry, R., Watson, L.K., Ernst, E. (2012). Is lavender an anxiolytic drug? A systematic review of randomized clinical trails. *Phtomedicine.* 19: pp 825–835.

2. Kasper, Siegfried, et al., (2010). Silexan, an orally administered Lavandula oil preparation, is effective in the treatment of 'subsyndromal' anxiety disorder: a randomized, double–blind, placebo controlled trial. *International Clinical Psychopharmacology.* 25(5): pp 277–287.

3. Vakilian, Katayon, et al., (2011). Healing advantages of lavender essential oil during episiotomy recover: A clinical trial. *Complimentary Therapies in Clinical Practice.* 17(1): pp 50–53.

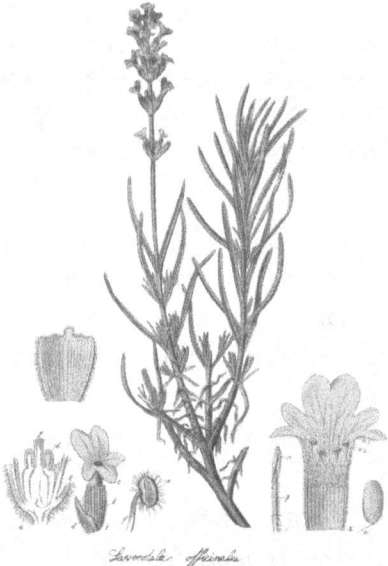

Lavandula officinalis

Rosemary

Rosmarinus officinalis L.

Lameaceae

Rosemarini officinalis folium

Chinese name: *mídiéxiāng* (迷迭香)

Favor and Qi: acrid, aromatic, warm

Channels entered: urinary bladder, stomach, heart

Actions: antioxidant, antidepressant, antispasmodic, hyperglycemic

Functions & Indications:

Dissipates cold, dispels wind, and warms and frees the channels and network vessels. Rosemary is used for headaches, muddled thinking, confusion, forgetfulness, pain in the teeth associated with external contraction of cold or vacuity cold conditions leading to stagnation of qi or congestion. Rosemary is acrid and warm, with acrid warmth it dissipates cold and dispels wind. Rosemary is also aromatic and with aroma penetrates the channels and network vessels. This combination of acridity, aroma, and warmth, along with its affinity for the head, make rosemary a very important herb for the treatment of headaches, especially associated with cold.

Moves and rectifies qi, and harmonizes the liver and stomach. Rosemary is used for liver qi over-acting on the stomach leading to fullness in the chest and abdomen, rib-side pain as well as digestive complaints such as bloating, painful flatus, stomach duct pain, and abdominal pain. Rosemary is acrid, aromatic, and warm, and like many other plants with these qualities it has a positive effect on the digestion when there is qi stagnation. Warm acridity can move qi and disperse. Rosemary courses the liver to resolve liver constraint; with aroma it opens the stomach and assist the stomach to move qi downward.

Dispels phlegm and opens the orifices of the heart. Rosemary is used for a variety of conditions associated with disturbance of the mind/spirit due to phlegm confounding the orifices of the heart. This herb is used for conditions such as muddled thinking, loss of speech, mania, epilepsy, and other mental/emotional disorders associated with these patterns. By its acridity and warmth it helps to free the channels, open the orifices and transform phlegm when treating the mind/spirit that has been disturbed by clouding, phlegm, rheum, dampness, and/or cold. This herb can be used in heat conditions if the main pathology is attributed to phlegm, but must be combined with heat clearing medicinals. When used for this function, an alcohol preparation or the essential oil is best.

Cautions:

Rosemary is also a culinary herb and is considered very safe. However, because of Rosemary's strong acrid and aromatic nature, caution should be exercised for those with yin vacuity, especially yin vacuity heat.

Dosage and Preparation:

Tincture 1–3ml; strong infusion 2–6g; essential oil 0.05–0.3ml (Use with caution internally)

Major Combinations:

This is an important medicinal to add to formulas for the treatment of wind–cold external invasion when there is headache present. Formulas such as *Guì Zhī Tāng*, *Má Huáng Tāng*, and the like will all benefit from this herb when there is pronounced headache. It can also be used to modify wind–heat external invasion formulas when headache is present.

Combine with *yuǎnzhì* and *shíchāngpú* for phlegm misting the mind/spirit with symptoms of dispondency, muddled thinking, forgetfulness, etc.

Commentary:

Rosemary is a commonly used culinary herb and has a long history of use as a medicinal plant. Rosemary is a perennial bush that is very easy to grow as long as there is not a very hard freeze. It is a native to the Mediterranean region, but is now grown in many places around the world. In places like California, USA (a Mediterranean climate) it is a very common garden plant and is often used in landscape architecture because it is easily manicured, has a pleasant fragrance, is drought tolerant, and offers a sweet light blue to purple bloom in the spring and summer.

Considering the long history of use of this plant, it is hard to believe that there is not an abundance of both ethnobotanical and modern laboratory research. There is ethnobotanical literature, but is is almost all part of larger studies that are looking at the uses of plants in a particular area and do not offer much insight into any particular plant in the listings. One interesting research study showed a dose dependant, but very significant, improvement of gastric ulcers induced by various means, including ethanol.[1] Its use as a preservative in food has also produced an enormous amount of research pertaining to its action as an antioxidant. Unfortunately the vast majority of the modern research done on this plant uses animal models in an attempt to explain or "understand" it's traditional uses. Thus, a traditional use such as antidepressant in Spain[2] yields research on rats and mice, subjecting them to forced swimming and being hung by their tail to show that, yes in fact, Rosemary seems to have an antidepressant action. Other studies show similar positive results based on reviewing the historical literature, but for our purposes, we will just stick to the literature that shows how Rosemary works on people.

One of the main indications for this medicinal is in the treatment of headaches and other congested pathologies of the head. Like *xìxīn* (*Asarum* sp.), Rosemary is acrid and warm and treats headaches. This is a commonality between them, although these medicinals are different in many other ways. Because of our more recent knowledge of aristolochic acid being present in most *xìxīn* and our understanding of its potential toxicity, not to mention that most Western countries have banned the sale of *xìxīn*, Rosemary is a good alternative to consider when you might have otherwise prescribed *xìxīn* in the treatment of headaches. Rosemary can be substituted in any formula where *xìxīn* is called for and will yield good results without the concern for exposing your patients to aristolochic acid; this is especially true for symptoms in the head. Rosemary is not as good as *xìxīn* for the treatment of nasal congestion or cough, but will have a positive effect on those symptoms as well. However, Rosemary must be used in full doses, or as a tincture, in order to get an effect one might be used to getting when using *xìxīn*.

Dioscorides (2000 *trans.*) states, "It is warming and cures jaundice." Dioscorides doesn't say much else about this medicinal, but there is little doubt that this medicinal had many other applications that he did not write about.

Gerard (1597) speaks highly of this medicinal, first noting its importance in "civil purposes." The civil purposes he is referencing are wedding, funerals, and other similar societal ceremonies. In discussing it's use in medicine he starts by saying, "...the warming and comforting heat thereof helpeth all cold diseases, both of the head, stomach, liver, and belly: the decoction thereof in wine helpeth the cold distillations of the brain into the eyes, etc. and all other cold diseases of the head and brain..." He goes on to mention most of the symptoms described in the monograph above. Gerard's discussion confirms the obvious warm/acrid nature of this medicinal, and shows us that this medicinal (and culinary herb) has been used for the same or similar applications for no less than 500 years!

Culpeper (1653) says, "it helpeth all cold diseases of the head, stomach, liver, and belly." Owing to its warmth and affinity for the head/brain he says, "The decoction in wine, helpeth the cold distillations of rheums into the eyes, and all other cold diseases of the head and brain, as the giddiness or swimmings therein, drowsiness or dullness of the mind and senses like a stupidness, the dumb palsy, or loss of speech, the lethargy and falling-sickness" Although Culpeper attributes these illnesses to cold, and there very well might be cold according to Chinese medicine, these types of illnesses are generally considered a pathology of phlegm confounding the orifices of the heart and congesting the channels. This is caused by phlegm turbidity.

Interestingly, the greatest moments of American herbal medicine (the Eclectic and Physiomedical traditions) essentially ignored this medicinal. It has only a cursory entry in Felter & Llody (1909) and is absent elsewhere. Like Thyme, Rosemary, as a medicinal plant, seems cursed by its place of significance in the culinary arts. However, in my opinion, it is worthy of a significant place in the materia medica.

Translation of Available Source Material:

The medicinal first appeared in the *Bēn Cǎo Shí Yí* (741). This book lists it as acrid, warm, and without toxicity; governs malign qi (恶气). The *Grand Dictionary of Chinese Medicinals* (2009) says it induces sweating, fortifies the spleen, quiets the spirit, and stops pain. Used to treat all kinds of headaches, and stops early hair loss. Decoction 4.5–9g for internal use or soaked in water for external use.

1. Corrêa, Patrícia, et al., (2010). Antiulcerogenic activity of crude hydroalcoholic extract of *Rosmarinus officinalis* L. *Journal of Ethnopharmacology*. 69(1): pp 57–62.

2. Heinrich, Michael, Kufer, Johanna, Marco, Leonti, Pardo–de–Santayana, Manuel (2006). Ethnobotany and ethnopharmacology—Interdisciplinary ling with the historical sciences. *Journal of Ethnopharmacology* 107(3): pp 157–160.

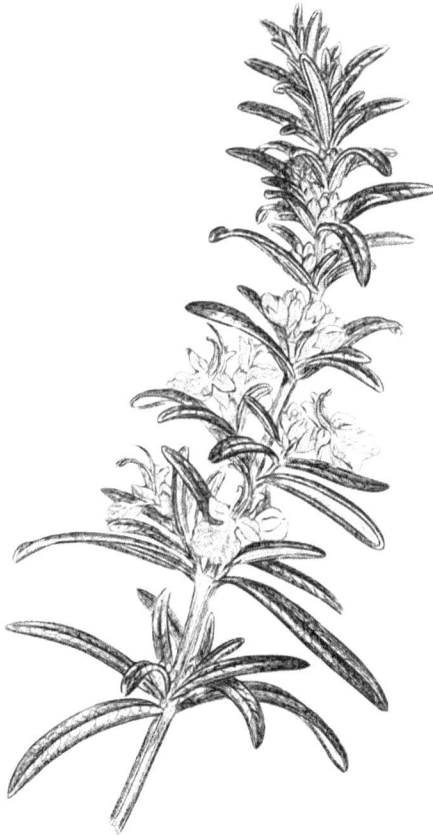

Rosmarinus officinalis

Medicinal	Nature	Flavor	Channels	Functions	Indications
Lavender	warm	acrid, bitter, slightly sweet	heart, liver	Disperses phlegm, eliminates vexation, and quiets the spirit; Moves qi and relieves constraint; Quickens blood and engenders flesh	anxiety, restlessness and sleeplessness; abdominal pain and menstrual pain, associated with headache and vexation due to liver constraint; external application burns and "degraded tissue"
Rosemary	warm	acrid, aromatic	urinary bladder, stomach, heart	Dissipates cold, dispels wind, and warms and frees the channels and network vessels; Moves and rectifies qi, and harmonizes the liver and stomach; Dispels phlegm and opens the orifices of the heart	headaches, muddled thinking, confusion, forgetfulness, pain in the teeth; fullness in the chest and abdomen, rib-side pain, bloating, painful flatus, stomach duct pain, and abdominal pain; muddled thinking, loss of speech, mania, epilepsy, and other mental/emotional disorders

外用薬

External Application Medicinals

The external application category of medicinals is a group of medicinals that are primarily used for application to the outer surface of the body. These medicinals are used from a wide range of ailments from acute trauma to sores due to either external damage or internal patterns that have led to external manifestations of sore, carbuncles, or other damage to the skin and flesh.

The medicinals in this category are often acrid and moving in nature because quickening the blood and moving qi are necessary for both relieving pain due to trauma and healing wounds. While these medicinals are primarily used externally they may also be used internally. Some, like Comfrey, are specific for engendering flesh and are important medicinals for treating wounds from any cause. And, while not placed in this category, medicinals like Calendula (found in the blood quickening category) are also used externally.

Pain is almost always associated with ailments treated by external application medicinals because whether acute trauma or external manifestations of internal patterns, most of these illnesses include pain as a symptom. Likewise, heat is a very common sign due to the fact that stagnation (the primary reason for pain) will eventually lead to heat, and many of the medicinals in this category clear heat.

In this materia medica Comfrey stands out as one of the most important medicinals world-wide for the treatment of trauma, but of the skin and flesh, and of the bones. This medicinal should be studied and well-understood by Chinese herbalists so that it can be assimilated into the practice of Chinese medicine; there is no medicinal in the Chinese materia medica that can rival Comfrey.

California Coast Sage

Artemisia californica Less.

Asteraceae

Artemisiae californicae herba

Favor and Qi: bitter, acrid, aromatic, cold

Channels entered: liver, gall bladder

Actions: digestive bitter, anthelmintic, diuretic, antiinflammatory, analgesic

Functions & Indications:

Stops pain and clears heat. California Coast Sage is used externally for traumatic injury or chronic painful conditions such as wind–damp impediment. California Coast Sage is a traditional external (and sometime internal) medicinal for pain syndromes (see *Commentary* for more details). Its strong acrid aroma and cold nature both moves qi and quicken the blood, as well as clearing heat, making this medicinal excellent for hot painful joints or other inflamed traumatic injuries.

Clears heat, resolves toxin, and stops pain. California Coast Sage is applied externally as a wash or other preparation and is used for traumatic wounds to the skin, welling–abscess, or other open sores that are red and swollen with or without pus. California Coast Sage is bitter and cold and can clear heat and resolve toxin; with acridity is moves qi and quickens the blood to relieve pain. Although this medicinal is primarily used externally for these conditions it can also be used internally.

Clears heat and drains dampness. California Coast Sage is used for damp–heat in the liver and gallbladder with symptoms of abdominal pain with fullness, rid–side pain, constipation or diarrhea, with possible vomiting; a red tongue with thick slimy yellow fur, and rapid (and possibly slippery or firm) pulse. California Coast Sage is bitter, acrid, and cold; with cold bitterness it clears heat and drains downward to help resolve pathogenic heat and dampness while utilizing aroma to assist the spleen and help to resolve dampness, and with acridity it moves qi and blood and relieves pain.

Cautions:

Although there are no noted cautions for this medicinal, due to its cold and acrid nature it is advisable to be use caution in patients with spleen/stomach cold conditions or other patterns where such medicinals are ill–advised.

Dosage and Preparation:

Decoction or infusion 2–6g; fresh plant tincture 1–3ml; prepared as either an oil or liniment for external application

Major Combinations:

Prepared as an external liniment using fresh plant tincture. Add Arnica, *hónghuā*, and Cayenne for an excellent initial response liniment. For chronic problems remove Arnica and add *mòyào* and *rǔxiāng*.

Combine with Oregon Grape Root for damp–heat in the liver and gallbladder.

Combine with *Lóng Dǎn Xiè Gān Tāng* for pronounced rib–side pain and abdominal fullness.

Combine with Calendula, St. John's Wort, and Goldenseal (or *huánglián*) for supporating open wounds or welling–abscesses.

Commentary:

California Coast Sage is a common coastal and coastal mountain shrub, growing from the northern part of the San Francisco Bay Area to soutn to Northern Baja Mexico. It is an integral part of these ecosystems, giving small animals protection from predators as well as protecting hillsides from erosion. Although it is called "sage" it is actually a member of the Asteraceae family within the genus *Artemisia*, which includes Mugwort (*àiyè*); true sages are in the Mint or Lamiaceae family.

Although this is one of the most common shrubs of the California coast, it has gained almost no traction as a medicinal plant among modern herbalists. The Kumeyaay people of Southern California and Northern Baja used the plant to wash sores or wounds, and taken internally to relieve pain related to the gall bladder and for digestive problems such as fullness in the abdomen, vomiting, or diarrhea.[1] The Costanoan people used it for similar medicinal applications as well as cough, colds, and asthma. The former ailment was treated with an accompanying application of a poultice of the plant to the chest and back.[2] The Chumash people of Southern California used this plant for chronic pain of arthritis and other muscle and joint problems. And, there are other accounts that reflect similar usage.

The use of this plant as an external liniment caught the attention of researchers and recent work into the chemistry and application of this medicinal as a liniment has proven to be very fruitful. Chemical analysis found 15 monoterpenes, many well known to relieve pain such as eucolyptol, borneol, and camphor; additional compounds known to have antiinflammatory properties were also isolated. Additionally, the researchers found that a tincture made with this medicinal gave significant relief to moderate to severe pain when applied to human subjects.[3]

This is a common plant with a significant range in the coastal mountains from the San Francisco Bay Area into northern Baja Mexico. Although it had wide native use and has a small body of positive modern research, California Coast Sage remains an uncommonly used plant worthy of more investigation.

Translation of Available Source Material:

There are many species of *Artemisia* used in Chinese medicine, and although there are some similarities of use between the medicinal in this monograph and *Artemisia capillaris* (yīnchén), the latter is a well-known medicinal and there are plenty of references available in English for its use.

1. Wilken, Michael Alan, Master's Thesis, 2012.
2. Rocek, Barbara R. (1984). *Economic Botany*, 38(2): pp 240–255.
3. Fontaine, Pauline, et al. (2013) *Journal of Pharmacognosy and Phytotherapy*, (5)1: pp 1–11.

Witch Hazel

Hamamelis virginiana L.
Hamamelidaceae
Hamameli virginici folium
Favor and Qi: acrid, astringent, warm
Channels entered: heart, spleen
Actions: astringent

Functions & Indications:

Quicken the blood, resolves stasis, and stops pain. Witch Hazel is used for various types of blood stasis associated with cold coagulation of the blood, static blood due to cold vacuity, or static blood as a secondary factor of damp accumulation or qi stagnation. This herb can be used for hemorrhoids, varicose veins (especially if painful), blood in the stool due to blood stasis, and bruises and pain from knocks and falls. Witch Hazel is acrid and warm and enters the heart channel, which controls the vessels; with warm acridity it quickens the blood and resolves stasis to stop pain. Although primarily used externally, this medicinal can be and is used internally for these patterns.

Warms the channels and frees the network vessels. Witch Hazel is used for soreness due to cold stagnation impeding the flow of blood and qi in the vessels. This can manifest in multiple patterns where the vessels have been impacted by cold combined with wind, dampness, or blood stasis causing sore muscles. Witch Hazel enters the spleen, which controls the flesh, and the heart, which controls the vessels. It is warm, acrid, astringent and thus can enter the channels and move with warm acridity, while utilizing warming astringency to assist the functioning of the vessels and flesh to resolve pathogenic factors such as wind and dampness.

Witch Hazel is often used internally as a gargle for lax gums with or without bleeding, sore throat of any etiology, and mouth sores. It is also used externally for application to the vagina and anus for prolapse (vaginal and anal) and hemorrhoids (anal) as well as vaginal infections and discharge (also applied as a douche). Witch Hazel's warm astringency offers a gentle but effective resolution to these symptoms.

Cautions:

None noted

Dosage and Preparation:

Fluid extract 1–3ml, tincture 3–6ml, decoction 6–12g

Major Combinations:

Externally combined the *bark* of Witch Hazel with Bay Berry bark makes for an outstanding stimulating astringent. The combination of these two barks is simply one of the best stimulating astringent combinations I know. I like to combine this base with a number of other herbs depending on the presentation; Goldenseal for damp–heat, Cayenne for cold impediment, *sānqì* for bleeding, Horse Chestnut for hemorrhoids and varicose veins, etc.

The distilled extract (readily available at your local drug store) can be used along with a diluted decoction of Goldenseal for pink eye. A simple home remedy is to soak a Chamomile tea bag in this extract and apply it to the eye, allowing it to stay for 10 or more minutes.

Combine with Golden Seal and *kǔshēn* as a vaginal wash or douche for malodorous vaginal discharge due to damp–heat with itching, redness, swelling, and heat of the external (or internal) vaginal area.

Commentary:

Witch Hazel is one of the first plants I ever used as medicine. When I first starting studying martial arts in the early 80's my teacher gave us all a bottle of Witch Hazel extract, and instructed us to use it after every class. Classes were pretty hard core and I always left sore and sweating. But after the application of the Witch Hazel, I felt less sore and the sweating always slowed or stopped before I actually left the building. At the time I never thought to ask why, now it seems pretty obvious. Of course, my teacher hoped to relieve some of the soreness in our muscles, but the need to close our pores, at least to some extent, before we went out into the harsh New England winter was critical for us to avoid getting invaded by Cape Cod's cold and damp wind.

This plant is native to North America and was used widely by Native Americans within its range, including the Cherokee, Iroquois, and Chippewa; among others. The family (Hamamelidaceae) is an interesting family of about 140 species with a wide distribution, having genera in Asia, Australia, and North, Central, and South America. The two most widely distributed genera are also both medicinal genera, *Hamamelis* (Witch Hazel) and *Liquidamber*,[1] the latter is represented in Chinese medicine by the medicinal *lùlùtōng*. From a biogeographical point of view this family, and the above mentioned genera, are of particular interest in the attempt to understand how plants have migrated and how speciation has occurred. Furthermore, based on family and genus relationships, we might be able to better understand how to apply the Chinese medical paradigm to this valuable North American plant.

Although the leaves are the primary source of this botanical medicine, the young twigs and bark are also employed. Most frequently the leaves and young twigs are harvested together. While there are different opinions on which is better, I could find no research literature to support any one of the three possibilities. That said, when considering the quotes below; please note that the author's are primarily referring to the leaves and young twigs of this plant.

Cook (1869) states:

> *"It is quite soothing in its influence; and is one in a small list of plants which combine diffusive relaxant properties with astringency. This fact gives it a peculiar action, and renders it one of the most available of all the astringents in the second stages of dysentery and diarrhea, in hemorrhage from the bowels and bladder, catarrh of the bladder, nursing sore mouth, gonorrhea, and similar difficulties. It soothes the bowels rather than excites them, as many astringents do; and is an admirable wash in leucorrhea, prolapsus uteri and ani, and purulent ophthalmia, especially when combined with hydrastis [Goldenseal]."*

The "diffusive relaxant properties" that Cook mentions above I take to mean, or allude to, Witch Hazel's blood quickening action. Notice that he suggests its use in various bowel disorders when there is bleeding. Bleeding is, by definition, blood stasis. The action of "quickening" the blood, does not necessarily mean to move it faster, but rather to "enliven" it and "harmonize" it within the vessels. Thus, by offering the bowels an astringent blood quickening medicinal, the action is to slow or stop the bleeding, thus improving the tone and action of the bowels, leading to an over–all improvement of symptoms.

Felter & Llody (1909) state, "Its most pronounced virtue is its stimulating and tonic action upon the venous coats, exhibited so markedly in its power over *varicoses, hemorrhoids, hemorrhages*, and other conditions due to relaxation of venous structures." This text also offers a number of example for using this medicinal for uterine hemorrhage (both from excessive menstrual bleeding and postpartum hemorrhage), relieving pain from trauma, used both internally and external. Moerman (1998) offers many references of Native American use that supports these latter indications.

Translation of Available Source Material:

A Chinese species *Hamamelis mollis* Oliv. *jīnlǚméi* (金縷梅) is listed in modern Chinese materia medicas like *Xīn Huá Běn Cáo Gāng Yào* (1988) and the *Quán Guó Zhōng Cǎo Yào Huì Biān* (2008). The former says that it is sweet, warm, and enters the spleen channel. It supplements the middle and boosts the spleen for spleen qi vacuity and weakness patterns. It is used in decoction 9-15g. The latter repeats the former but adds that it can be used externally for knife wounds and can be drenched in alcohol, decocted with water and taken with brown sugar, a solution which should be taken before each meal. The small tree is native to central China from Zhejiang to Sichuan Provinces growing in thickets and forests from 300-800 meters. It has been under cultivation for many years and several varieties have been selected for their flowers. What is special about this genus, although not the only one, is that it blooms in the early spring before the leaves emerge, giving it a key place in gardens and landscapes.

1. Jianhua Li, A. Linn Bogle and Anita S. Klein (1999). Phylogenetic relationships of the Hamamelidaceae inferred from sequences of internal transcribed spacers (ITS) of nuclear ribosomal DNA. *American Journal of Botany*. 86(7): pp 1027–1037.

Comfrey

Symphytum officinalis L.
Boraginaceae
Symphyti radix et folium
Favor and Qi: bitter, sweet, cool
Channels entered: stomach, lung, liver, kidney
Actions: antiinflammatory, antitussive, wound healer

Functions & Indications:

Clears heat, disperses swelling, and engenders flesh. Comfrey is used externally and internally (see *Cautions* regarding internal use) for all types of external wounds to the flesh. Comfrey is bitter and cool. Bitter can clear and drain, and coolness can clear heat. The combination of bitter and cool of this medicinal very effectively clear heat, reduce swelling and engender flesh; quite possibly better than any other plant on the planet.

Promotes bone growth when used externally and internally. Comfrey is used for fractures due to knocks and falls. Bone growth and healing is governed by the kidney. Comfrey supplements the kidney essence with sweetness to hasten the repair of broken bones. No other medicinal known to me has such a profound affect on bone healing.

Cools the blood, clears heat, nourishes yin, stops bleeding and engenders flesh. Comfrey is used internally to treat either replete heat or yin vacuity heat that has damaged the lung, stomach, and intestines leading to dryness, bleeding, ulcers, etc. Comfrey is bitter, sweet, and cool. Sweet can nourish, while bitter can drain and coolness can clear heat. Internal bleeding can be from a variety of causes, the most prominent of those are heat entering the blood aspect and heat damaging the vessels. In either situation there is repletion heat, but there is also often yin vacuity, which is particularly true in the case of heat entering the blood aspect since the transformation of an external pattern to the deepest aspect of the blood generally necessitates a long-standing illness. In either case, although there may not be overt yin vacuity, the yin fluids are being damaged by the heat pathogen and must be preserved in order to protect the body from further damage. This medicinal is particularly effective for the treatment of coughing of blood and blood in the stool caused by heat damage.

Cautions:

Comfrey is known to contain paralyzadine alkoloids, some of which are known to be toxic to the liver (see commentary for more information). Although this medicinal has a long history of use internally, this medicinal is not recommended for internal use for patients with liver diseases, and, in fact, I do not recommend its use internally by untrained individuals; caution is advised. When using this medicinal externally for deep wounds, it is important to be careful not to allow the wound to heal over but rather allow it to heal from the inside out (see paragraph below regarding combination with Cayenne).

Dosage and Preparation:

External: fresh root mashed and applied as a plaster; dried root ground to a powder and mixed with water and applied as a plaster; dried root infused in oil and used as a salve (leaf can also be used). Internal: infusion 2–6g

Major Combinations:

Combine with Plantain, Calendula, *dāngguī*, and *zǐcǎogēn* for external application to swollen scrapes and cuts due to knocks and falls. Add *mòyào* and *rǔxiāng* if there is swelling and pain. This combination is applied as a plaster or can be prepared as a salve.

Combine with Yarrow and *dàhuáng* for swollen, red, and painful wounds. This combination is applied externally as a plaster.

Combine with Cayenne for deep wounds. The Cayenne in this formula helps the wound to heal from the inside out.

Commentary:

Although Comfrey sometimes gets a "bad rap" for containing peralyzadine alkaloids, it simply is, to the best of the author's knowledge, the best herb for healing external wounds, broken bones, and treating knocks and falls. Comfrey leaf has a long history as a fodder for animals and also has been eaten by humans. It does indeed have a rich mineral composition. Today, due to the known presence of peralyzadine alkaloids, I get the benefits of this high mineral content by composting the leaves and using that material to grow my food and herbs. Furthermore, the leaves can be made into a "tea" for application to plants as a liquid foliar feeding solution similar to the way Stinging Nettles can be used.

One of the old names for Comfrey is "bone-knit," which comes from its ability to heal fractures. Indeed, this medicinal is exceptionally good for healing bones. Although it was historically used internally and externally, today it is prudent to only use it externally, although I have used it internally on myself. It is likely safe to use for short periods of time (5–15 days) at moderate dosages by those with no liver disease and who are of relatively strong health. Allen and Hatfield (2004) report that in the British Isles and Ireland (where this old name comes from), it was widely used for these purposes according to the ethnobotanical literature. The primary use in those records is for sprains, then fractures, then other external wounds.

Dioscorides (2000 *trans.*) does not give this herb a long monograph, but it is one of our oldest records for the use of this herb. He states that the internal part of the root is to be used (other sources also say to peel the root, but those sources quite likely relied on Dioscorides) and "Pounded into small pieces (and taken in a drink) they are good for bloodspitters and hernias. Applied, they close up new wounds. Boiled, they join pieces of flesh together. They are smeared on for inflammations—most usefully for those in the perineum—with leaves of *Senecio*." The first indication (spitting of blood) is still widely considered appropriate, but because of the alkaloid content mentioned in other parts of this monograph, most avoid this use. However, the external uses for the flesh and bone are still widely accepted and used.

Parkinson (1640) says:

> *"The great Comfrey is as some say, cold in a temperate degree, and others say hot, which is not held true, but drying and binding in a greater measure, for it helpeth those that spit blood, or that bleed at the mouth, or that make a bloody urine: as also for all inward hurts, bruises and wounds, and helpeth the ulcers of the lungs, coughing the phlegm that oppresseth them, to be easily spit forth, the root being boiled in water or wine..."*

What is most interesting is that Parkinson says this medicinal is cold, which makes sense in the Chinese way of looking at it. However, he says that it is "drying and binding in a great measure," which is curious until one looks closely at how he was using it to stop bleeding. Because of this action, he says it dries and binds, but then he goes on to say that it is good for oppressive phlegm and [loosens] it to allow it to be expectorated. This indication is still a common use for this medicinal and if one applies the theories of Chinese medicine such a medicinal would be classified as moistening; i.e. *màiméndōng* or *tiānhuāfěn*, which moisten and cool the lungs for thick difficult to expectorate phlegm. These herbs would also be used for abscesses in the lungs or any other bleeding in the lung, which would almost always be considered a condition of heat.

Parkinson, in his discussion of Comfrey's external application for broken bones or damaged tissue, had this very interesting (if not funny) bit to say, "The roots being outwardly applied, helpeth fresh wounds or cuts immediately; being bruised thereto, by gluing together their lips, and is especially good for ruptures and broken bones; it is said to be so powerful to consolidate or knit together, whatsoever needs knitting, that if they be boiled with severed pieces of flesh in a pot, it will join them together again."

Although I think we can safely say that putting Comfrey in a pot to boil with two pieces of flesh is not likely to yield very positive results, it is telling that this plant was given nearly magical powers by people; and Parkinson thought so highly of the plant as to recite this anecdote in his book.

Culpeper (1653) says, "The root boiled in water or wine, and the decoction drank, helps all inward hurts, bruises, wounds, and ulcers of the lungs, and causes the phlegm that oppresses them to be easily spit forth." Like Parkinson, Culpeper also considered this medicinal to be cold, this suggested that this medicinal would be applicable to either damage by heat, or damage by cold that has transformed into heat. Culpeper also says, "The roots being outwardly applied, help fresh wounds or cuts immediately, being bruised and laid thereto; and is especially good for ruptures and broken bones;" This is likely the most common use of this medicinal today. It is used in a variety of preparations to be applied externally, from salves to liniments. I have used this medicinal to help heal my own fractured patella. The use of this medicinal reduced my healing time to approximately half of the estimate according to the orthopedic physician I was seeing at the time. I was lucky to have been living in Oregon, where I had a large herb garden and was able to harvest the root fresh and apply it to my knee every day. There is no doubt in my mind that this therapy contributed immensely to the healing of my patella. I also used an internal formula that that contained Comfrey, among other herbs.

This formula was designed by my friend and colleague Brian Weissbach at KW Botanicals in California, USA:

Eliminates Wind and Damp

Shen Jin Cao	Lycopodium (Club Moss)

Tonifies Yin

Sphaeralcea	Yerba de la Negrita, also Tonifies Yang
Symphytum	Comfrey Plant

Tonifies Yang

Gu Sui Bu	Drynaria Rhizome
Bu Gu Zhi	Psoralea
Ba Ji Tian	Morinda Root

Vitalizes Blood

Yan Hu Suo	Corydalis (Turkey Corn Tuber)
Commiphora	Gugul Gum, also Astringent
Yang Qi Cao	Achillea (Yarrow), also Clears Heat
Chuan Xiong	Ligusticum (Osha), also Clears Heat
Xi Zang Hong Hua	Crocus (Saffron)
Tu Bie Chong	Eupolyphagia

Hemostatic

Ji Cai	Capsella (Shepherd's Purse)
Tian Qi	Panax notoginseng (Pseudoginseng)
Xian He Cao	Agrimonia (Agrimony)
Ai Ye	Artemisia (Mugwort), also Vitalizes Blood

Astringent

Wu Wei Zi	Schisandra (Five Flavor Fruit)

Tonifies Blood

Urtica	Stinging Nettles Leaf, also Activates Yang

Regulates Qi

Tan Xiang	Santalum (Sandalwood)

This formula uses a combination of Chinese and Western herbs but employees Chinese medical theory. Brian is a master formulator with some 40 plus years of experience. Not only did I use this formula to heal my patella, but I have used in numerous times over the years with very good success. It helps to both relieve pain and hasten the healing process.

Salmon (1710) states:

> *"The powder of the root. Being taken inwardly to one dram in a little of the syrup, it stops inward bleeding, heals wounds in the stomach and thorax, as also ulcers in the lungs. If it is applied to green wounds, as soon as the wound is made, it conglutinates or joins the lips thereof together, and causes it speedily to be healed mixed with the syrup, and applied to the hemorrhoids or piles, it cools the inflammation, and represses their over much bleeding, and allays the heat of the parts adjacent, taking away, and easing all the pain."*

There is little doubt about the effectiveness of this medicinal, unfortunately the presence of the potentially toxic alkaloids render this medicinal questionable for internal application. However, Comfrey is also an excellent external medicinal and can be used as such with little concern for toxicity. In a study done in Germany using an external product, "After 2–3 days of application of the study medication a highly significantly and clinically relevantly faster initial reduction of wound size [was found]."[1] While a study in Georgia on a different species that also has a long history of use as the species listed in this monograph. *S. asperum* was found to not only heal both wounds and burns faster than controls (a 2.5% allantoin ointment), but it also left no scar where the skin had been damaged.[2] It should be noted here that allantoin is NOT inert; it is a known constituent of Comfrey (as well as Plantain, see Garran 2008), is well researched and has been proven to increase cell proliferation.

There are a multitude of other studies similar to those above. In addition, there has been very positive results using the external application of Comfrey cream in the treatment of osteoarthritis (OA). In one study done in the USA, Smith & Jacobson (2011) concluded that, "Both active topical Comfrey formulations were effective in relieving pain and stiffness and in improving physical functioning and were superior to placebo in those with primary OA of the knee without serious adverse effects."[3] And, another study done in Germany, concluded that, "The results suggest that the comfrey root extract ointment is well suited for the treatment of osteoarthritis of the knee. Pain is reduced, mobility of the knee improved and quality of life increased."[4]

1. Barna M, Kucera A, Hladícova M, Kucera M. (2007) Wound healing effects of a Symphytum herb extract cream (Symphytum x uplandicum NYMAN:): results of a randomized, controlled double-blind study. *Wien Med Wochenschr.* 157(21–22): pp 569–74. *article in German.*

2. Vakhtang Barbakadze, Karen Mulkijanyan, Lali Gogilashvili, Lela Amiranashvili, Maia Merlani, Zhana Novikova, Marine Sulakvelidze. (2000). Allantoin–and Pyrrolizidine Alkaloids–Free Wound Healing Compositions from *Symphytum asperum. Bulletin of the Georgian National Academy of Sciences.* 3(1).

3. Smith, Doug B. & Jacobson, Bert H. (2011). Effect of a blend of comfrey root extract (*Symphytum officinale* L.) and tannic acid creams in the treatment of osteoarthritis of the knee: randomized, placebo-controlled, double-blind, multiclinical trials. *Journal of Chiropractic Medicine.* 10: pp 147–156.

4. Grube B, Grünwald J, Krug L, Staiger C. (2007). Efficacy of a comfrey root (Symphyti offic. radix) extract ointment in the treatment of patients with painful osteoarthritis of the knee: results of a double–blind, randomised, bicenter, placebo-controlled trial. *Phytomedicine.* Jan;14(1): pp 2–10.

Chickweed

Stellaria media (L.) Vill.
Caryophyllaceaea
Stellariae mediae herba
Chinese Name: *fánlǚ* (繁縷)
Favor and Qi: bitter, bland, slightly sweet, cool
Channels entered: stomach, lung, kidney
Actions: diuretic, tonic, vulnerary, expectorant

Functions & Indications:

Clears heat and cools the blood. Chickweed is used for external application to a variety of skin conditions where there is heat or fire. This medicinal can be applied when the fluids have been scorched and the condition is dry, or when the condition is complicated by dampness and there is swelling and/or pus. Chickweed is bitter and cool and acts directly on the skin to clear heat and resolve toxin. Although a relatively gentle herb, Chickweed acts to reinforce the actions of other herbs when used in a formula. It also has a dual function of soothing and moistening the skin when there is local dryness due to heat-toxin. This is important as a supporting herb in an external formula because most herbs that are used in these cases are quite drying and tend to damage the skin. The fresh juice is an excellent method of applying this medicinal.

Clears heat and percolates dampness. Chickweed is used for damp-heat in the lower burner with scant dark-yellow urine. Chickweed's bland and bitter flavor drain dampness and disinhibit urination, and its coolness clears heat. As mentioned above, Chickweed has a mild moistening effect and as such can be used in cases of localized tissue damage due to heat damaging the fluids.

Clears heat and nourishes yin humors. Chickweed is used for yin and blood vacuity heat patterns with symptoms of scant, dark, and/or reddish urination, dry cough, dry skin (especially with itching), and dry stool. Chickweed is bitter and cool and clears vacuity heat, but also nourishes with sweetness. This herb can be either eaten as a salad green or taken as a tea to gently nourish yin and blood.

Clears heat and engenders flesh for external application to scrapes and cuts. Chickweed is commonly employed as an herb in external preparations for scrapes and cuts, generally in the form of a salve and usually as an assisting herb rather than a lead herb, with some exceptions.

Cautions:

None noted. This is a very safe herb and can be eaten as a spring green when it is fresh and tender.

Dosage and Preparation:

Infusion or decoction 10–30g; up to 60g may be used (fresh is best)

Major Combinations:

Combine with Calendula, Comfrey, and Plantain prepared as an oil extraction and finished with bees wax to make a salve. This is a very common combination used for external application to scraps, chapped lips, cracked dry skin, and other similar minor conditions.

Commentary:

Chickweed is a member of the Caryophyllaceae or Pink family and is a found on every continent except Antartica, although it is found on the subantarctic islands in the Southern Hemisphere.[1] This led to the following comment by one author:

> *"Common chickweed is an excellent example of 'speed and agility' over 'size and strength.' An individual plant may not impress the casual observer or threaten a gardener, but the sheer numbers, rapid growth, and widespread occurrence of the weed around the world is legendary. Perhaps the most notable trait of common chickweed was its ability to support and follow another successful pioneering and cosmopolitan species–Homo sapiens."[2]*

The family is relatively large with some 3000 species grouped into over 80 genera. The family boasts a number of medicinal plants other than Chickweed including the Chinese medicinals *qúmài* and *wángbùliúxíng*. Chickweed is a common weed and might be found in any disturbed area. Apparently the seeds can live for up to 50 years in the soil, so if it is in your garden, it is most like going to stay there. It is easily recognized by its slender root, white flower, and the single row of hairs that run up the stem.

Although Chickweed is used by many folk herbalists, it is used much less in professional practice. The reason for this, in my opinion, is not because of its lack of efficacy, but because in order for it to have a reasonable therapeutic action in professional practice, the dosage must be much higher than what most Western herbalists are accustomed to using. Although I have seen it recommended at dosages from one teaspoon to one tablespoon, this amount is unlikely to have much of an effect beyond a very mild action. Thus, when I have used it internally, I have employed much higher dosages, and found it of reasonable therapeutic usefulness. However, as mentioned in the primary monograph, I would not consider it a lead herb in a formula, but rather an assistant.

A study done in Russia seems to support the idea of higher dosing along with clear therapeutic effect. The study was done on rats but the dose was 100mg/kg, an unusually high dosage in experimental animals. However, at that dosage the researchers, while studying toxic hepatitis, found: "...reduction of inflammatory and degenerative processes in hepatocytes, stimulated the regenerative potential of hepatic tissue, promoting stabilization of hepatocyte membranes and inhibiting the release of enzymes into the blood (ALT and AST activities did not differ from the control. Hence, the treatment promoted hepatocyte normalization."[3]

Chickweed is thought to have a rich complex of minerals, amino acids, and vitamins by many folk herbalists; however the literature does not support this, or is at least conflicted. There are a number of reports on the nutritional value of Chickweed, but there is so much variation that citing any article, or even several articles does not do the literature justice. This inconsistency is most likely due to growing conditions, soil types, etc. Therefore, although Chickweed *may* be of high nutritional value, it frequently does not compare with other weed species such as Dandelion or Stinging Nettle, but is generally better than common cultivated species such as the lettuces. It is a nourishing plant and quite refreshing, which is why it is well-known as a spring salad green. I would suggest that these qualities make a strong case for its use in yin vacuity patterns. Although I don't generally like to make these types of connections between chemistry and Chinese medicine (specifically in the case of yin and other vacuity patterns because they are so poorly understood from the biomedical perspective), this may be a reasonable explanation for why this plant acts positively in cases of yin vacuity. This herb is widely used in folk herbalism as a nourishing tonic made into a vinegar preparation, often with other herbs such as Stinging Nettle and Dandelion (see recipe below), and then used to dress salads or simply consumed "as is" in small quantities for its mineral richness.

Simple recipe:
Place equal parts Chickweed, Stinging Nettle, and Dandelion leaf in a jar, as much as you can fit, and cover with apple cider vinegar. Place the jar in a pot of water and slowly bring to a boil. Heat for 15–20 minutes with the lid loosely closed. Soak the cooked herbal mixture for 2 weeks, then strain and enjoy. This can be modified with herbs like Lemon Balm, Basil, Garden Sage, Rosemary, etc. for whatever desired flavor you prefer.
Use this vinegar as an addition to salad dressings, sauces, or any other cooking preparation you desire.

Gerard (1597) says that, "Chickweed is cold and moist, and of a waterish substance; and therefore it cools without astriction or binding, as Galen saith." While it is unclear if this quote is entirely from Galen, or just the latter portion, nevertheless it does clearly show a very long history of energetic understanding. After discussing its medicinal use, Gerard sums up his comments with the following: "In a word, it comforts, digests, defends, and suppurates very notably." Again, as noted above, this medicinal clearly seems to have value according to the old authors and I would argue that they were likely using it in relatively large doses, although they never state dosage.

Parkinson (1640) writes at length on this medicinal, but the following quote, which is preeceded by invoking several Greek authors, is most telling of Chickweed's internal application: "It severes therefore for all manner of heat whether inward or outward, to cool and temper the blood inflamed in Agues, or the heat of the stomach and liver breaking out into the lips, and to procure an appetite being lost or becoming weak, and is used in hectic feavers, and to asswage the heat of the back and urine." Here was have a clear look at how Parkinson and other authors of his time were viewing internal heat (of the stomach and liver) and how it might manifest as observable symptomology in the form of cracked lips. According to Wiseman & Ye (1998), cracked lips come from two etiologys, 1) exuberant spleen–stomach heat and 2) effulgent yin vacuity fire. The first is obvious as a reference to heat in the stomach mentioned above. The second, effulgent yin vacuity fire is liver and kidney yin vacuity leading to fire. Thus, although Parkinson may not have used the same terminology as we do in Chinese medicine, he clearly recognized the connection between heat in the stomach and liver and the external manifestation of cracked lips.

Culpeper (1653) says of Chickweed, "...is of good effect to ease pains from the heat and sharpness of the blood in the piles, and generally all pains in the body that arise of heat. It is used also in the hot and virulent ulcers and sores in the privy parts, or on the legs, or elsewhere." It is unclear if Culpeper was applying this externally or using it internally. However, I would guess that this is primarily for external application, and he is mostly likely using the fresh pressed juice, although a decoction would also work. We can see that, according to Culpeper, there is no doubt that this medicinal is a cooling agent.

Salmon (1710) says Chickweed is "cold and moist in the second degree." Of the juice he says:

> "It is good for all heat and redness of the eyes, being dropped into them; also put into the ears warm, it eases their pain and proceeding from a hot cause. The piles [hemorrhoids] bathed, or fomented therewith, it abates their pain, and takes away their heat and sharpness, and eases all other pains of the body preceeding from heat and sharpness of humors. It is good against hot and virulent sores and ulcers in the privy parts, legs, or elsewhere, they being often washed therewith."

And, of the infused oil he says:

> "Made by boiling the herb in olive oil until crisp, and repeating it three or four times with fresh herb, it heals sore legs, ulcers, wheals, pushes, scabs, and the like; and being anointed upon shrunk up sinews, it extends them eases their pains, and makes them pliable again."

Salmon clearly sees this medicinal as a very cooling herb to clear heat, primarily by applying externally. But more than just clearing heat, by stating [of sinews] "makes them pliable again." Is suggesting a nourishing action of either yin or blood. Salmon also gives an interesting, if not unusual "compound oil" recipe.

"Take green [fresh] Chickweed, fresh Red Rose leaves, of each two handfuls; oil of trotters [pigs lard], two pounds. Boil till they are crisp, and strain out; repeat this boiling with fresh Chickweed and Red Rose Leaves, twice more: strain out, and keep it for use. Being anointed warm, and well rubbed in upon sinews which are strained, it is a most excellent thing. Let it be used morning and evening, and in little time the patient will be cured."

To this last formula I might suggest adding *dānguī*, *mòyào*, and *rŭxiāng* to help with both pain and healing of strained sinews.

Translation of Available Source Material:

According to the *Grand Dictionary of Chinese Medicinals* (2009), this herb first appeared in the *Map of the Materia Medica* (1061). I have been unable to find the specific reference in what remains of that book, which is for all intents and purposes lost and only existing in other books as quotations, although it has been reconstructed. However, there are abundant references to this medicinal in Chinese, and although there is agreement on most aspects of this medicinal, there are some books that differ a great deal.

Here is what the *Grand Dictionary of Chinese Medicinals* says: slightly bitter, sweet, sour, and cool; enters the liver and large intestine channels. Clears heat and transforms toxin, cools the blood and disperses welling–abscess, quickens the blood and stops pain, and promotes lactation. It is used to treat dysentery, intestinal welling-abscess, pulmonary welling-abscess, mammary welling-abscess, clove-sore swelling and toxin, hemorrhoids with swelling and pain, bleeding, injury from knocks and falls, postpartum abdominal pain due to stasis and stagnation, and breast milk stoppage. Internally it is used in decoction at 15–30 gram dosages.

The *Běn Căo Yuán Mìng Bāo* (1331) specifically mentions it for dysenteric diarrhea in children, and the *Yunnan Materia Medica* (1470) says it supplements the center and boosts qi, disperses phlegm, stops headache, "head and eyes dizziness," and disinhibits urine.

The *Gui Zhou Collection of Herbal Folk Remedies* (1978) says this medicinal resolves heat and disinhibits urine, and is used for high fever, urinary blockage, child *gān* accumulation, child fright wind, innominate toxin swelling, and clove flat abscess.

1. Defelice, Michael, S. (2004). Common Chickweed, *Stellaria media* (L.) Vill.—"Mere Chicken Feed?" *Weed Technology.* 18(1): pp 193–200.

2. ibid

3. Gorina, Ya. V., et al, (2013). Evaluation of Hepatoprotective Activity of Water-Soluble Polysaccharide Fraction of *Stellaria media* L. *Bulletin of Experimental Biology and Medicine.* 154(5): pp 645–648. (trans. *original article in Russian*).

Medicinal	Nature	Flavor	Channels	Functions	Indications
California Coast Sage	cold	bitter, acrid, aromatic	liver, gallbladder	Clears heat and drains dampness; Stops pain and clears heat; Clears heat, resolves toxin, and stops pain	abdominal pain w/ fullness, rid-side pain, constipation or diarrhea, w/ possible vomiting; hot painful joints or other inflamed traumatic injuries; traumatic wounds to the skin, welling-abscess, or red & swollen open sores
Witch Hazel	warm	acrid, bitter, astringent	heart, spleen	Quicken the blood, resolves stasis, and stops pain; Warms the channels and frees the network vessels	hemorrhoids, varicose veins (especially if painful), blood in the stool due to blood stasis, and bruises and pain from knocks and falls; sore muscles
Comfrey	cool	bitter, sweet	stomach, lung, liver, kidney	Clears heat, disperses swelling, & engenders flesh; Promotes bone growth; Cools the blood, clears heat, nourishes yin, stops bleeding & engenders flesh	chronic cough with weakness, dry cough, and panting; oppressive sensation in the chest, cough, panting and wheezing, and shortness of breath
Chickweed	cool	bitter, bland, slightly sweet	stomach, lung, kidney	Clears heat and cools the blood; Clears heat and percolates dampness; Clears heat and nourishes yin humors; Clears heat and engenders flesh	Dry cracked skin, heat-toxin sores; scant dark-yellow urine; scant, dark, and/or reddish urination, dry cough, dry skin (especially with itching), and dry stool; scrapes & cuts

驅

蟲

藥

Eliminate Parasites Medicinals

The eliminate parasites category is a relatively small group of medicinals that has largely been replaced by modern day anti-parasitic drugs. These medicinals are generally toxic to one degree or another and should be used carefully. The medicinals are used for two primary groups of parasites; parasites in the intestines and skin parasites. The single medicinal in this materia medica, Epazote, is used for the former.

Once a common problem, intestinal parasites are all but absent from modern practice in developed countries, however they remain a significant problem in other countries and those who travel to those countries frequently return home with parasitic infections. That said, intestinal parasites remain a small but difficult illness throughout the world, and parasites such as Borrelia burgdorferi, transmitted by ticks and known as Lyme Disease, have become a very significant problem in North America.

The single medicinal in this materia medica has a long history of use in Mexico and the southern United States and is primarily used for intestinal parasites. Common symptoms of intestinal parasite infections include loss of weight, lack of appetite or significantly increased appetite but with weight loss, abdominal pain, diarrhea, and a withered yellow facial complexion. While some parasites, such as pin worms are little more than a discomfort, other parasites can be significant health concerns.

Epazote

Dysphania ambrosioides (L.) Mosyakin & Clemants
Chenopodeaceae
Dysphaniae ambrosioidi herba cum semen
Other Names: Wormseed, Mexican Tea
Chinese Name: *tǔjīngjiè* (土荆芥)
Favor and Qi: acrid, bitter, aromatic, warm
Channels entered: large intestine, bladder, gallbladder, stomach
Actions: anthelmintic, carminative

Functions & Indications:

Kills parasites. Epazote is used for many different types of parasites, particularly intestinal parasites. This primary function of Epazote is well-known and effective. Epazote's warm, bitter aroma penetrates the intestines and strongly acts to kill worms and other parasites.

Warms the spleen, aromatically transforms dampness, and move the qi. Epazote is used for spleen cold and dampness accompanied by qi stagnation causing fullness, bloating, diarrhea with undigested food in the stool, pain that is relieved by warmth. Epazote is warm, acrid, aromatic and can warm the spleen and aromatically transform dampness while moving qi with acridity.

Cautions:

The essential oil of this medicinal should not be used without extreme caution. Although the herb itself is generally safe, it should not be used in excessive doses or for those with kidney and liver disease. Use caution when administering to children.

Dosage and Preparation:

Infusion or light decoction 2–6g

Commentary:

Epazote is a member of the *Dysphania* genus, which has about 32 species, mostly centered in the deserts of Australia. Epazote is native to the Americas, but has become a widespread weed in the tropics, including China. A related genus *Chenopodium* has at least one important crop, Quinoa (*C. quinoa*). The family is known as the Chenopodiaceae or

Goosefoot family and is considered an ancient family of plants. The family is mostly found in the desert areas of Eurasia and Australia and has 100 genera with approximately 1500 species. Other important food crops in the family are chard and beet.

I learned about this herb when I was first studying herbs in the Bay Area and working in a professional kitchen. First, a friend took me to meet her teacher, a Native American man who lived in San Jose, CA. When I walked in the house the smell of Epazote was very strong, there was a lot of herbs hanging all over the room, and I being a curious young and budding herbalist asked what the smell was. The man laughed, as my friend giggled a bit. He waved his hand around the room and said, "Epazote! What do you think?" I had no idea what it was, but it seemed pretty clear it was important. Later, the man told me he treated a lot of intestinal worms and that it was the best thing he knew to use. About a year later, after harvesting it and wondering if I would ever get the chance to use it, I went to work and found my Executive Chef hanging a huge bundle of this herb in the dry storage room. I asked what she was doing with it, since I only knew it as an herb to kill worms. She told me that we would be using it in a new menu item, which I believe ended up in the book we did (*The Fog City Diner Cookbook*) while I worked there. The herb is a staple in Mexican bean dishes and the flavor is something for which there is no substitute.

While this herb is well known for killing parasites it is also used extensively in Mexican cooking, and frankly beans aren't quite the same without it, in my opinion. As noted in the translation from Chinese literature below, the Chinese can't seem to decide how to label this herb as far as toxicity, let alone flavor and qi. And, although this herb has some toxicity I would suggest it is safer when taken as a decoction, while more care should be used when using it as a tincture, especially if using it with children or very weak individuals. That said, while I could find no references to human death caused by this plant, animal death has been documented, and it is likely that when the oil was commonly used in the early 1900's there were some deaths.

Translation of Available Source Material:

This medicinal is known as *tǔjīngjiè* (土荊芥) in Chinese medicine and was first found in the *Shēng Cǎo Yào Xìng Bèi Yào* (1711). It is considered acrid, bitter, slightly warm, with significant toxicity. Different sources have varying opinions about the flavor and qi of this herb, as well as the toxicity. While most sources agree that it is acrid, only a few say it is bitter. Also, the qi of the herb varies between cool and warm, with several sources saying it is neutral. Finally, no one can agree on its toxicity, with the range from no mention at all of toxicity to significant toxicity (above) and everything in between (see commentary for more information on this). This phenomenon is not uncommon, and not just because this is not a native plant to China. I point this out, to again, show that there is NO standard when it comes to flavor and nature. As discussed earlier in the text, the agreed upon flavors and natures of medicinals has only really become codified since the 1950's and 1960's and we can speculate that this has more to do with the political climate during that time than any "fact" that doctors and authors necessarily agreed upon.

It has the functions of dispelling wind and expelling dampness, killing parasites and stopping itch, quickening the blood and dispersing swelling. It is used to treat ancylostonmiasis, round worm, pinworm, pediculosis capitis, eczema, scab and lichen, wind–dampness impediment pain, menstrual block, painful menstruation, acute sores in the mouth or on the tongue, swollen and painful throat, injuries from knocks and falls, and bites by snakes and insects.

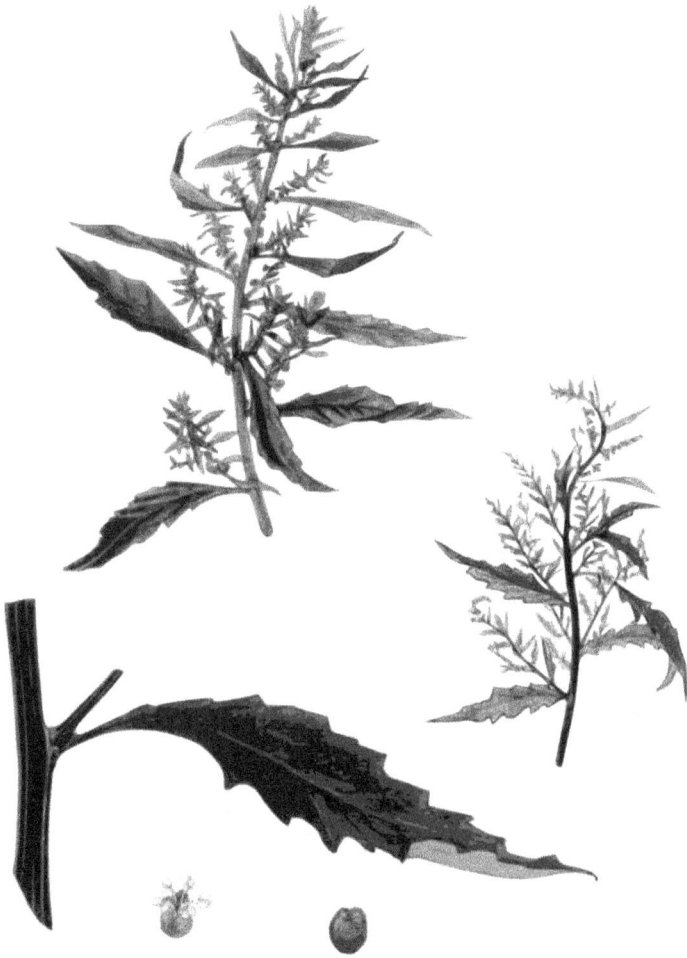

CHENOPODIUM ANTHELMINTICUM L. 1784

Appendix I
Additional Information to the First Volume

Additional information, from the Chinese literature, that has become available regarding the medicinals in the first volume. Unless otherwise noted, the source for all this material is the *Grand Dictionary of Chinese Medicinals* (2009).

Cleavers
Galium aparine
bāxiāncǎo (八仙草) or *zhūyāngyāng* (豬殃殃)
Acrid, slightly bitter, slightly cold
Enters *shàoyáng* and *tàiyīn* channels
Clears heat and resolves toxin, disinhibits urination and frees strangury, and disperses swelling and stops pain.

Used for toxic swollen flat and welling-abscess, mastitis, appendicitis, water swelling, heat effusion associated with influenza or the common cold, dysentery, urinary tract infection, blood in the urine, bleeding from the gums, and bleeding due to knife wounds. Used in decoction 15-30g, also used externally applied to wounds as a powder.

In a formula for appendicitis: Cleavers 90g, *Bidens pilosa* 30g, *Shuteria pampaniniana* 30g. Taken as a decoction. The middle herb has a monograph in this volume. The third herb is from South China, is bitter and cool, and enters the liver and gallbladder channels.

Another formula for heat pattern bleeding: Cleavers 30, *dìyú* 12g, *xiǎojì* 12g, taken as a decoction. (*Sichuan Journal of Chinese Medicinals* 四川中藥志 1979).

Meadowsweet
Filipendula ulmaria (L.) Maxim.
héyèzǐ (和葉子)
Slightly sour, astringent, neutral
Promotes contraction and lower high blood pressure.
The root is used at 15g combined with *chúnxiāngcǎo* (唇香草) 6g and *dàhuáng* 2.4g to treat high blood pressure.

Milk Thistle
*Silybum marianum*L.
shuǐfēijì (水飛薊)
Bitter and cool
Clears heat and resolves toxin, protects the liver, disinhibits the gallbladder

The entirety of what the books say about this herb in Chinese is Western medicine based, showing a strong bias toward Western medicine in China. There is essentially no classical Chinese medicine understanding of this plant in any literature I can find, but lots about its functions from a biomedical point of view, which is easily available in English

Appendix II
Medicinal Plants Used in Chinese Medicine Growing in the West or Related Species

Abies sp.

Under the name *pòsōngshí* (朴松實) there are two species, *A. chensiensis* and *A. fargesii*.They both grow in what is geographically Central China. The former has a more narrow elevation range (2300–3000m) with smaller, more elongated cones (7–11cm long, 3–4cm around); while the former grows from 1500–3700m with shorter cones (5–8cm long, 3–4cm around). They are collectively considered sweet, astringent, slightly acrid, and neutral. They have the function to calm the liver, regulate the menses and stop bleeding, and stop vaginal discharge. They are used for high blood pressure (modern), headache, dizziness, disquieted heart-spirit, irregular menses, flooding and leaking (inappropriate menstrual bleeding), and vaginal discharge. Dosage is 6–9g in decoction.

A. delavayi (*lěngshānguǒ* 冷杉果) grows in the Western mountains of Sichuan, Yunnan, and Tibet in the elevation range of 2800–4400m with a cone that ranges from 6–10cm long and is 3–4cm around. It is considered warm, acrid and without toxicity. It rectifies qi and dissipates cold and treats "sand" qi pain, cold pain in the chest and abdomen and small intestine mounting qi (this is similar to, if not the same as hernia in Western medicine), and other similar types of ailments. It is used in 9–12g doses in decoction.

Abies nephrolepis (*chòulěngshān* 臭冷杉) is different in that the bark and leaves are used, similar to the how we use our Abies in the West. These species grows in the provinces of Shanxi, Beijing, Hebei, Heilongjiang, Jilin, North Korea, and Eastern Russia in the elevation range of 300–2100m. Since this species grows near where I live in China, I will make it a point to find it and report back in the future. There is scant traditional information available, although there is some modern research. Traditionally it is used to treat lower back and leg pain, as a decoction. Modern research on the plant has covered several types of pain, cough, antiinflammatory, etc.

Anaphalis margaritacea L.
dàyèbáitóuwēng (大葉白頭翁)
Bitter, acrid, cool
Clears heat, dries dampness. Used to treat dysentery, toothache, mammary sores, scrophula, and ulceration of the lower leg.
Decoction: 10–30g; externally made into a poultice.
This is a common plant found throughout most of North America, with the exception of the Southeastern United States. In Chinese medicine the entire plant is used either fresh or dried. Some Western herbalists use this medicinal, primarily for lung complaints.

Aster tataricus L.
This is the well-known *zǐwǎn* commonly used in Chinese medicine. It is present throughout much of the Eastern part of the United States and has been reported in adjacent parts of Canada.

There are at least 7 other species of Aster used in Chinese medicine; mostly they are used either exactly like, or very similarly to the uses of the above medicinal. Interestingly, in Tibet both the root and the flower of at least three species are used. The flower is said to be used the same way as the root; to stop coughing and expel phlegm, as well as clear heat and resolve toxin (*Commonly Used Medicinals of Tibet* 1971).

Chelidonium majus L.
báiqūcài (白屈菜)
First appeared in the *Jiù Huāng Běn Cǎo* (救荒本草 1406)
It is considered bitter, cool, and toxic, however of the four sources I have available to me that have flavor and qi, none of them agree on the qi ranging from slightly warm to cold, all say it is bitter, one says sour

and another says acrid. It has the functions of settle pain and stop cough, and disinhibit urination and resolve toxin. It is used to treat stomach and abdominal pain; intestinal inflammation in dysenteric disorders; chronic cough; yellow jaundice; edema and ascites; scab, lichen, sores and swelling; snake and insect bites. The Chinese only use the herbaceous parts of the plant (see commentary for more information about the difference between the herb and the root) and use it in 3–6g dosages in decoction.

This medicinal didn't quite make the cut for this volume. This is a very commonly found plant and is used by a good percentage of Western herbalists, primarily as a stimulant bitter for all manner of liver diseases, jaundice, headaches, hemorrhoids, and for pain due to gallbladder complaints. It has also been used for rheumatic complaints and the fresh latex (sap) can be applied to warts with good success.

Gelsemium elegans Benth.
gōuwěn (钩吻)
First appeared in the *Shén Nóng Běn Cǎo Jīng*
Acrid, bitter, warm, toxic

Expels wind and attacks toxin, scatters binds, stops pain. Used to treat scab and "lai" diseases, eczema, scrofula, swollen welling–abscess, clove sores, traumatic injury, wind–dampness impediment pain, and nerve pain. Mostly used externally as a paste or powder. When used internally 0.5–2g is the dosage.

Not recommended unless trained by an experienced practitioner, the plant is toxic and has been used to kill people as recently as 2011 in a very high profile case where a billionaire in China was allegedly killed by adding some of this herb to a stew he ate.

This herb is very closely related to *Gelsemium sempervirens* used in Western herbal medicine. In Western herbal medicine it has a history of about 200 years of use among American herbalists, primarily. There are only three species in the genus, they all grow in sub–tropical to tropical areas. Two grow in the Americas, and the other is the species mentioned in this brief monograph. These plants are beautiful plants and are sometimes found planted in yards and other plantings.

Gossypium sp.
miánhuā (棉花)

First appeared in the *Commonly Used Chinese Medicinals of Shanghai* (1970) and lists four separate species; *G. herbaceum*, *G. hirsutum* L., *G. barbadense* L., *G. arsboreum* L. This is not surprising since several species are also used interchangeably in the West. The *Grand Dictionary of Chinese Medicinals* says it is sweet and warm and enters the lung channel. It stops coughing and calms panting, frees the channels and stops pain. It is used to treat cough, asthma, menstruation not regulated, and flooding and spotting. They list it at 15–30g as a decoction. The *Hu Bei Journal of Chinese Herbal Medicine* (1982) lists it at acrid and warm and treats mounting qi, breast milk not free, flooding and spotting, and associated conditions.

This is another medicinal that didn't quite make the cut for this book. This is a medicinal that has a long history of use in Western herbal medicine, many say that it was the slaves of the Southern United States that first taught the white Europeans how to use it. This medicinal is primarily used for dysmenorrhea and excessive menstrual bleeding or hemorrhaging after giving birth. Western herbalists primarily use it as a tincture, which is better for quickening blood and relieving pain, while decoctions are at least as good or better for stopping hemorrhage.

Hedychium coronarium Koen.
lùbiānjiāng 路邊姜
First appeared in the Sichuan Journal of Chinese Medicinal (1981)

The rhizome is used in Sichuan. It is spicy and warm and used to promote sweating for common cold etc.; sinew and bone pain; arthritis type pain associated with wind, cold, and dampness; and for pain caused by cold in the abdomen. It is also used for pain due to physical trauma. There are several names, but the main name listed is *lùbiānjiāng*, which literally translates to "ginger beside the road." The dried rhizome is used in 9–15g dosages/day in decoction (with other herbs).

Hyoscyamus niger L.
tiānxiānzǐ (天仙子)
First appeared in the *Běn Cǎo Tú Jīng* (本草圖經 Song Dynasty 1061)
Bitter, acrid, warm, toxic
Enters the heart, stomach, and liver channels

Resolves tetany and stops pain, calms the spirit and stabilizes epilepsy. Used to treat abdominal pain, wind–damp impediment pain, "wind–worm" toothache, pain due to traumatic external injuries, unstoppable panting and coughing, dysentery with prolapse rectum, mania and withdrawal, fright epilepsy, and toxic swollen welling abscesses.

The seed is used in decoction 0.6–1.2g or the powder in 0.06–0.6g; also ground and used externally, as well as the tea can be used externally.

This medicinal is used by some more experienced Western herbalists in tincture form. This is a Eurasian plant known as Henbane, and has a long history of use in Europe and the North America. The seeds were official in the US Pharmacopeia in 1870, but were primarily used to produce a singular alkaloid, hyoscyamine, which has long been used to relieve pain. Although this is clearly a toxic medicinal, it was favored over opium for children and the elderly because it is considered less toxic, does not cause constipation, and death from overdose is rare. Although it has been used for a wide variety of ailments associated with pain and spasms including cough and dysmenorrhea, I have found it most valuable for very difficult cases of pain such as herpes zoster and interstitial cystitis. However, this medicinal should be used carefully and patients should be made aware that they should never exceed the recommended dosage.

Magnolia denudate Desr.
yùlán (玉蘭) aka *xīnyíhuā* (辛夷花)

This is a very common medicinal in Chinese medicine to treat wind–cold patterns and to free the orifice of the now. This plant is mentioned several times in the text including in the Ambrosia monograph.

The species here is one of three species listed as main species for this medicinal and is cultivated in North America in yards and parks. There are at least 15 other species of Magnolia in the United States alone, and I suspect there are other species that can be used as this medicinal. Species are not very difficult to identify, but the key is if those buds smell of camphor.

Mentha spicta L.
liúlánxiāng (留蘭香)
acrid and slightly warm

Resolves the exterior, harmonizes the middle, moves qi. Used to treat common cold, cough, headache, sore throat, read eyes, bleeding from the nose, stomach pain, abdominal distention, sudden turmoil with vomiting and diarrhea, menstrual pain, numbness of the limbs, pain and swelling due to external traumatic injury, sores, and chapped skin.

Dosage: 3–9g or 15–30g of the fresh herb. Externally the fresh herb can be pounded to form a poultice or the juice expressed for use.

Menyanthes trifoliate L.

shuìcài or *shuìcàigēn* (睡菜 或 睡菜根)

First appeared in the *Běn Cǎo Gāng Mù* 1590

Sweet, slightly bitter, cold

Herb: Clears heat and disinhibits dampness, calms the spirit. Used to treat stomach duct pain, acute stomach inflammation, damp–heat jaundice, rib–side pain, water swelling, disquietude of essence–spirit, palpitations, and insomnia.

Dosage: 10–15g in decoction or juiced fresh.

Root: Moistens the lung and stops cough, disinhibits urine and disperses swelling. Used to treat cough, water swelling, and wind–damp impediment.

Dosage: 10–15g, 30g of the fresh root; or juiced fresh.

This is a circumboreal plant of the Northern Hemisphere and is used in Western herbal medicine, primarily as a bitter tonic for digestive problems.

Metaplexis japonica (Thunb.) Makino

luómó 萝藦

First appeared in the *Běn Cǎo Jīng Jí Zhù* (本草經集注 Tang Dynasty 480–498)

Sweet, acrid, and neutral

Supplements essence and boosts qi, resolves toxin and disperses swelling. Used for vacuity–detriment taxation damage, impotence, seminal emission and white vaginal discharge, insufficient breast milk, cinnabar toxin, scrofula, clove sore, and snake and insect bites.

Although the entire plant is used, it appears that the root is the primary medicinal. This is a common weed throughout much of China and is currently found in at least the state of Iowa in the US where it is considered a weed in corn fields. The genus is part of the Asclepiadaceae family and there is but this one plant within the genus.

Opuntia dillenii Haw. and ***O. vulgaris*** Mill.
xiānrénzhǎng 仙人掌

Bitter and cold; Moves qi and quickens blood, cools blood and stops bleeding, resolves toxin and disperses swelling. This medicinal is used in Chinese medicine to treat stomach pain, glomus lump (concretions, conglomerations, accumulations, and gatherings), dysentery, throat pain, lung heat coughing, pulmonary consumption with expectoration of blood, spitting blood, bleeding hemorrhoids, abscesses and sores, mammary abscesses, mumps, lichen, injury from snake or insect bites, burns, and frostbite.

One of my teachers also uses this medicinal externally for herpes zoster as part of a larger external formula.

Related species have been used in the Southwestern United States and Mexico for diabetes. The pads are also a regular food in Mexican cooking, and the fruit is a delicious treat, just be careful of those pesky spines!

Appendix III
Medicinals in this materia medica listed by Common Name

Common Name	Latin Binomial	*Pínyín*	漢子
Achyranthes	*Achyranthes aspera*	*niúxī*	怀牛膝
Aconite	*Aconitum columbianum*	*běiměifùzǐ*	北美附子
Ambrosia	*Ambrosia dumosa, A. trifida, A. artemesiifolia, A. psilostachya*	*túncǎo*	豚草
Amur Corktree Bark	*Phellodendron chinensis*	*huángbǎi*	黄柏
Angelica, Brewer's	*Angelica breweri*		
Angelica, Chinese	*Angelica dahurica*	*báizhǐ*	白芷
Angelica, European	*Angelica archangelica*	*ōubáizhǐ*	歐白芷
Angelica, Pubescent	*Angelica pubescens*	*dúhuó*	獨活
Apricot kernel	*Armeniaca sibirica*	*xìngrén*	杏仁
Arnebia	*Arnebia euchroma*	*zǐcǎogēn*	紫草根 -新疆
Arnica	*Arnica sp.*	*shānjīnchē*	山金車
Astragalus (unprocessed)	*Astragalus membranaceus*	*shēnghuángqí*	生黄芪
Astragalus, Honey Mix-fried	*Astragalus membranaceus*	*zhìhuángqí*	炙黄芪
Atractylodes, Red	*Atractylodes lancea*	*cāngzhú*	蒼術
Atractylodes, White	*Atractylodes macrocephala*	*báizhú*	白術
Aucklandia	*Aucklandia lappa*	*mùxiāng*	木香
Balloon Flower	*Platycodon grandiflorus*	*jiégěng*	桔梗
Beebalm	*Monarda citriodora*	*měiguóbòhe*	美國薄荷
Bethroot	*Trillium sp.*	*yánlíngcǎo*	延齡草
Bidens	*Bidens pilosa*	*guǐzhēncǎo, mángchángcǎo*	鬼針草, 盲腸草
Bitter Sophora	*Sophora flavescens*	*kǔshēn*	苦参
Bittersweet	*Solanum dulcamara*	*kǔqié*	苦茄
Black Cohosh	*Actaea racemosa*	*hēishēngmá*	黑升麻
Black Haw	*Viburnum prunifolium*	*hēijiápéng*	黑莢蓬
Bleeding Hearts, Pacific	*Dicentra formosa*		
Blessed Thistle	*Centaurea benedicta*		
Blue Cohosh	*Caulophyllum thalictroides*	*lánzǐhóngmáoqī*	藍籽紅毛七
Blue Curls	*Trichostema lanceolatum, T. laxum*		
Blueberry	*Vaccinium sp.*	*lánméi*	藍莓
British Yellowhead	*Inula britannica*	*xuánfùhuā*	旋複花
Bugleweed	*Lycopusvirginicus*	*měizhōudìsǔn*	北洲地筍

Bupleurum	*Bupleurum chinensis*	*cháihú*	柴胡
Calamus	*Acorus calamus*	*shíchāngpú*	石菖蒲
Calendula	*Calendula officinalis*	*jīnzhǎnjú*	金盏菊
California Coast Sage	*Artemesia californica*	*jiāzhōuhāo*	加州蒿
California Coffee Berry	*Rhamnus californica*	*jiāzhōushǔlǐ*	加州鼠李
California Poppy	*Eschscholtzia californica*	*huālíngcǎo*	花菱草
Catnip	*Nepeta cataria*	*māobòhe*	貓薄荷
Cayenne	*Capsicum sp.*	*Làjiāo*	辣椒
Cedar	*Thuja occidentalis*	*běiměixiāngbǎi*	北美香柏
Chameleon	*Houttuynia cordata*	*yúxīngcǎo*	魚腥草
Chamomile	*Matricaria chamomilla*	*mǔjú*	母菊
Chaparral	*Larrea tridentata*	*shítànsuānguànmù*	石炭酸灌木
Chickweed	*Stellaria media*	*fánlǚ*	繁缕
Chinese Corkbark	*Phellodendron chinensis*	*huángbái*	黃柏
Chysanthemum	*Chrysanthemum morifolium*	*júhuā*	菊花
Cleavers	*Galium aparine*	*bāxiāncǎo*	八仙草
Cogon Grass	*Imperata cylindrical*	*báimáogēn*	白茅根
Coix	*Coix lacroyma-jobi*	*yìyǐrén*	薏苡仁
Coltsfoot	*Tussilago farfare*	*kuǎndōnghuā*	款冬花
Comfrey	*Symphytum officinale*	*jùhécǎo*	聚合草
Coptis	*Coptis chinensis*	*huánglián*	黃連
Corydalis, Chinese	*Corydalis yanhusuo*	*yánhúsuǒ*	延胡索
Cotton Root bark	*Gossypium sp.*	*miánhua*	棉花
Cramp Bark	*Viburum opulus*	*ōuzhōujiámí*	歐洲莢蒾
Curcuma, Aromatic	*Curcuma wenyujin*	*yùjīn*	鬱金
Cyperus	*Cyperus rotundus*	*xiāngfù*	香附
Dandelion	*Taraxicum officinale*	*ōuzhōupúgōngyīng*	歐洲蒲公英
Dang Gui	*Angelica sinensis*	*dāngguī*	當歸
Devil's Club	*Opolopanax horrididum*		
Dill Seed	*Anethum graveolens*	*shíluózǐ*	莳萝子
Dwarf Turf Lily	*Ophiopogon japonicus*	*màiméndōng*	麥門冬
Echinacea	*Echinacea purpurea, E. angustifolium, etc.*	*zǐzhuījú*	紫锥菊
Elecampane	*Inula helenium*	*tǔbáizhú*	土白術
Epezoté	*Dysphania ambrosioides*	*tǔjīngjìe*	土荆芥
Eucalyptus	*Eucalyptus globulus*	*ānyè*	桉葉
Eucommia	*Eucommia ulminoides*	*dùzhòng*	杜仲
Fennel seed	*Foeniculum vulgare*	*huíxiāngzǐ*	茴香籽

Fenugreek	*Trigonella foenum-graecum*	*húlúbā*	葫蘆巴
Feverfew	*Tanacetum officinale*	*àijú*	艾菊
Field Mint	*Mentha canadensis*	*bòhé*	薄荷
Figwort, California	*Scrophularia californica*	*jiāzhōuxuánshēn*	加州玄參
Figwort, Chinese	*Scrophularia ningpoensis*	*xuánshēn*	玄參
Five Flavor Berry (Schizandra)	*Schizandra chinensis*	*wǔwèizǐ*	五味子
Forsythia	*Forsythia suspensa*	*liánqiáo*	連翹
Foxglove, Chinese	*Rehmannia glutinosa*	*shēngdìhuáng*	生地黃
Frankincense	*Boswellia sacra*	*rǔxiāng*	乳香
Fritillary, Sichuan	*Fritillaria cirrhosa*	*chuānbèimǔ*	川貝母
Fritillary, Thunberg	*Fritillaria thunbergii*	*zhèbèimǔ*	浙貝母
Gardenia	*Gardenia jasminoides*	*shānzhīzǐ*	山梔子
Gardenia, Carbonized	*Gardenia jaminoides*	*tànshānzhīzǐ*	炭山梔子
Gentian	*Gentiana sp.*	*lóngdǎn*	龍膽
Ginger, dry	*Zingiber officinale*	*gānjiāng*	干姜
Ginger, fresh	*Zingiber officinale*	*shēngjiāng*	生姜
Ginseng, American	*Panax quinquefolium*	*xīyángshēn*	西洋參
Ginseng, Asian	*Panax ginseng*	*rénshēn*	人參
Ginseng, Prince	*Pseudostellaria heterophylla*	*tàizǐshēn*	太子參
Ginseng, Tian Qi	*Panax notoginseng*	*sānqī*	三七
Ginseng, White	*Panax ginseng*	*báirénshēn*	白人參
Glehnia, Coastal	*Glehnia littoralis*	*shāshēn (běi)*	沙參（北）
Goldenrod	*Solidago canadensis*	*jiānádàyīzhīhuánghuā*	加拿大一枝黃花
Goldenseal	*Hydrastis canadensis*	*báimáogèn*	白毛莨
Gotu Kola	*Centella asiatica*	*jīxuěcǎo*	積雪草
Grindelia	*Grindelia sp.*	*yàoyònggānjiāocǎo*	藥用干膠草
Hedge Nettle	*Stachys sp.*	*shuǐsū*	水蘇
Hops	*Humulus lupulus*	*píjiǔhuā*	啤酒花
Horehound	*Marrubium vulgare*	*ōuxiàzhìcǎo*	歐夏至草
Horny Goat Weed	*Epimidium sp.*	*yínyánghuò*	淫羊藿
Horse Chestnut	*Aesculus hippocastanum*	*suōluózǐ*	娑羅子
Hyssop	*Hyssopus officinalis*	*shénxiāngcǎo*	神香草
Sicklepod Senna	*Senna obtusifolia*	*juémíngzǐ*	決明子
Juniper	*Juniperus communis*	*ōucìbǎi*	歐刺柏
Kava	*Piper methysticum*	*kǎwǎhújiāo*	卡瓦胡椒
Lavender	*Lavendula spica, L. angustifolia*	*xūnyīcǎo*	薰衣草
Lemon Balm	*Melissa officinalis*	*níngméngxāingfēngcǎo*	檸檬香蜂草

Leopard Lily	*Belamcanda chinensis*	*shègān*	射干
Licorice Fern	*Polypodium glycyrrhiza*		
Licorice, Chinese	*Glycrrhiza uralensis*	*gāncǎo*	甘草
Ligusticum, Chinese	*Ligusticum chuanxiong*	*chuānxiōng*	川芎
Lobelia	*Lobelia inflata*	*běiměishāngěngcài*	北美山梗菜
Lousewort, Pine	*Pedicularis semibarbata*	*mǎxiānhāo (sōng)*	馬先蒿（松）
Lycium Fruit (goji)	*Lycium barbarum*	*gǒuqǐzi*	枸杞子
Lycopus, Chinese	*Lycopus lucidus*	*zélán*	澤蘭
Magnolia bark	*Magnolia officinalis*	*hòupò*	厚樸
Magnolia buds	*Magnolia denudata*	*xīnyíhuā*	辛夷花
Marshmallow root	*Althea officinalis*	*yàoshǔkuí*	藥蜀葵
Milkwort, Chinese	*Polygala tenuifolia*	*yuǎnzhì*	遠志
Motherwort	*Leonorus cardiac*	*ōuzhōuyìmǔcǎo*	歐洲益母草
Motherwort, Chinese	*Leonorus siberica*	*yìmǔcǎo*	益母草
Mullein (leaf)	*Verbascum thapsus*	*dàmáoyè*	大毛葉
Myrrh	*Commiphora myrrha*	*mòyào*	沒藥
Notopterygium	*Notopterygium incisum*	*qiānghuó*	羌活
Ocotillo	*Fourquaria splendens*	*làzhúmū*	蠟燭木
Orange, Bitter	*Poncirus trifoliata*	*zhǐshí*	枳實
Oregon Grape root	*Berberis aquifolium*	*élègāngpúpao*	俄勒岡葡萄
Osha	*Ligusticum porteri, L. grayii*		
Ox-eye Daisy	*Chrysanthemum leucanthemum, Leucanthemun vulgare*	*bīnjú*	濱菊
Parley root	*Petroselinum crispum*	*ōuqíngēn*	歐芹跟
Partridgeberry	*Mitchella repens*	*wànhǔcì*	蔓虎刺
Pasque Flower	*Anemone occidentalis, A. patens*	*yínliánhuā*	銀蓮花
Pedicularis	*Pedicularis densiflora, P. groenlandica, etc.*	*mǎxiānhāo*	馬先蒿
Peppermint	*Mentha piperita*	*ōuzhōubóhe*	歐洲薄荷
Pinellia	*Pinellia ternata*	*bànxià*	半夏
Pinellia, ginger-processed	*Pinellia ternata*	*jiāngbànxià*	姜半夏
Plantain (leaf)	*Plantago sp.*	*chēqiányè*	車前葉
Plantain seed, Chinese	*Plantago asiatica*	*chēqiánzǐ*	車前子
Pleurisy Root	*Asclepias tuberosa*	*kuàigēnmǎlìjīn*	塊根馬利筋
Poria	*Poria coccos*	*fúlíng*	茯苓
Processed Rehmannia	*Rehmannia glutinosa*	*shúdìhuáng*	熟地黃
Red Baneberry	*Actaea rubra*	*hónglèiyèshēngmá*	紅類葉升麻
Red Peony, Chinese	*Paeonia rubra*	*chìsháo*	赤芍

Red Root	*Ceanothus americanum*	*měizhōuchá*	美洲茶
Red Sage root, Chinese	*Salvia miltorrhiza*	*dānshēn*	丹參
Rhubarb	*Rhuem sp.*	*dàhuáng*	大黃
Rosemary	*Rosmarinus officinalis*	*mídiéxiāng*	迷迭香
Safflower	*Carthamus tinctorius*	*hónghuā*	紅花
Sage Brush	*Artemisia tridentata*	*sānchǐhāo*	三齒蒿
Shepherd's Purse	*Capsella bursa-pastoris*	*jìcài*	薺菜
Skullcap	*Scutellaria lateriflora*	*cèhuāhuángqín*	側花黃芩
Skullcap, Chinese	*Scutellaria baicalensis*	*huángqín*	黃芩
St. John's Wort	*Hypericum perfoliatum*	*guànyèliánqiào*	貫葉連翹
Starwort root	*Stellaria dichotoma*	*yíncháihú*	銀柴胡
Stemona	*Stemona sp.*	*báibù*	百部
Stinging Nettle Seed	*Urtica dioica*	*cìqiánmá*	刺蕁麻
Teasel, Chinese	*Dipsacus asperoides*	*xùduàn*	續斷
Vervain	*Verbena officinalis*	*mǎbiāncǎo*	馬鞭草
Vitex, Chinese	*Vitex trifolia*	*mànjīngzǐ*	蔓荊子
Walnut, Black	*Juglans nigra, J. regia*	*hēihétao*	黑核桃
Wax Gourd	*Trichosanthus kirilowii*	*tiānhuāfěn*	天花粉
Wax Gourd (peel)	*Trichosanthes kirilowii*	*guālóupí*	瓜蔞皮
Wax Gourd (whole)	*Trichosanthus kirilowii*	*guālóu*	瓜蔞
White Peony, Chinese	*Paeonia alba*	*báisháo*	白芍
White Willow	*Salix album*	*bái liǔ*	白柳
Wild Cherry bark	*Prunus virginicus*	*fújíníyàlǐ*	佛吉尼亞李
Wild Lettuce	*Lactuca virosa*	*dúwōjù*	毒萵苣
Wild Yam	*Dioscorea villosa*	*chángróumáoshǔyù*	長柔毛薯蕷
Witch Hazel	*Hamamelis virginiana*	*běiměijīnlǚměi*	北美金縷梅
Yarrow	*Achillea millifolium*	*ōushīcǎo*	歐蓍草
Yellow Pond Lily	*Nuphar luteum, N. polysepala*	*ōuyápíngpéng*	歐亞萍蓬
Yerba Mansa	*Anemopsis californica*	*běiměijiǎyínliánhuā*	北美假銀蓮花
Yerba Santa	*Eriodictyon californica*		
Yucca	*Yucca sp.*	*sīlán*	絲蘭

Appendix IV

Medicinals in this materia medica listed by Latin Binomial

Latin Binomial	Common Name	Pínyín	漢字
Achillea millifolium	Yarrow	*ōushīcǎo*	歐蓍草
Achyranthes aspera	Achyranthes	*niúxī*	怀牛膝
Aconitum columbianum	Aconite	*běiměifùzǐ*	北美附子
Acorus calamus	Calamus	*shíchāngpú*	石菖蒲
Actaea racemosa	Black Cohosh	*hēishēngmá*	黑升麻
Actaea rubra	Red Baneberry	*hónglèiyèshēngmá*	紅類葉升麻
Aesculus hippocastanum	Horse Chestnut	*suōluózǐ*	娑罗子
Althea officinalis	Marshmallow root	*yàoshǔkuí*	藥蜀葵
Ambrosia dumosa, A. trifida, A. *artemesiifolia, A. psilostachya*	Ambrosia	*túncǎo*	豚草
Anemone occidentalis, A. patens	Pasque Flower	*yínliánhuā*	銀蓮花
Anemopsis californica	Yerba Mansa	*běiměijiǎyínliánhuā*	北美假銀蓮花
Anethum graveolens	Dill Seed	*shíluózǐ*	蒔萝子
Angelica archangelica	Angelica, European	*ōubáizhǐ*	歐白芷
Angelica breweri	Angelica, Brewer's		
Angelica dahurica	Angelica, Chinese	*báizhǐ*	白芷
Angelica pubescens	Angelica, Pubescent	*dúhuó*	獨活
Angelica sinensis	Dang Gui	*dāngguī*	當歸
Armeniaca sibirica	Apricot kernel	*xìngrén*	杏仁
Arnebia euchroma	Arnebia	*zǐcǎogēn*	紫草根 -新疆
Arnica sp.	Arnica	*shānjīnchē*	山金車
Artemesia californica	California Coast Sage	*jiāzhōuhāo*	加州蒿
Artemisia tridentata	Sage Brush	*sānchǐhāo*	三齒蒿
Asclepias tuberosa	Pleurisy Root	*kuàigēnmǎlìjīn*	塊根馬利筋
Astragalus membranaceus	Astragalus (unprocessed)	*shēnghuángqí*	生黃芪
Astragalus membranaceus	Astragalus, Honey Mix-fried	*zhìhuángqí*	炙黃芪
Atractylodes lancea	Atractylodes, Red	*cāngzhú*	蒼術
Atractylodes macrocephala	Atractylodes, White	*báizhú*	白術
Aucklandia lappa	Aucklandia	*mùxiāng*	木香
Belamcanda chinensis	Leopard Lily	*shègān*	射干
Berberis aquifolium	Oregon Grape root	*élègāngpúpao*	俄勒岡葡萄
Bidens pilosa	Bidens	*guǐzhēncǎo, mángchángcǎo*	鬼針草-盲腸草
Boswelliasacra	Frankincense	*rǔxiāng*	乳香

Bupleurum chinensis	Bupleurum	*cháihú*	柴胡
Calendula officinalis	Calendula	*jīnzhǎnjú*	金盞菊
Capsella bursa-pastoris	Shepherd's Purse	*jìcài*	薺菜
Capsicum sp.	Cayenne	*làjiāo*	辣椒
Carthamus tinctorius	Safflower	*hónghuā*	紅花
Caulophyllum thalictroides	Blue Cohosh	*lánzǐhóngmáoqī*	藍籽紅毛七
Ceanothus americanum	Red Root	*měizhōuchá*	美洲茶
Centaurea benedicta	Blessed Thistle		
Centella asiatica	Gotu Kola	*jīxuěcǎo*	積雪草
Chrysanthemum leucanthemum,	Ox-eye Daisy	*bīnjú*	濱菊
Leucanthemun vulgare			
Chrysanthemum morifolium	Chysanthemum	*júhuā*	菊花
Coix lacroyma-jobi	Coix	*yìyǐrén*	薏苡仁
Commiphora myrrha	Myrrh	*mòyào*	沒藥
Coptis chinensis	Coptis	*huánglián*	黃連
Corydalis yanhusuo	Corydalis, Chinese	*yánhúsuǒ*	延胡索
Curcuma wenyujin	Curcuma, Aromatic	*yùjīn*	鬱金
Cyperus rotundus	Cyperus	*xiāngfù*	香附
Dicentra formosa	Bleeding Hearts, Pacific		
Dioscorea villosa	Wild Yam	*chángróumáoshǔyù*	長柔毛薯蕷
Dipsacus asperoides	Teasel, Chinese	*xùduàn*	續斷
Dysphania ambrosioides	Epezoté	*tǔjīngjìe*	土荊芥
Echinacea purpurea, E.	Echinacea	*zǐzhuījú*	紫錐菊
angustifolium, etc.			
Epimidium sp.	Horny Goat Weed	*yínyánghuò*	淫羊藿
Eriodictyon californica	Yerba Santa		
Eschscholtzia californica	California Poppy	*huālíngcǎo*	花菱草
Eucalyptus globulus	Eucalyptus	*ānyè*	桉葉
Eucommia ulminoides	Eucommia	*dùzhòng*	杜仲
Foeniculum vulgare	Fennel seed	*huíxiāngzǐ*	茴香籽
Forsythia suspensa	Forsythia	*liánqiáo*	連翹
Fourquaria splendens	Ocotillo	*làzhúmū*	蠟燭木
Fritillaria cirrhosa	Fritillary, Sichuan	*chuānbèimǔ*	川貝母
Fritillaria thunbergii	Fritillary, Thunberg	*zhèbèimǔ*	浙貝母
Galium aparine	Cleavers	*bāxiāncǎo*	八仙草
Gardenia jaminoides	Gardenia, Carbonized	*tànshānzhīzǐ*	炭山梔子
Gardenia jasminoides	Gardenia	*shānzhīzǐ*	山梔子
Gentiana sp.	Gentian	*lóngdǎn*	龍膽

Glehnia littoralis	Glehnia, Coastal	*Shāshēn (běi)*	沙参（北）
Glycrrhiza uralensis	Licorice, Chinese	*gāncǎo*	甘草
Gossypium sp.	Cotton Root bark	*miánhua*	棉花
Grindelia sp.	Grindelia	*yàoyònggānjiāocǎo*	藥用干膠草
Hamamelis virginiana	Witch Hazel	*běiměijīnlǚměi*	北美金縷梅
Houttuynia cordata	Chameleon	*yúxīngcǎo*	魚腥草
Humulus lupulus	Hops	*píjiǔhuā*	啤酒花
Hydrastis canadensis	Goldenseal	*báimáogèn*	白毛茛
Hypericum perfoliatum	St. John's Wort	*guànyèliánqiào*	貫葉連翹
Hyssopus officinalis	Hyssop	*shénxiāngcǎo*	神香草
Imperata cylindrical	Cogon Grass	*báimáogēn*	白茅根
Inula britannica	British Yellowhead	*xuánfùhuā*	旋複花
Inula helenium	Elecampane	*tǔbáizhú*	土白術
Juglans nigra, J. regia	Walnut, Black	*hēihétao*	黑核桃
Juniperus communis	Juniper	*ōucìbǎi*	歐刺柏
Lactuca virosa	Wild Lettuce	*dúwōjù*	毒萵苣
Larrea tridentata	Chaparral	*shítànsuānguànmù*	石炭酸灌木
Lavendula spica, L. angustifolia	Lavender	*xūnyīcǎo*	薰衣草
Leonorus cardiac	Motherwort	*ōuzhōuyìmǔcǎo*	歐洲益母草
Leonorus siberica	Motherwort, Chinese	*yìmǔcǎo*	益母草
Ligusticum chuanxiong	Ligusticum, Chinese	*chuānxiōng*	川芎
Ligusticum porteri, L. grayii	Osha		
Lobelia inflata	Lobelia	*běiměishāngěngcài*	北美山梗菜
Lycium barbarum	Lycium Fruit (goji)	*gǒuqǐzi*	枸杞子
Lycopus lucidus	Lycopus, Chinese	*zélán*	澤蘭
Lycopus virginicus	Bugleweed	*měizhōudìsǔn*	北洲地筍
Magnolia denudata	Magnolia buds	*xīnyíhuā*	辛夷花
Magnolia officinalis	Magnolia bark	*hòupò*	厚樸
Marrubium vulgare	Horehound	*ōuxiàzhìcǎo*	歐夏至草
Matricaria chamomilla	Chamomile	*mǔjú*	母菊
Melissa officinalis	Lemon Balm	*níngméngxāingfēngcǎo*	檸檬香蜂草
Mentha canadensis	Field Mint	*bòhé*	薄荷
Mentha piperita	Peppermint	*ōuzhōubóhe*	歐洲薄荷
Mitchella repens	Partridgeberry	*wànhǔcì*	蔓虎刺
Monarda citriodora	Beebalm	*měiguóbòhe*	美國薄荷
Nepeta cataria	Catnip	*māobòhe*	貓薄荷
Notopterygium incisum	Notopterygium	*qiānghuó*	羌活

Nuphar luteum, N. polysepala	Yellow Pond Lily	*ōuyápíngpéng*	歐亞萍蓬
Ophiopogon japonicus	Dwarf Turf Lily	*màiméndōng*	麥門冬
Opolopanax horrididum	Devil's Club		
Paeonia alba	White Peony, Chinese	*báisháo*	白芍
Paeonia rubra	Red Peony, Chinese	*chìsháo*	赤芍
Panax ginseng	Ginseng, Asian	*rénshēn*	人參
Panax ginseng	Ginseng, White Chinese	*báirénshēn*	白人參
Panax notoginseng	Ginseng, Tian Qi	*sānqī*	三七
Panax quinquefolium	Ginseng, American	*xīyángshēn*	西洋參
Pedicularis densiflora, P. groenlandica, etc.	Pedicularis	*mǎxiānhāo*	馬先蒿
Pedicularis semibarbata	Lousewort, Pine	*mǎxiānhāo (sōng)*	馬先蒿 （松）
Petroselinum crispum	Parley root	*ōuqíngēn*	歐芹跟
Phellodendron chinensis	Amur Corktree Bark	*huángbǎi*	黃柏
Phellodendron chinensis	Chinese Corkbark	*huángbái*	黃柏
Pinellia ternata	Pinellia	*bànxià*	半夏
Pinellia ternata	Pinellia, Ginger-processed	*jiāngbànxià*	姜半夏
Piper methysticum	Kava	*kǎwǎhújiāo*	卡瓦胡椒
Plantago asiatica	Plantain seed, Chinese	*chēqiánzǐ*	車前子
Plantago sp.	Plantain (leaf)	*chēqiányè*	車前葉
Platycodon grandiflorus	Balloon Flower	*jiégěng*	桔梗
Polygala tenuifolia	Milkwort, Chinese	*yuǎnzhì*	遠志
Polypodium glycyrrhiza	Licorice Fern		
Poncirus trifoliata	Orange, Bitter	*zhǐshí*	枳實
Poria coccos	Poria	*fúlíng*	茯苓
Prunus virginicus	Wild Cherry bark	*fújíníyàlǐ*	佛吉尼亞李
Pseudostellaria heterophylla	Ginseng, Prince	*tàizǐshēn*	太子參
Rehmannia glutinosa	Foxglove, Chinese	*shēngdìhuáng*	生地黃
Rehmannia glutinosa	Processed Rehmannia	*shúdìhuáng*	熟地黃
Rhamnus californica	California Coffee Berry	*jiāzhōushǔlǐ*	加州鼠李
Rhuem sp.	Rhubarb	*dàhuáng*	大黃
Rosmarinus officinalis	Rosemary	*mídiéxiāng*	迷迭香
Salix album	White Willow	*bái liǔ*	白柳
Salvia miltorrhiza	Red Sage root, Chinese	*dānshēn*	丹參
Schizandra chinensis	Five Flavor Berry (Schizandra)	*wǔwèizǐ*	五味子
Scrophularia californica	Figwort, California	*jiāzhōuxuánshēn*	加州玄參
Scrophularia ningpoensis	Figwort, Chinese	*xuánshēn*	玄參

Scutellaria baicalensis	Skullcap, Chinese	*huángqín*	黃芩
Scutellaria lateriflora	Skullcap	*cèhuāhuángqín*	側花黃芩
Senna obtusifolia	Sicklepod Senna	*juémíngzǐ*	決明子
Solanum dulcamara	Bittersweet	*kǔqié*	苦茄
Solidago canadensis	Golden Rod	*jiānádàyīzhīhuánghuā*	加拿大一枝黃花
Sophora flavescens	Bitter Sophora	*kǔshēn*	苦參
Stachys sp.	Hedge Nettle	*shuǐsū*	水蘇
Stellaria dichotoma	Starwort root	*yíncháihú*	銀柴胡
Stellaria media	Chickweed	*fánlǚ*	繁縷
Stemona sp.	Stemona	*báibù*	百部
Symphytum officinale	Comfrey	*jùhécǎo*	聚合草
Tanacetum officinale	Feverfew	*àijú*	艾菊
Taraxicum officinale	Dandelion	*ōuzhōupúgōngyīng*	歐洲蒲公英
Thuja occidentalis	Cedar	*běiměixiāngbǎi*	北美香柏
Trichosanthes kirilowii	Wax Gourd (peel)	*guālóupí*	瓜蔞皮
Trichosanthus kirilowii	Wax Gourd	*tiānhuāfěn*	天花粉
Trichosanthus kirilowii	Wax Gourd (whole)	*guālóu*	瓜蔞
Trichostema lanceolatum, T. laxum	Blue Curls		
Trigonella foenum-graecum	Fenugreek	*húlúbā*	葫蘆巴
Trillium sp.	Bethroot	*yánlíngcǎo*	延齡草
Tussilago farfare	Coltsfoot	*kuǎndōnghuā*	款冬花
Urtica dioica	Stinging Nettle Seed	*cìqiánmá*	刺蕁麻
Vaccinium sp.	Blueberry	*lánméi*	藍莓
Verbascum thapsus	Mullein (leaf)	*dàmáoyè*	大毛葉
Verbena officinalis	Vervain	*mǎbiāncǎo*	馬鞭草
Viburnum prunifolium	Black Haw	*hēijiápéng*	黑莢蓬
Viburum opulus	Cramp Bark	*ōuzhōujiámí*	歐洲莢蒾
Vitex trifolia	Vitex, Chinese	*mànjīngzǐ*	蔓荊子
Yucca sp.	Yucca	*sīlán*	絲蘭
Zingiber officinale	Ginger, dry	*gānjiāng*	干姜
Zingiber officinale	Ginger, fresh	*shēngjiāng*	生姜

Appendix V

Medicinals in this materia medica listed by pínyín

Pínyín	Latin Binomial	Common Name	漢子
àijú	*Tanacetum officinale*	Feverfew	艾菊
ānyè	*Eucalyptus globulus*	Eucalyptus	桉葉
bái liǔ	*Salix album*	White Willow	白柳
báibù	*Stemona sp.*	Stemona	百部
báimáogèn	*Hydrastis canadensis*	Goldenseal	白毛茛
báimáogēn	*Imperata cylindrical*	Cogon Grass	白茅根
báirénshēn	*Panax ginseng*	Ginseng, White Chinese	白人參
báisháo	*Paeonia alba*	White Peony, Chinese	白芍
báizhǐ	*Angelica dahurica*	Angelica, Chinese	白芷
báizhú	*Atractylodes macrocephala*	Atractylodes, White	白術
bànxià	*Pinellia ternata*	Pinellia	半夏
bāxiāncǎo	*Galium aparine*	Cleavers	八仙草
běiměifùzǐ	*Aconitum columbianum*	Aconite	北美附子
běiměijiǎyínliánhuā	*Anemopsis californica*	Yerba Mansa	北美假银莲花
běiměijīnlǚměi	*Hamamelis virginiana*	Witch Hazel	北美金縷梅
běiměishāngěngcài	*Lobelia inflata*	Lobelia	北美山梗菜
běiměixiāngbǎi	*Thuja occidentalis*	Cedar	北美香柏
bīnjú	*Chrysanthemum leucanthemum, Leucanthemun vulgare*	Ox-eye Daisy	滨菊
bòhé	*Mentha canadensis*	Field Mint	薄荷
cāngzhú	*Atractylodes lancea*	Atractylodes, Red	蒼術
cèhuāhuángqín	*Scutellaria lateriflora*	Skullcap	側花黃芩
cháihú	*Bupleurum chinensis*	Bupleurum	柴胡
chángróumáoshǔyù	*Dioscorea villosa*	Wild Yam	長柔毛薯蕷
chēqiányè	*Plantago sp.*	Plantain (leaf)	車前葉
chēqiánzǐ	*Plantago asiatica*	Plantain seed, Chinese	車前子
chìsháo	*Paeonia rubra*	Red Peony, Chinese	赤芍
chuānbèimǔ	*Fritillaria cirrhosa*	Fritillary, Sichuan	川貝母
chuānxiōng	*Ligusticum chuanxiong*	Ligusticum, Chinese	川芎
cìqiánmá	*Urtica dioica*	Stinging Nettle Seed	刺蕁麻
dàhuáng	*Rhuem sp.*	Rhubarb	大黃
dàmáoyè	*Verbascum thapsus*	Mullein (leaf)	大毛葉
dāngguī	*Angelica sinensis*	Dang Gui	當歸
dānshēn	*Salvia miltorrhiza*	Red Sage root, Chinese	丹參

dúhuó	*Angelica pubescens*	Angelica, Pubescent	獨活
dúwōjù	*Lactuca virosa*	Wild Lettuce	毒萵苣
dùzhòng	*Eucommia ulminoides*	Eucommia	杜仲
élègāngpúpao	*Berberis aquifolium*	Oregon Grape root	俄勒岡葡萄
fánlǚ	*Stellaria media*	Chickweed	繁缕
fújíníyàlǐ	*Prunus virginicus*	Wild Cherry bark	佛吉尼亞李
fúlíng	*Poria coccos*	Poria	茯苓
gāncǎo	*Glycrrhiza uralensis*	Licorice, Chinese	甘草
gānjiāng	*Zingiber officinale*	Ginger, dry	干姜
gǒuqǐzi	*Lycium barbarum*	Lycium Fruit (goji)	枸杞子
guālóu	*Trichosanthus kirilowii*	Wax Gourd (whole)	瓜蔞
guālóupí	*Trichosanthes kirilowii*	Wax Gourd (peel)	瓜蔞皮
guànyèliánqiào	*Hypericum perfoliatum*	St. John's Wort	貫葉連翹
guǐzhēncǎo, mángchángcǎo	*Bidens pilosa*	Bidens	鬼針草－盲腸草
hēihétao	*Juglans nigra, J. regia*	Walnut, Black	黑核桃
hēijiápéng	*Viburnum prunifolium*	Black Haw	黑莢蓬
hēishēngmá	*Actaea racemosa*	Black Cohosh	黑升麻
hónghuā	*Carthamus tinctorius*	Safflower	紅花
hónglèiyèshēngmá	*Actaea rubra*	Red Baneberry	紅類葉升麻
hòupò	*Magnolia officinalis*	Magnolia bark	厚樸
huālíngcǎo	*Eschscholtzia californica*	California Poppy	花菱草
huángbái	*Phellodendron chinensis*	Chinese Corkbark	黃柏
huángbǎi	*Phellodendron chinensis*	Amur Corktree Bark	黃柏
huánglián	*Coptis chinensis*	Coptis	黃連
huángqín	*Scutellaria baicalensis*	Skullcap, Chinese	黃芩
huíxiāngzǐ	*Foeniculum vulgare*	Fennel seed	茴香籽
húlúbā	*Trigonella foenum-graecum*	Fenugreek	葫蘆巴
jiānádàyīzhīhuánghuā	*Solidago canadensis*	Golden Rod	加拿大一枝黃花
jiāngbànxià	*Pinellia ternata*	Pinellia, ginger-processed	姜半夏
jiāzhōuhāo	*Artemesia californica*	California Coast Sage	加州蒿
jiāzhōushǔlǐ	*Rhamnus californica*	California Coffee Berry	加州鼠李
jiāzhōuxuánshēn	*Scrophularia californica*	Figwort, California	加州玄參
jìcài	*Capsella bursa-pastoris*	Shepherd's Purse	薺菜
jiégěng	*Platycodon grandiflorus*	Balloon Flower	桔梗
jīnzhǎnjú	*Calendula officinalis*	Calendula	金盞菊
jīxuěcǎo	*Centella asiatica*	Gotu Kola	積雪草
juémíngzǐ	*Senna obtusifolia*	Sicklepod Senna	決明子
jùhécǎo	*Symphytum officinale*	Comfrey	聚合草

júhuā	*Chrysanthemum morifolium*	Chysanthemum	菊花
kǎwǎhújiāo	*Piper methysticum*	Kava	卡瓦胡椒
kuàigēnmǎlìjīn	*Asclepias tuberosa*	Pleurisy Root	塊根馬利筋
kuǎndōnghuā	*Tussilago farfare*	Coltsfoot	款冬花
kǔqié	*Solanum dulcamara*	Bittersweet	苦茄
kǔshēn	*Sophora flavescens*	Bitter Sophora	苦參
Làjiāo	*Capsicum sp.*	Cayenne	辣椒
lánméi	*Vaccinium sp.*	Blueberry	藍莓
lánzǐhóngmáoqī	*Caulophyllum thalictroides*	Blue Cohosh	藍籽紅毛七
làzhúmū	*Fourquaria splendens*	Ocotillo	蠟燭木
liánqiáo	*Forsythia suspensa*	Forsythia	連翹
lóngdǎn	*Gentiana sp.*	Gentian	龍膽
mǎbiāncǎo	*Verbena officinalis*	Vervain	馬鞭草
màiméndōng	*Ophiopogon japonicus*	Dwarf Turf Lily	麥門冬
mànjīngzǐ	*Vitex trifolia*	Vitex, Chinese	蔓荊子
māobòhe	*Nepeta cataria*	Catnip	貓薄荷
mǎxiānhāo	*Pedicularis densiflora, P. groenlandica, etc.*	Pedicularis	馬先蒿
mǎxiānhāo (sōng)	*Pedicularis semibarbata*	Lousewort, Pine	馬先蒿（松）
měiguóbòhe	*Monarda citriodora*	Beebalm	美國薄荷
měizhōuchá	*Ceanothus americanum*	Red Root	美洲茶
měizhōudìsǔn	*Lycopus virginicus*	Bugleweed	北洲地筍
miánhua	*Gossypium sp.*	Cotton Root bark	棉花
mídiéxiāng	*Rosmarinus officinalis*	Rosemary	迷迭香
mòyào	*Commiphora myrrha*	Myrrh	沒藥
mǔjú	*Matricaria chamomilla*	Chamomile	母菊
mùxiāng	*Aucklandia lappa*	Aucklandia	木香
níngméngxāingfēngcǎo	*Melissa officinalis*	Lemon Balm	檸檬香蜂草
niúxī	*Achyranthes aspera*	Achyranthes	怀牛膝
ōubáizhǐ	*Angelica archangelica*	Angelica, European	歐白芷
ōucìbǎi	*Juniperus communis*	Juniper	歐刺柏
ōuqíngēn	*Petroselinum crispum*	Parley root	歐芹跟
ōushīcǎo	*Achillea millifolium*	Yarrow	歐蓍草
ōuxiàzhìcǎo	*Marrubium vulgare*	Horehound	歐夏至草
ōuyápíngpéng	*Nuphar luteum, N. polysepala*	Yellow Pond Lily	歐亞萍蓬
ōuzhōubòhe	*Mentha piperita*	Peppermint	歐洲薄荷
ōuzhōujiámí	*Viburum opulus*	Cramp Bark	歐洲莢蒾
ōuzhōupúgōngyīng	*Taraxicum officinale*	Dandelion	歐洲蒲公英

ōuzhōuyìmǔcǎo	*Leonorus cardiac*	Motherwort	歐洲益母草
píjiǔhuā	*Humulus lupulus*	Hops	啤酒花
qiānghuó	*Notopterygium incisum*	Notopterygium	羌活
rénshēn	*Panax ginseng*	Ginseng, Asian	人參
rǔxiāng	*Boswellia sacra*	Frankincense	乳香
sānchǐhāo	*Artemisia tridentata*	Sage Brush	三齒蒿
sānqī	*Panax notoginseng*	Ginseng, Tian Qi	三七
shānjīnchē	*Arnica sp.*	Arnica	山金車
shānzhīzǐ	*Gardenia jasminoides*	Gardenia	山梔子
Shāshēn (běi)	*Glehnia littoralis*	Glehnia, Coastal	沙參（北）
shègān	*Belamcanda chinensis*	Leopard Lily	射干
shēngdìhuáng	*Rehmannia glutinosa*	Foxglove, Chinese	生地黃
shēnghuángqí	*Astragalus membranaceus*	Astragalus (unprocessed)	生黃芪
shēngjiāng	*Zingiber officinale*	Ginger, fresh	生姜
shénxiāngcǎo	*Hyssopus officinalis*	Hyssop	神香草
shíchāngpú	*Acorus calamus*	Calamus	石菖蒲
shíluózǐ	*Anethum graveolens*	Dill Seed	蒔萝子
shítànsuānguànmù	*Larrea tridentata*	Chaparral	石炭酸灌木
shúdìhuáng	*Rehmannia glutinosa*	Processed Rehmannia	熟地黃
shuǐsū	*Stachys sp.*	Hedge Nettle	水蘇
sīlán	*Yucca sp.*	Yucca	絲蘭
suōluózǐ	*Aesculus hippocastanum*	Horse Chestnut	娑罗子
tàizǐshēn	*Pseudostellaria heterophylla*	Ginseng, Prince	太子參
tànshānzhīzǐ	*Gardenia jaminoides*	Gardenia, Carbonized	炭山梔子
tiānhuāfěn	*Trichosanthus kirilowii*	Wax Gourd	天花粉
tǔbáizhú	*Inula helenium*	Elecampane	土白術
tǔjīngjìe	*Dysphania ambrosioides*	Epezoté	土荊芥
túncǎo	*Ambrosia dumosa, A. trifida, A. artemesiifolia, A. psilostachya*	Ambrosia	豚草
wànhǔcì	*Mitchella repens*	Partridgeberry	蔓虎刺
wǔwèizǐ	*Schizandra chinensis*	Five Flavor Berry (Schizandra)	五味子
xiāngfù	*Cyperus rotundus*	Cyperus	香附
xìngrén	*Armeniaca sibirica*	Apricot kernel	杏仁
xīnyíhuā	*Magnolia denudata*	Magnolia buds	辛夷花
xīyángshēn	*Panax quinquefolium*	Ginseng, American	西洋參
xuánfùhuā	*Inula britannica*	British Yellowhead	旋覆花
xuánshēn	*Scrophularia ningpoensis*	Figwort, Chinese	玄參
xùduàn	*Dipsacus asperoides*	Teasel, Chinese	續斷

xūnyīcǎo	*Lavendula spica, L. angustifolia*	Lavender	薰衣草
yánhúsuǒ	*Corydalis yanhusuo*	Corydalis, Chinese	延胡索
yánlíngcǎo	*Trillium sp.*	Bethroot	延齡草
yàoshǔkuí	*Althea officinalis*	Marshmallow root	藥蜀葵
yàoyònggānjiāocǎo	*Grindelia sp.*	Grindelia	藥用干膠草
yìmǔcǎo	*Leonorus siberica*	Motherwort, Chinese	益母草
yíncháihú	*Stellaria dichotoma*	Starwort root	銀柴胡
yínliánhuā	*Anemone occidentalis, A. patens*	Pasque Flower	銀蓮花
yínyánghuò	*Epimidium sp.*	Horny Goat Weed	淫羊藿
yìyǐrén	*Coix lacroyma-jobi*	Coix	薏苡仁
yuǎnzhì	*Polygala tenuifolia*	Milkwort, Chinese	遠志
yùjīn	*Curcuma wenyujin*	Curcuma, Aromatic	鬱金
yúxīngcǎo	*Houttuynia cordata*	Chameleon	魚腥草
zélán	*Lycopus lucidus*	Lycopus, Chinese	澤蘭
zhèbèimǔ	*Fritillaria thunbergii*	Fritillary, Thunberg	浙貝母
zhìhuángqí	*Astragalus membranaceus*	Astragalus, honey mix-fried	炙黃芪
zhǐshí	*Poncirus trifoliata*	Orange, Bitter	枳實
zǐcǎogēn	*Arnebia euchroma*	Arnebia	紫草根（新疆）
zǐzhuījú	*Echinacea purpurea, E. angustifolium, etc.*	Echinacea	紫錐菊

Appendix VI
Chinese formulas found in this book.

Pínyín	**English**	**漢字**
Bǎo Hé Wán	Preserve Harmony Pill	保和丸
Bí Yán Piàn	Nose Inflammation Pill	鼻炎片
Bǔ Zhōng Yì Qì Tāng	Tonify the Middle to Augment the Qi Decoction	補中益氣湯
Cāng'Ěr Zǐ Sān	Xanthium Powder	蒼耳子散
Chái Hú Shū Gān Sǎn	Bupleurum Powder to Dredge the Liver	柴胡疏肝散
Dà Chái Hú Tāng	Major Bupleurum Decoction	大柴胡湯
Dú Huó Jì Shēng Tāng	Pubescent Angelica and Taxillus Decoction	獨活寄生湯
Fú Líng Tāng	Poria Decoction	茯苓湯
Gù Běn Zhǐ Bēng Tāng	Stabilize the Root & Stop Excessive Uterine Bleeding Decoction	固本止崩湯
Gǔ Qì Tāng	Stabilize Qi Decoction	固氣湯
Guì Zhī Fú Líng Tāng	Cinnamon Twig and Poria Docoction	桂枝茯苓湯
Guì Zhī Tāng	Cinnamon Twig Decoction	桂枝湯
Jīng Fáng Bài Dú Sǎn	Schizonepeta and Saposhnikovia Powder to Overcome Pathogenic Influences	荊防敗毒散

Juān Bì Tāng	Remove Painful Obstruction Decoction	蠲痹湯
Liù Jūn Zǐ Tāng	Six-Gentleman Decoction	六君子湯
Lóng Dǎn Xiè Gān Tāng	Gentian Decoction to Drain the Liver	龍膽瀉肝湯
Má Huáng Tāng	Ephedra Decoction	麻黃湯
Qīng Shǔ Yì Qì Tāng	Clear Summerheat and Augment the Qi Decoction	清暑益氣湯
Sāng Jú Yǐn	Mulberry Leaf and Chrysanthemum Drink	桑菊飲
Sì Jūn Zǐ Tāng	Four-Gentlemen Decoction	四君子湯
Sì Nì Sǎn	Frigid Extremities Powder	四逆散
Suān Zǎo Rén Tāng	Sour Jujube Decoction	酸棗仁湯
Tòng Xiè Yào Fāng	Important Formula for Painful Diarrhea	痛瀉藥方
Wēn Dǎn Tāng	Warm Gallbladder Decoction	溫膽湯
Xiǎo Chái Hú Tāng	Minor Bupleurum Decoction	小柴胡湯
Xiǎo Qīng Lóng Tāng	Minor Bluegreen Dragon Decoction	小青龍湯
Xiāo Yáo Sǎn	Rambling Powder	逍遙散
Yín Qiáo Sàn	Honeysuckle and Forsythia Powder	銀翹散

Bibliography

Adams, Francis, trans. *The Works of Hippocrates and Galen*. London: Encyclopaedia Britannica 1952.

Allen, David E. & Hatfield, Gabrielle. *Medicinal Plants in Folk Tradition: An Ethnobotany of Britain & Ireland*. Portland, OR: Timber Press Inc. 2004.

Baldwin, Bruce G. et al. (Ed.). *The Jepson Manual: Vascular Plants of California, Second Edition, Thoroughly Revised and Expanded / Edition 2*. Berkeley, CA: University of California Press, 2012.

Bocek, Barbara R. *Ethnobotany of Costanoan Indians, California*, Based on Collections by John P. Harrington. 1984.

Burton, Robert, *The Anatomy of Melancholy*. Originally published in 1621, Reprinted by Ex-classics Project, 2009. Accessed at http://www.exclassics.com

Chén Xiū-yuán, *Shén Nóng Běn Cǎo Jīng Dú*. Reprint, ed. Lín Huì-guāng. Beijing: China's Chinese Medicinal Publisher, 1999, *in Chinese*.

Chrubasik, Sigrun, Eisenberg, Elon, Balan, Edith, Weinberger, Tuvia, Luzzati, Rachel, Conradt, Christian. Treatment of Low Back Pain Exacerbations with Willow Bark Extract: A Randomized Double-Blind Study. *The American Journal of Medicine*. 109(1): pp. 9-14. 2000.

Cook, William H. *The Physio-Medical Dispensatory: A Treaties on Therapeutics, Materia Medica, and Pharmacy, in Accordance with the Principles of Physiological Medication*. 1869. Repreint, Portland, OR: Eclectic Institute, 1985.

——. *A Compendium of the New Materia Medica Together with Additional Descriptions of Some Old Remedies*. Chicago: William H. Cook, 1896.

Clavey, Steven. *Fluid Physiology and Pathology in Traditional Chinese Medicine*, 2nd Edition. London: Churchill Livingstone, 2003.

Felter, Harvey Wickes. *The Eclectic Materia Medica, Pharmacology and Therapeutics*. 1922.

Felter, Harvey Wickes & Lloyd, John Uri. *King's American Dispensatory* Vol. I & II, 19th Ed., 3rd Revision. Cincinnati: The Ohio Valley Company, 1905.

Ellingwood, Finley, and John Uri Lloyd. *American Materia Medica, Therapeutics and Pharmacognosy*. 1919. Reprint, Sandy, OR: Eclectic Medical Publications, 1983.

Flora of North America Editorial Committee, eds. 1993+. *Flora of North America North of Mexico*. 16+ vols. New York and Oxford.

Garran, Thomas Avery, *Western Herbs According to Traditional Chinese Medicine: A Practitioners Guide*. Healing Arts Press, 2008.

Gerard, John, *The Herball or Generall Historie of Plantes*. London: John Norton, 1597.

Grieve, M. *A Modern Herbal*. 1931. Reprint, New York: Dover Publications, 1971.

Gunther, E. *Ethnobotany of Western Washington*. Seattle, WA. University of Washington Press, 1973.

Hickman, James C., ed. *The Jepson Manual: Higher Plants of California*. Berkeley: Univ. of California Press, 1993.

Homsher, R. D., Calendula officinalis – A Study, Comparison, and Local Uses, *Ellingwood's Therapeutist* Vol 2:11. Chicago: 1908.

Huáng Zhào-shèng, ed. *Zhōng Yào Xué*. 11th ed. Beijing: People'e Medical Publishing House, 2002, *in Chinese*.

Jones, W. H. S. (trans.). *Hippocrates* (4 Vol.). Harvard University Press, 1957.

K'Eogh, Job. *Botanalogia Universalis Hibernica, Or A General Irish Herbal*. Corke, Printed and folded at the corner of Meeting House Lane, 1735.

Lǐ Jīng-wěi, Yú Yíng-áo, Cài Jǐng-fēng, Zhāng Zhì-bīn, Ōu Yǒng-xīn, Dèng Tiě-tāo, Ōu Míng, eds. *Grand Dictionary of Chinese Medicine*, 2nd ed. Beijing: People's Medicinal Publishing House, 2009, *in Chinese*.

Lǐ Shí-zhēn, *Běn Cǎo Gāng Mù*. 1590. Reprint, ed. Liǔ Zhǎng-huá. Beijing: China's Chinese Medicinal Publisher, 1999, *in Chinese*.

Moerman, Daniel E. *Native American Ethnobotany*. Portland, OR: Timber Press, 1998.

——. Online database version of *Native American Ethnobotany* http://herb.umd.umich.edu/

Moore, Michael. *Medicinal Plants of the Pacific West*. Santa Fe, NM: Red Crane Books, 1993.

——. *Medicinal Plants of the Mountain West*, 2nd Edition. Santa Fe, NM: Museum of New Mexico Press, 2003.

Mou Hong-yi (牟鸿彝). *Natural Sciences of Chinese Medicinals/Guó Yào De Lǐ Xué* (國藥的理學). North Shanghai New Publishing House, 1952, in Chinese.

Parkinson, John. *Theatrum Botanicum: The Theater of Plants. Or An Herball of A Large Extent*. London, 1640.

Salmon, William. *Botanologia: The English Herbal: or, History of Plants*. London: printed by I. Dawks for H. Rhodes and J. Taylor, 1710.

Smith, Arthur Weir. *Medicinal Plants of North America* Vol. 1. Berwyn, Illinois, 1914.

Shěn Jīn-áo, *Zá Bìng Yuán Liú Xī Zhú* 杂病源流犀烛 (1774), *in Chinese.*

Sòng Sū-sòng, *Map of the Materia Medica. Běn Cǎo Tú Jīng,* 本草圖經 . http://www.zysj.com.cn/lilunshuji/bencaotujing/ 1061, *in Chinese.*

Sū Jìng, *Newly Revised Materia Medica, Xīn Xīu Běn Cǎo.* 新修本草 . 659, *in Chinese.*

Sūn Sī-miǎo, *A Thousand Gold Pieces Emergency Formulary* Vol. 1 translated by Sabine Wilms. circa 650.

Thomson, Samuel, *A New Guide to Health; Or Botanic Family Physician*, 2nd Ed. Boston, MA, 1825.

Tíng Xiù. *Yunnan Materia Medica Diān Nán Běn Cǎo.* 滇南本草 . 1470, *in Chinese.*

Unknown. *A Compilation of Commonly Used Folk Medicines.* Sichuan People's Publishing House, 1959, *in Chinese.*

Unknown. *Folk Medicines of Gui Zhou.* Guizhou People's Publishing House, 1965, *in Chinese.*

Unknown. *Frequently Used Chinese Medicinals of Tibet.* Tibet People's Publishing House, 1971, *in Chinese.*

Unknown. *Gansu Handbook of Chinese Medicinals/Gān Sù Zhōng Yào Shǒu Cè* 甘肅中藥手冊 . Gansu People Publishing House, 1959, *in Chinese.*

Unknown. *Gui Zhou Collection of Herbal Folk Remedies* (贵州民间方药集). Guizhou People Publishing House. 1978, *in Chinese.*

Unknown. *Handbook of Frequently Used Chinese Medicinals from Northern China.* Beijing: People's Medical Publishing House. 1971, *in Chinese.*

Unknown. *Journal of Medicinal Plants of the Northeast* [China] (东北药用植物志), 图书出版社：科学 1959, *in Chinese.*

Unknown. *Selected Medicinals from Yunnan.* Yunnan People's Publishing House, 1971, *in Chinese.*

Unknown. *Selected Medicinals from Shanxi, Gan Su, Ning Xia, and Qing Hai.* Compiled by Lanzhou Military District Logistics and Health Department, 1971, *in Chinese.*

Unknown. *The Luxuriant Materia Medica of Yunnan/Běn Cǎo Yuán Mìng Bāo.* 本草元命苞 . 1331, *in Chinese.*

Unknown. *Wàn Xiàn Zhōng Běn Cǎo* 萬縣中本草 , 1977, *in Chinese.*

Weiss, Rudolf Fritz. *Herbal Medicine.* Trans. A. R. Meuss. Beaconsfield, UK: Beaconsfield Publishers Ltd., 1988.

Wiseman, Nigel & Feng Ye. *A Practical Dictionary of Chinese Medicine.* Brookline, MA: Paradigm Publications, 1998.

Wood, Horatio C. & Joseph P. Remington. *The Dispensatory of the United States of America*, 20th ed. Philadelphia: J. B. Lippincott and Company, 1918.

Xiè Zōng-wan, Ed. *National Chinese Herbal Medicine Compilation* (全国中草药汇编), Peoples Medical Publishing House, 2012, *in Chinese.*

Xú Míng, ed. *Commonly Used Paired Medicinals.* Fuzhou: Fu Jiang Science and Technology Press, 2007, *in Chinese.*

Yán Zhèng-huá (顏正華) *Study of Chinese Medicinals, Zhōng Yào Xué* 中藥學. Beijing, People's Medical Publishing House, 2009, *in Chinese.*

Ye Ding-hong & Yuan Si-tong (Ed.) *Dictionary of Preparation of Chinese Medicinals, Zhōng Yào Páo Zhì Xué Cí Diǎn* (中藥炮製學辭典). Shanghai Science and Technology Pulishers, 2005, *in Chinese.*

Yè Tiān-shì (葉天士). *Treaties on Warm-Heat, Wēn Rè Lùn* 溫熱論. 1777. Reprint, ed. Fuzhou, Fujian Science and Technology Press, 2010, *in Chinese.*

Yè Tiān-shì (葉天士). *Yè Tiān-shì Quán Shū / Yè Tiān-shì's Complete Works.* Reprint, ed. Huáng Yīng-zhì. Beijing: Chinese Medical Publishing House, 1999, *in Chinese.*

Zhāng Jǐng-yuè, *Jìng Yuě Quán Shū/ Jìng Yuě's Complete Works.* 1624. Reprint, ed. Lǐ Zhì-yōng. Beijing: Chinese Medical Publishing House, 1999, *in Chinese.*

Zhāng Xī-chún, *Yī Xuē Zhōng Zhōng Cān Xī Lù.* Collection of papers originally published 1918 - 1934, published as one book in 1957. Reprint. Beijing: Chinese Medicine Science and Technology Press, 2011, *in Chinese.*

Zhào Guó-píng, Dài Shèn, Chén Rén-shòu, eds. *Grand Dictionary of Chinese Medicinals*, 2nd ed. Shanghai: Shanghai Science and Technology Press, 2009, *in Chinese.*

Zhū Dān-xī, *Dān-xī Xīn Fǎ/Zhū Dān-xī's Heart Methods.* 1481. Reprint, ed. Wáng Guó-chén. Beijing: China's Chinese Medicinal Publisher, 1996, *in Chinese.*

Index

Bolded entries represent plants with monographs in the text.

www.ingramcontent.com/pod-product-compliance
Lightning Source LLC
Chambersburg PA
CBHW052117230326
41598CB00080B/3804